Praise for Lawrence A. Kane and Kris Wilder...

"The forms of a given system are the "books" which contain all relev[...]
Unfortunately, many of today's martial arts enthusiasts are unable to [...]
you how to read your forms and extract the information which is conc[...]
"This book is an absolute must for any serious practitioner of traditional karate, tae kwon do, or kung-fu. In my many years of practicing and teaching martial arts, I have never seen a text like this; a work which clearly outlines the theories and principles of interpreting forms. This book has been sorely needed by the martial arts community for generations.
"For those who think the practice of traditional form (kata) is worthless and has no value insofar as real combat is concerned, read this book! You'll see your forms and your chosen martial art in a completely different light. This book will act as a torch to light the path which will lead you to the secrets of the traditional martial arts; information which has been hidden for many decades!
"Now if you'll excuse me, I've got to get back to studying my forms..."

– Philip Starr, Founder of Yiliquan;
Inside Kung Fu Hall of Fame Member

"For years, karateka have needed a manual to bridge the gap between their training and real violence. This book is a pioneering step in fulfilling that need. In so many real encounters, I would do something that I later recognized in my wife's karate kata. Not once did any karate instructor, when explaining that move, come even close to what I had actually done. It left me feeling that karate, at its root, was devastatingly effective, but that as it is commonly taught it was little more than a joke. This book will help an intelligent karateka find the combat system inside the dojo dance."

– Sgt. Rory Miller, tactical team leader;
Use of Force Policy and close quarters combat
instructor for law enforcement officers.

"I found this to be a comprehensive book that bridges the gap between form and application in a realistic, easy-to-read and easy-to-apply manner. It's packed with profound insight into the true meaning of kata, while at the same time identifying street-worthy technique as well as valuable tips for sparring competition. This book is loaded with fascinating history, street fighting wisdom, sparring tips, insight into well-known kata, and invaluable quotes and tips from a host of martial arts masters. It will increase your knowledge of the depth and wisdom of forms, and in the process make you a better fighter."

– Loren Christensen (www.lwcbooks.com), 7th
degree black belt, retired military and civilian
police officer, author of 29 books on martial arts.

"*The Way of Kata* demonstrates the practical uses of kata, relates the traditional and modern aspects of fighting, and brings meaningful information to today's martial arts practitioners."

– Martina Sprague (www.modernfighter.com),
author of five books on martial arts.

"*The Way of Kata* is a thoughtful, thorough and informative analysis of the 'hidden' fighting applications of kata. This superb book is essential reading for all those who wish to understand the highly effective techniques, concepts and strategies that the kata were created to record!"

– Iain Abernethy, (www.iainabernethy.com),
author of 4 books on applied karate, a former UK
national level kata judge, member of the Combat
Hall of Fame, and the holder of a 5th Dan in
applied karate from the British Combat
Association (one of the world's leading groups for
close-quarter combat and practical martial arts).

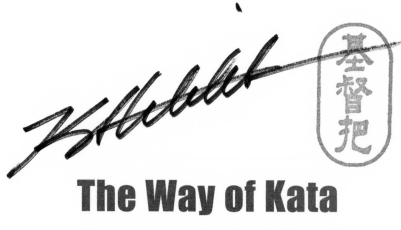

The Way of Kata

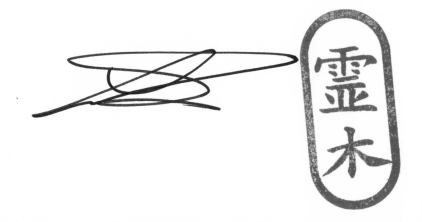

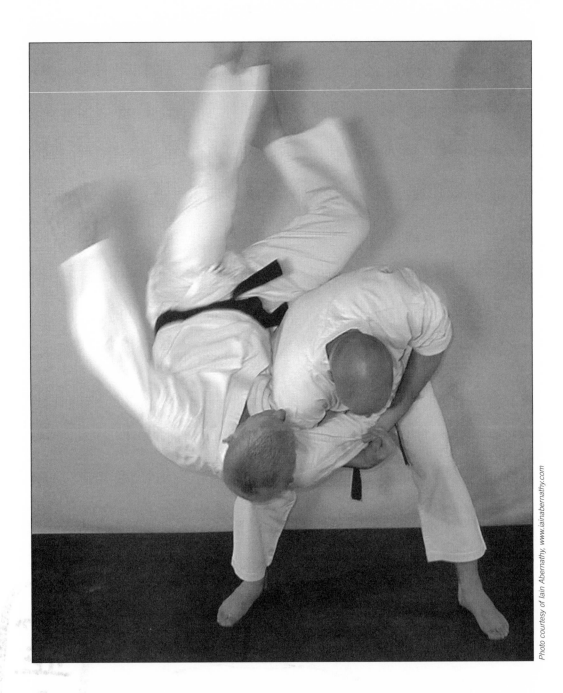

KUSHANKU THROW. EVEN THOUGH KARATE IS PRIMARILY A STRIKING ART, IT CONTAINS MANY GRAPPLING AND THROWING TECHNIQUES. HERE, IAIN ABERNETHY APPLIES A THROW FROM KUSHANKU (KANKU-DAI) KATA. THE RECIPIENT IS GARY HERBERT.

The Way of Kata

A Comprehensive Guide to Deciphering Martial Applications

LAWRENCE A. KANE AND
KRIS WILDER

YMAA Publication Center
Boston, Mass. USA

YMAA Publication Center, Inc.
Main Office
4354 Washington Street
Boston, Massachusetts, 02131
1-800-669-8892 • www.ymaa.com • ymaa@aol.com

Editor: Eleanor K. Sommer
Cover Design: Katya Popova
Illustrated by Kris Wilder

ISBN-10: 1-59439-058-4
ISBN-13: 978-1-59439-058-6

10   9   8   7   6   5   4   3   2   1

Publisher's Cataloging in Publication

Kane, Lawrence A.

The way of kata : a comprehensive guide to deciphering martial
applications / Lawrence A. Kane and Kris Wilder. -- 1st ed. --
Boston, Mass. : YMAA Publication Center, 2005.

   p. ; cm.

Includes bibliographical references, glossary, and index.
ISBN: 1-59439-058-4
ISBN-13: 978-1-59439-058-6

1. Martial arts. 2. Martial arts--Psychological aspects. 3. Hand-
to-hand fighting, Oriental. I. Wilder, Kris. II. Title.

GV1102.7.P75 K36 2005   2005930892
796.815--dc22   0509

Warning: Studying these materials may give you, or cause you to acquire, a certain degree of power that you did not previously possess. The authors and publisher expect you to use that power responsibly. Readers are encouraged to be aware of all appropriate local and national laws relating to self-defense, reasonable force, and the use of martial techniques in conflict situations and act in accordance with all applicable laws at all times. Neither the authors nor the publisher assume any responsibility for the use or misuse of information contained in this book.

All martial arts are, by their very definition, warlike and dangerous. Training should always be undertaken responsibly, ensuring every available precaution for the safety of all participants. No text, no matter how well written, can substitute for professional hands-on instruction. Consequently these materials should be used *for academic study only*.

Printed in Canada.

Dedication

To Joey and Jackson, two of the smallest guys that make the biggest difference.

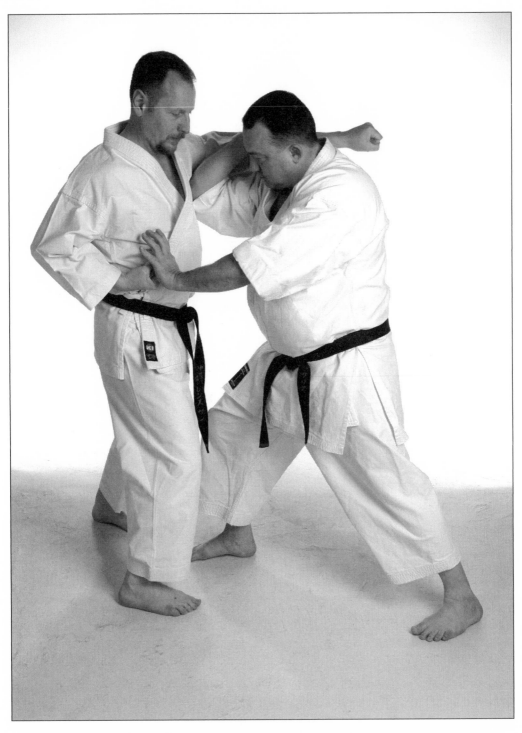

SHISOCHIN ELBOW STRIKE/FIST JAM. THIS IS A SIGNATURE MOVEMENT OF SHISOCHIN KATA WHEREIN THE PRESS BLOCK KEEPS THE
OPPONENT'S FOLLOW-ON PUNCH FROM GETTING STARTED. BLOCKS PERFORMED THIS CLOSE TO AN OPPONENT'S BODY ARE VERY
EFFECTIVE AT JAMMING AND DISRUPTING A PERSON'S TECHNIQUES.

Table of Contents

Foreword—Dr. Jeff Cooper   xi

Foreword—Iain Abernethy   xiii

Preface   xvii

Acknowledgments   xix

Introduction   xxi

CHAPTER 1   Background Fundamentals   1

  What is a *Kata?*   1

  Chinese Kung Fu   2

  Okinawan Martial Arts   3

  Kanryo Higashionna *(Naha Te)*   4

  Chojun Miyagi *(Goju Ryu)*   5

  Origin of *Kata* in the West   9

  Kata as a Textbook   12

  Types of Applications   14

  Types of "Fighting"   16

  Why Applications are Not Readily Discernable in *Kata*   *20*

  More Than One Proper Application Exists   24

  Hidden Applications between *Kata* Movements   27

  Summary   28

CHAPTER 2   Strategy and Tactics   35

  Effective Applications Must Be Grounded in a System's Strategy   35

  Strategy vs. Tactics   37

  Do Not Confuse the Quality of the Strategy with the Skill of the Fighter   40

  Once You Have a Strategy, Use It   41

  The Decision Stick   43

  Strategy of *Goju Ryu*   45

  Principles of Enforcement   51

  Tactics of *Goju Ryu*   60

  Forms of Compliance   60

  Summary   63

CHAPTER 3   Principles   67

  1. There is More Than One Proper Interpretation of Any Movement   68

  2. Every Technique Should Be Able to End the Fight Immediately   69

  3. Strike to Disrupt; Disrupt to Strike   70

  4. Nerve Strikes are "Extra Credit"   74

  5. Work with the Adrenaline Rush, Not Against It   79

CHAPTER 3   Principles *(continued)*

    6. Full Speed and Power 81
    7. It Must Work on an "Unwilling" Partner 83
    8. Strive to Understand *Why* It Works 86
    9. Deception Is Not Real 88
    10. If You Are Not There, You Cannot Get Hit 90
    11. Cross the T to Escape 93
    12. Stances Aren't Just for *Kata* 95
    13. Don't Forget to Breathe 97
    14. Use Both Hands 100
    15. A Lock or Hold is Not a Primary Fighting Technique 102
    Summary 103

CHAPTER 4   Rules 109

    1. Do Not Be Deceived by the Enbusen Rule 110
    2. Advancing Techniques Imply Attack, While Retreating Techniques Imply Defense ... 112
    3. There is Only One Enemy at a Time 113
    4. Every Movement in Every *Kata* Has Martial Significance 116
    5. A Hand Returning to Chamber Usually Has Something in It 118
    6. Utilize the Shortest Distance to Your Opponent 120
    7. Control an Opponent's Head and You Control the Opponent 122
    8. There is No Block 126
    9. *Kata* Demonstrate the Proper Angles 130
    10. Touching Your Own Body in *Kata* Indicates Touching Your Opponent ... 133
    11. Contour the Body—Strike Hard to Soft and Soft to Hard 134
    12. There is No Pause. 136
    Summary 139

CHAPTER 5   Physics, Physiology, and Other Considerations 145

    Characteristics of Violence 147
    Physiological Threat Response 158
    Brain Activity in Combat 160
    Non-diagnostic Response 162
    Levels of Response 163
    Catching Bullets 164
    Stealing Time 166
    Speed Kills! 167
    Vital Points *(Kyushu)* 171
    Summary 177

CHAPTER 6   Process   181
   Bringing It All Together   181
   Dojo Practice   186
   Cooperative Performance   187
   Formula   188
   Summary   191

CHAPTER 7   Kata Examples   193
   Saifa   194
   Seiyunchin   198
   Seisan   202
   Saipai   206
   Shisochin   210
   Kururunfa   212
   Sanseiru   218
   Suparinpei   222
   Gekisai (Dai Ni)   226
   Summary   228

CONCLUSION   231
   Summary   232

APPENDIX A   Bubishi Poem—Eight Precepts of Kempo   239

APPENDIX B   Kata of Goju Ryu   241

APPENDIX C   Kata Application Evaluation Checklist   245

Notes   247
Glossary   251
Glossary of Terms   251
Glossary of Techniques   258
Bibliography   269
Index   271
About the Authors   277

Foreword
by Dr. Jeff Cooper

My karate teacher, John Roseberry (a pioneer of Okinawan martial arts in America—9th degree black belt in karate, 7th degree black belt in judo and 3rd degree black belt in aikido), used to say of *kata*, "*Kata* is our textbook." He would similarly state, "It's all in there."

The problem for me was that although I could go through the motions of the *kata*, I apparently was having a difficult time "reading" the text. Through my association with Kris Wilder, Lawrence Kane, and others (e.g., Marcus Davila, Scott Schweitzer, Kelly Worden to name just a few) I have been taught how to read the textbook.

Although many people have learned to read, it is Mr.'s Wilder and Kane that have taken the time to put all the reading lessons together in one place. The authors of this book have taken their practice of traditional *Goju Ryu* karate and delved deeply for meaning to its strong emphasis on *kata*.

"Why practice kata?"

"Is kata just dance?"

"How does kata enhance my ability to defend myself?"

These are just a few of the questions posed regarding the practice of *kata*. This book presents concepts that can help any practitioner gain more meaning from form practice. Looking at the techniques presented in a form, one starts to extract the underlying tactics and, from them, to understand the strategies from which those tactics spring. Once those strategies are identified and understood, the *kata* of a system become rich in meaning and in usefulness as further tactics and techniques are extracted.

The gaining of the strategic and tactical concepts of one's system is the reward of the approach put forward by Mr.'s Wilder and Kane. Modern defensive tactics systems and "reality-based" systems have largely excluded *kata*. This book offers students of systems that include form practice a guide to understanding the meaning of the forms. It provides guidance regarding the strategy and tactics within the forms. This book helps to bridge the gap between traditional, form-based martial arts and the modern, eclectic defensive systems, which do not choose to include or emphasize form training.

Readers from either side of that gap will reap gains from this book regarding the application of strategic and tactical thinking, training, and principles common to all the combative arts. Basically, it's a damn good book.

– Jeffrey Cooper, MD

Jeffrey Cooper, M.D., is a fellow of the American Academy of Emergency Medicine and a clinical instructor of emergency medicine. He has been involved in the martial arts for some 25 years, achieving the rank of yodan *(4th degree black belt) in* Goju Ryu *karate. As tactical medical director of Toledo (Ohio) SWAT, he has received advanced training in hostage extraction, hand-to-hand combat, firearms, and knife fighting. Dr. Cooper is also a commander in the US Naval Reserve Medical Corps.*

Foreword

by Iain Abernethy

There are many differing views on the value of *kata*. *Kata* is regarded by some as the very "soul" of the martial arts. By others, it is regarded as a complete waste of time. To my mind, both views have merit depending upon what is meant by *kata* and how it is approached.

One thing I think all martial artists can agree on is that the study of *kata* is definitely not a prerequisite for combative effectiveness. There are many highly effective martial arts that do not include *kata* on their curriculum. If *kata* training is not critical to developing fighting skill, why do so many "traditional systems" like karate make such a big deal about it?

To fully explore this question, we need to understand why *kata* were created in the first place. Someone somewhere must have firmly believed that *kata* served a useful purpose or it never would have come into being in the first place. Further, if *kata* was not useful, it certainly would not have lasted very long after its inception.

By way of example, let's discuss the creation of the karate *kata Chinto* (renamed *Gankaku* in *Shotokan*). *Chinto kata* is named after a Chinese martial artist and sailor of the same name. During the 1800s, Chinto became shipwrecked on Okinawa and set up home in a cave. Finding himself stranded without resources, Chinto began to steal food and livestock from the locals at night in order to sustain himself. This unwelcome behavior was reported to the Okinawan king who sent Sokon Matsumura—his chief bodyguard and a legendary karate master in his own right—to deal with the situation.

Matsumura was a very skilled fighter who normally defeated his opponents with ease. When Matsumura confronted him, however, Chinto fought back with exceptional skill and Matsumura quickly found himself equally matched. Always keen to further enhance his formidable skills, Matsumura made a deal with Chinto; he would take care of him in exchange for instruction in Chinto's fighting method. Upon Chinto's return to China, Matsumura formulated a *kata*—named after the originator of the system it contained—to ensure Chinto's methods were recorded and passed on to future generations. Many other *kata* were also developed by an individual's students in order to record what they had been taught.

What has eventually become known as karate is in fact a mix of many different fighting systems (cross-training is nothing new). The past masters used *kata* as a means to record the lessons they had learnt from various individuals and fighting systems and to then pass those lessons on to others.

From the example of Chinto and Matsumura, we can see that *kata* were developed to ensure that the most effective methods of a particular individual or style were not lost. *Kata* can therefore be defined as "a way to record and summarize the key combative techniques and principles of a fighting style."

As a way to record techniques, drills, and principles, *kata* certainly works. Hundreds of years after Chinto finished teaching Matsumura his fighting method, we modern *karateka* have a record of the key points of Chinto's teaching. However, over time *kata* has drifted away from being viewed as a record of highly potent fighting methods, to instead being generally considered as an athletic or aesthetic pursuit that has little relation to actual combat. Regardless of how *kata* may be perceived today, for *karateka* with an interest in the original civilian fighting system, *kata* provides a living link back to that system.

To practice karate as a pragmatic system, *kata* needs to be actively studied, as opposed to just "practiced." Gichin Funakoshi (the founder of *Shotokan* karate) considered the practice of *kata* useless unless one learned how to apply it in actual self-defense situations (*Karate-do Kyohan*). I wholeheartedly agree with his sentiments. Without in-depth study of *bunkai* (*kata* application), *kata* practice loses all meaning. The information contained in this book will ensure that your *kata* practice has meaning and is relevant to real life situations.

Kata is a record of the fighting systems that combined to form karate; the original syllabus if you will. *Karateka* who ignore the lessons of *kata* inadvertently practice karate as a partial art. Without an understanding of *kata bunkai*, karate is a grossly inadequate and incomplete system. When modern day practitioners of any martial art choose not to bother with *kata*, they often do so in the name of realism. What they fail to appreciate is that by abandoning *kata* they have effectively abandoned the very syllabus of their original fighting system. Without *kata*, all that remains is a shell of the original martial art.

Kata has great value when correctly approached. It ensures that the martial art you practice is a workable system. That is where this superb book by Lawrence Kane and Kris Wilder proves so invaluable to pragmatically minded *budoka*. *The Way of Kata* will give you the vital information you need to approach *kata* in the 'correct' way and to practice your art as a functional, holistic, and pragmatic martial system. Enjoy!

– Iain Abernethy

Iain Abernethy holds a godan *(5th degree black belt) in applied karate from the British Combat Association, one of the world's leading groups for close-quarter combat and practical martial arts. He is also a* yodan *(4th degree black belt) in Wado-Ryu* *karate (English Karate Governing Body), a member of the Combat Hall of Fame, and a former national level* kata *judge in the UK. He is the author of four books on applied* karate: Bunkai-Jutsu: The Practical Application of Karate Kata; Throws for Strikers: The Forgotten Throws of Karate, Boxing, and Taekwondo; Karate's Grappling Methods; *and* Arm-Locks for All Styles. *Sensei Abernethy has produced numerous DVDs and videos on applied* karate *and* kata bunkai *and is a regular contributor to all of UK's leading martial arts magazines. His Web site address is www.iainabernethy.com.*

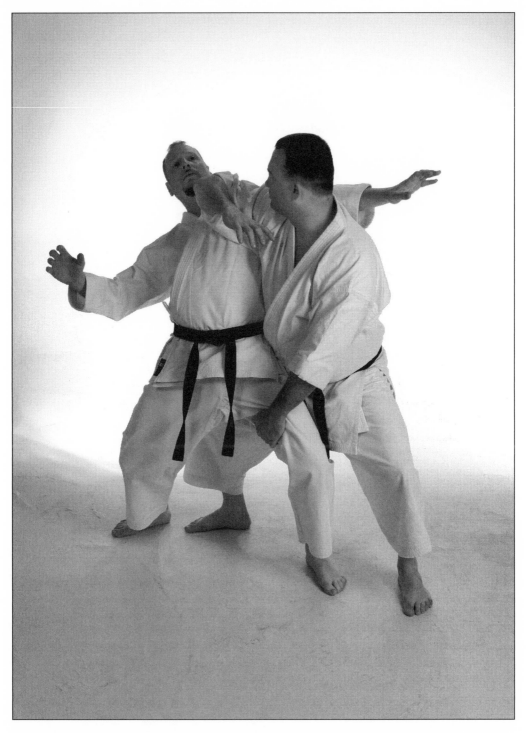

SAIPAI LEG HOOK/ELBOW STRIKE. IN THIS APPLICATION FROM *SAIPAI KATA*, KRIS SHIFTS IN SIMULTANEOUSLY STRIKING WITH HIS ELBOW AND HOOKING HIS OPPONENT'S LEG TO KNOCK LAWRENCE TO THE GROUND.

Preface

"I only expected to be in this country for three months; however, when I came to Spokane (Washington) and saw the deplorable level of Goju Ryu there, I took time and great pains to correct it. After six months—twice the length of time I had planned to stay—I realized that it would be easier to start from scratch than to fix the problems. It's usually better to rebuild a house than to remodel it!

"The Goju Ryu that I saw when I finally visited dojos across the country was very poor, but I knew it wasn't anybody's fault. I understood there had been many teachers before, many bridges, and the messages often got crossed. There was such a gap between those practitioners and me! I didn't want to make any instructor uncomfortable.

"My job first was to encourage people, not discourage them. I started correcting the basics and built the kata on them. Once we had some common ground, I could build on it. It was harder working with the instructors than with the beginners, because they had high rank and their pride prevented them from training with me in front of their students. And sometimes their students were better than they! But I understood the situation. So I gave them private instruction whenever I could, usually during breaks." [1]

– Teruo Chinen

When new martial artists begin their training, they find they have to relearn basic concepts like breathing, standing, and walking. They are taught how to breathe through their diaphragm rather than solely with their lungs, introduced to a variety of uncomfortable stances and foreign postures, and shown how to move in unusual new ways. Balance and coordination take on a new meaning. And that's just the beginning.

Soon they are introduced to *kata*, the dancelike movements in which the ancient masters hid the secrets of their unique fighting systems. Almost all Asian martial systems have *kata* of one type or another, from arnis to kung fu, karate to judo, and tae kwon do to tai chi. A *kata* is simply a pattern of movements containing a logical series of offensive and defensive techniques that are performed in a particular order. Its origins can be found in the nature of fighting, more than a thousand years of trial and error based on practical experience as well as keen observations about combat between animal and animal, between animal and man, and man-to-man.

According to Morio Higaonna,* "The true meaning and spirit of karate are imbedded in *kata* and only by the practice of *kata* can we come to understand them." Individuals who learn an art's strategy and diligently practice its *kata* can learn real-world fighting applications that they may use to defend themselves.

While each *kata* is supposed to be performed the same way every time, there are a plethora of applications, or *bunkai,* from every *kata,* movements that can be applied in a real fight. Some applications, especially simple, straightforward ones, are easier to decipher than others. Unfortunately, such applications are not always the best interpretation of a given movement, nor are they the most likely to succeed in actual combat. Anything less than the best is simply not good enough if your life is on the line.

Kata is not dance practice nor is it aerobic training.† It is the fundamental basis of a fighting art. Like a textbook, it contains all the applications you need to defend yourself in mortal combat. To get the most out of your martial art, you simply need to know how to "read" your *kata* like a book.

Ah, but that's the rub isn't it? How does one learn how to read the *kata* textbook? The answer to that question is, of course, contained herein. We wrote these materials to help you do just that.

The theory of deciphering applications from *kata* is called *kaisai.* Since it offers guidelines for unlocking the true meaning of each *kata* movement, *kaisai no genri* (the theory of *kaisai*) was once a great mystery revealed only to trusted disciples of the ancient masters in order to protect the secrets of their systems. Using the rules of *kaisai no genri,* practitioners can decipher the original intent of *kata* movements by logically analyzing each specific movement to find its *okuden waza* (hidden technique).

This book helps practitioners understand the strategy behind whatever martial art they have chosen to study so that they can utilize its tactics wisely. Our efforts will show you how to analyze your *kata* to determine the best applications for a given situation. The heart of these materials covers fifteen general principles for identifying effective techniques as well as twelve discrete rules for deciphering applications from *kata.*

---

* Morio Higaonna, Hanshi (9th dan black belt), is the chief instructor of the International Okinawan Goju Ryu Karate-Do Federation (IOGKF)

† Though physical conditioning is certainly a side benefit of practicing it.

Acknowledgments

We would like to express our sincere appreciation for Hiroo Ito's guidance and counseling. Thank you for sharing your vast knowledge with us. We would also like to recognize Mike Canonica, who modeled for our illustrations, along with Iain Abernethy, Loren Christensen, and Franco Sanguinetti who contributed photographs for this work. Special thanks as well to Lumina Photography (www.LuminaPhotography.com), David Ripianzi, Tim Comrie, Ellie Sommer, and Laura Vanderpool who helped us with this project.

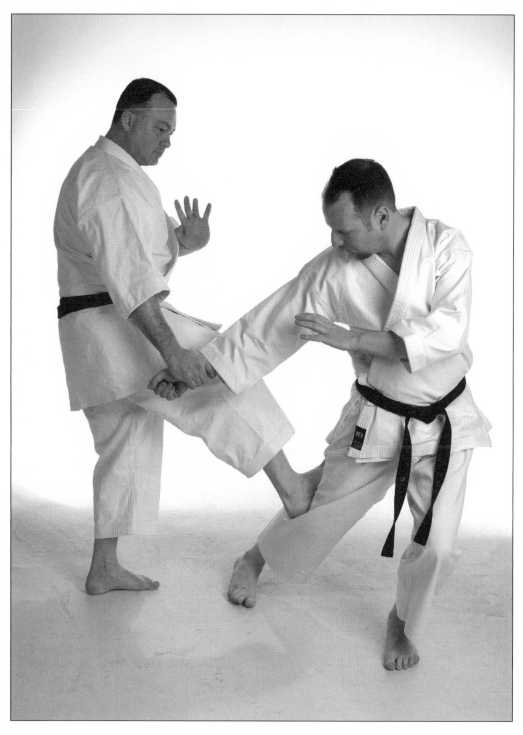

KENSETSU GERI. THIS JOINT KICK IS ESPECIALLY EFFECTIVE BECAUSE THE GRAB
POSTS THE OPPONENT'S WEIGHT ON THE LEG KRIS IS ATTACKING WITH HIS KICK.

Introduction

"Despite a lack of complete understanding, one should not assume that the movements have no meaning or function. I advise performing the movements, thinking about them, and interpreting them in your own way, concentrating heart and soul. This is practice."[2]

– Shigeru Egami

Following a time honored tradition of *kakidameshi* (dueling), *budoka* (martial artists) in ancient Okinawa routinely tested each other's fighting skills through actual combat. Like the feudal *samurai* before or the Old West gunfighter that would follow, the more famous the practitioner, the more often he was challenged to combat by those seeking fame. Such fights were often to the death. Even when the loser survived, his degradation was so considerable that his humiliated relatives rarely considered revenge.

Such challenges even took the form of sudden ambush or sneak attacks. Consequently, while the masters of such arts had to ensure that their forms would work in actual combat, they jealously guarded the secrets of their style. In many cases they taught the secrets of deciphering their *kata* orally to a single student, a sole successor who promised never to reveal these *okuden waza*, or secret techniques, to the public.

In Japanese, martial arts understanding can be classified in two ways: *omote* and *ura waza*. *Omote* signifies the outer or surface training, while *ura waza* can be translated to denote the inner or subtle way. *Omote* is the most common and well understood. *Ura waza*, on the other hand, is the subtle details that make the obvious succeed. Practitioners who never learn these crucial details lack essential tools required to make the most of their martial art.

While *kata* is the foundation of most Asian martial disciplines, numerous misunderstandings continue to prevail regarding the true intent of such forms. A common example is that many practitioners are led to believe that defensive techniques, called *uke* in Japanese, should be thought of as "blocks." A more accurate translation of the word *uke* would be "receive," a term implying active ownership. Once a practitioner owns an aggressor's attack, he or she may redirect it as needed to put an end to the confrontation, often without even striking an "offensive" blow. Seen in this light, defensive postures can take on an entirely new meaning. You will learn more about this in chapter 4 where the rules of *kata* are outlined.*

Traditional study of martial systems presumes the ability to perform techniques in actual combat. Sport and conditioning applications are more or less fringe bene-

---

* Please note that we will refer to these rules (chapter 4) and to a set of principles (chapter 3) from time to time prior to those chapters.

fits associated with such study. A student whose primary reason for studying a martial art is to get into shape might be better off pursuing aerobics, yoga, weightlifting, Jazzercise, Pilates, or similar activities. Such arts focus on the fitness aspects and are far less painful to learn. If you really want to gain the skills necessary to defend yourself, however, martial pursuits are the right path to take.

By the time you finish reading this book, you will have developed comprehensive knowledge needed to decipher the hidden meaning of your own *kata* and get the most out of your martial art. We would like to preview what you will learn with the following example:

In *seiyunchin kata,** a *Goju Ryu* karate form, there are two sections showing forward-moving *gedan uke* (down blocks) performed in *shiko dachi* (sumo or straddle stance). In one case the practitioner's right hand is in chamber (at his or her side) while the left hand executes the downward block. One might consider it somewhat odd to step forward in such a low, immovable stance while blocking downward.

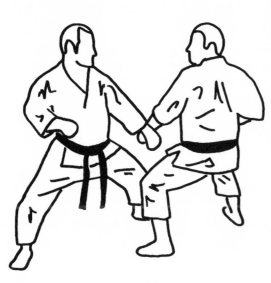

SEIYUNCHIN KATA: BASIC SHIKO DACHI (SUMO STANCE) WITH GEDAN UKE (DOWN BLOCK). THE DEFENDER IS ON THE LEFT.

The most commonly attributed application or *bunkai* for this movement would be a simple down block. Using *henka waza* (variation technique), the movement would more than likely be shown retreating rather than advancing as performed in the *kata*. This is because blocking while moving forward is somewhat counterintuitive (later on we'll discuss more about the fallacy of even considering defensive techniques "blocks" at all).

There is nothing wrong with this example. Indeed, it is a viable, if basic, technique. In almost every case there is more than one "correct" interpretation for any movement in a *kata*. While this simple explanation may be correct, however, it falls far short of being all it could be.

A variety of principles and rules outlined in this book will help practitioners identify the *okuden waza* found in their *kata*. These secret techniques offer much more powerful interpretations of such movements. Let's face it, if all you do is block, a

* Which translates as "pull off balance and fight."

determined opponent will continue to attack until he or she either lands enough solid blows to crush you, or you do something better than basic blocking to stop him or her. Logic dictates that the simplest interpretation of this sequence is, at best, sub-optimal.

Let's analyze this combination in more depth to figure out what this *kata's* inventor was really trying to tell us. Applying some of the rules and principles outlined later in this book illuminates our example:

- Moving forward implies offensive technique,[*] so what we perceive as a down block must really be a strike.[†] Since we have selected a *Goju Ryu kata* as our example, it is important to note that this assertion also fits within *Goju Ryu's* overall strategy of closing distance with an opponent and disrupting him or her.[‡] One way to validate that your interpretation of *kata* technique is suitable is to ensure that it fits within your system's overall strategy. In this case our enhanced interpretation passes that crucial test.

- The strength of *shiko dachi* is in uprooting an opponent.[§] *Shiko dachi* is also the least mobile stance in karate (or any martial art for that matter). It must, therefore, imply close body contact to an opponent in order to crash and disrupt his or her balance. At proper range the *shiko dachi* stance alone affords us an opportunity to attack an opponent's legs with our feet and knees while closing the distance.

- Since the technique is performed in *shiko dachi*, the range shown in Figure 1 is really too far away, placing the practitioner at a distinct disadvantage. When the distance is closed up, the downward strike clearly aims for the groin (*kinteki*)—if you are on the inside or kidneys (*ushiro denko*) if you are on the outside—both of which are vital areas.[||]

- Since the right hand is closed and in chamber, the practitioner most likely has his or her opponent's arm captured and held within it.[¶] This not only distracts the adversary, but helps keep him or her in place long enough to be hit, an important advantage with a relatively immobile stance.

- Because it is necessary to disrupt before striking,[**] there is very likely an additional hidden application[††] performed between the more obvious upward and downward movements of the *gedan uke*.[‡‡] In this case that hidden application is most likely a concussive ear slap.

- Since the "block" is actually a strike,[§§] the *kata* is in fact demonstrating a blow to the groin or possibly kidney. Either way, this causes physiological damage to a vital area—a core tenet of the *Goju Ryu* strategy.[||||] Performed correctly, a solid blow to either of those vital areas can immediately end a fight.[¶¶]

---

[*] See Rule 2—advancing implies attack.
[†] See Rule 8– there is no "block."
[‡] See Strategy of *Goju Ryu* in chapter 2 for more information.
[§] See Principle 12– stances aren't just for kata.
[||] See Principle 2– every technique should be able to end the fight immediately, and Rule 11—contour the body.
[¶] See Rule 5—hand in chamber usually has something in it.
[**] See Principle 3—strike to disrupt; disrupt to strike.
[††] See Hidden Applications Between Kata Movements.
[‡‡] Also see Rule 6—utilize the shortest distance to your opponent.
[§§] See Rules 2 and 8.
[||||] See Strategy of *Goju Ryu* in chapter 2. The strategy of almost every martial art includes striving for physiological damage to defeat an adversary.
[¶¶] See Principle 2—every technique should be able to end the fight immediately.

• Using a combination of rules and principles we have uncovered a much stronger set of techniques from what first appeared to be a simple block. Combined, these movements affect the opponent's legs and/or feet, groin or kidney, and head, working the whole body.* As deciphered, they are indeed quite powerful, much more so than the most simple and commonly held interpretation would imply.

Here is how our newfound interpretation might look:

Now that we have whet your appetite, here is a summary of the major points covered in each chapter of this book:

Chapter 1—Background Fundamentals. A Japanese word meaning "formal exercise," *kata* contain logical sequences of movements consisting of practical offensive and defensive techniques that are performed in a particular order. The ancient masters imbedded the secrets of their unique fighting systems in their *kata*. There are almost unlimited combat applications or *bunkai* hidden within each movement. Such applications can even be hidden *between* the movements of a *kata*.

While the basic movements of *kata* are widely known, advanced practical applications and sophisticated techniques frequently remain

* See Principles of Enforcement in chapter 2.

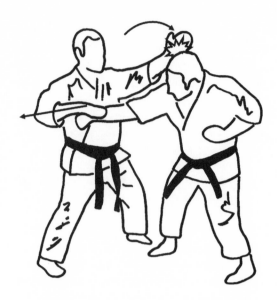

SEIYUNCHIN KATA: TRANSITIONAL EAR SLAP (A HIDDEN TECHNIQUE NOT TRADITIONALLY SHOWN DURING PERFORMANCE OF THE KATA).

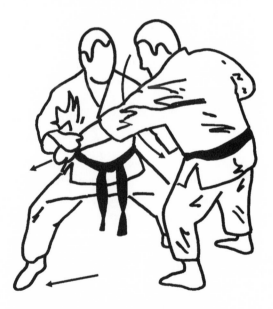

SEIYUNCHIN KATA: PROPER SHIKO DACHI (SUMO STANCE) WITH DOWN BLOCK/GROIN STRIKE.

hidden from the casual observer. Historically there was often a two-track system of martial arts instruction not only in Okinawa, but in Japan, China, and Korea as well. The outer circle of students learned basic fundamentals; unknowingly receiving modified *kata* where critical details or important principles were omitted. The inner circle that had gained a master's trust and respect, on the other hand, could be taught *okuden waza*, the secret applications of *kata*.

Even within this inner circle, the rules and principles for deciphering all of a system's *kata* frequently were taught to only a single student, the master's chosen successor, rather than to the group as a whole. Often this instruction was withheld until the master became quite old or very ill, shortly before his death. On occasion the master waited too long to pass along this vital knowledge and it was lost altogether.

In modern times *kata* was spread from Okinawa to the rest of the world, primarily by American GIs and Allied troops who learned karate during the occupation of Japan at the end of World War II. Although many *budo** masters were willing to teach the Westerners as a means to earn a living, most foreigners were not initiated into their inner circles. Further, even when instructors wished to share their secrets, language barriers often inhibited comprehensive communication.

Later on, as *budo* was opened-up to society at large, it frequently was taught to schoolchildren. Many dangerous techniques were hidden from these practitioners simply because they were not mature enough to handle them responsibly. Consequently, much of what made it to the outside world was intermediate-level martial arts, devoid of principles and rules necessary to understand and employ hidden techniques.

Chapter 2—Strategy and Tactics. A deep understanding of strategy and tactics is a necessary prerequisite for comprehending and properly deciphering *kata*. Strategy is a plan of action. In martial arts as in war, it is what you do to prepare for engagement with an enemy long before the fight begins. Tactics, on the other hand, are expedient means of achieving an end, in this case defeating an adversary. Tactics are selected during the heat of battle.

Like a house without a solid foundation, tactics without strategy will ultimately fail. If the strategic foundation is strong, on the other hand, appropriate tactics can be employed automatically without conscious thought, instantly reacting to most any situation. In actual combat, understanding and adhering to your strategy may mean the difference between victory and defeat. History is strewn with the corpses of those who forgot this essential lesson.

In *Goju Ryu* karate, for example, the essential strategy is to close distance, imbalance, and use physiological damage to incapacitate an opponent. Looking at its core *kata*, an easy way to ascertain the tactics of an art form, you will find that they include about 70 percent hand techniques, 20 percent foot techniques, 5 percent throws, and

---

* Martial ways or arts.

5 percent groundwork. While everything is included therein, karate is primarily a striking art. Every useful martial art is built around a strategic framework.

In a real fight, decisions must be made in an instant. To survive, practitioners must be engaged in the moment of now. Responses take the form of a "decision stick," rather than a decision tree. They are uncomplicated and straightforward, relying less on what an opponent does than on what the practitioner's strategy requires him or her to do.

Chapter 3—Principles. The following fifteen principles are necessary for analyzing *kata*. They form the strategic framework within which practitioners can identify valid interpretations of *bunkai*,* *henka waza*,† and even *okuden waza*‡ in the *kata* they practice:

1. There is more than one proper interpretation of any movement.

2. Every technique should be able to end the fight immediately.

3. Strike to disrupt; disrupt to strike.

4. Nerve strikes are "extra credit."

5. Work with the adrenaline rush, not against it.

6. Techniques must work at full speed and power.

7. It must work on an "unwilling" partner.

8. Strive to understand why it works.

9. Deception is not real.

10. If you are not there, you cannot get hit.

11. Cross the T to escape.

12. Stances aren't just for *kata*.

13. Don't forget to breathe.

14. Use both hands.

15. A lock or hold is not a primary fighting technique.

Chapter 4—Rules. Although there are numerous "correct" interpretations for each movement of every *kata*, techniques are typically stylized with their actual applications obscured. The work to uncover hidden applications in *kata* is called *kaisai* in Japanese. Since it offers guidelines for unlocking the secrets of each *kata*, *kaisai no genri*§ was once a great mystery revealed only to trusted disciples of the ancient masters in order to protect the secrets of their system.

Using the principles of *kaisai no genri* practitioners can decipher the original intent of *kata* techniques by logically analyzing each specific movement to find its hidden meaning. The first three conventions are called *shuyo san gensoko*, meaning "main" or "basic" rules. Rules 4 through 12 are called *hosoku joko*, which translates as supplementary or advanced rules:

* Applications.
† Variation techniques.
‡ Hidden or secret techniques.
§ The theory of kaisai.

1. Do not be deceived by the *enbusen* rule.

2. Advancing techniques imply attack, while retreating techniques imply defense.

3. There is only one enemy at a time.

4. Every movement in *kata* has martial meaning/significance and can be used in a real fight.

5. A hand returning to chamber usually has something in it.

6. Utilize the shortest distance to your opponent.

7. Control an opponent's head and you control the opponent.

8. There is no "block."

9. *Kata* demonstrates the proper angles.

10. Touching your own body in *kata* indicates touching your opponent.

11. Contour the body—strike hard to soft and soft to hard.

12. There is no pause.

Chapter 5—Physics, Physiology, and Other Considerations. Every movement in kata has practical self-defense applications. If one accurately strikes or grabs an attacker's vital area, he or she can elicit pain, temporary paralysis, dislocation or hyperextension of a joint, knockout, or possibly even death. Whoever lands the first solid blow to a vital area during a real fight will undoubtedly be victorious. In combat, speed and accuracy are paramount.

Part of what makes practitioners fast, is the ability to react in a non-diagnostic manner. They do not think—they simply do. In the old days, traditional practitioners would spend many years learning a single *kata*. Although many of the ancient masters learned only two or three *kata*, each contained a fully effective and comprehensive fighting system providing everything they really needed to know. They would study these *kata* in great depth, learning all the subtle nuances and internalizing the movements until they became second nature. Applications could be launched instantly without conscious thought.

Threat responses work like rungs on a ladder. The lowest rung, or base foundation, is built upon our natural neurological reactions, taking advantage of hardwired fight or flight responses. Tactics and strategy, the next higher rungs in ascending order, must work synergistically with the body's natural physiological reactions. Control is the highest form of response. By control we mean adapting strategy and choosing tactics as appropriate for a given situation. The ancient masters took such things into consideration as they built their *kata*. In deciphering applications, we must understand them as well.

The best self-defense, of course, is avoiding a fight altogether. Even if a person legitimately uses force in order to escape an imminent and unavoidable danger, he or she will still have to live with the physiological and psychological results of doing so. Further, he or she must be prepared to face the very real prospect of subsequent litigation by the defeated opponent and/or the government. A good understanding of the characteristics of violence and insight into the criminal mind can help practitioners avoid dangerous confrontations.

Once a conflict occurs, however, you must do everything you can to end it quickly. You have to be at least as ruthless and violent as your attacker(s). Unlike sparring in the *dojo*, vital areas are most certainly not off limits. They are the only targets that matter, required knowledge for survival.

Chapter 6—Process. The simplest interpretation of most any *kata* sequence is bound to be sub-optimal. When practitioners adopt the principles, rules, and strategic guidelines we have outlined in this book, they will have the power to get the most out of their martial art. Using a technique called cooperative performance, *budoka* can work with others in their *dojo* to experiment with their own *kata*, identify what they believe are hidden applications, and ascertain whether or not they will work in a self-defense situation.

Although a practitioner may be able to perform a *kata* and understand its various applications and hidden techniques, he or she may still not want to rely on it in actual combat. Everyone is better at some things than others. It is essential that practitioners understand how to personalize techniques, instinctively applying applications for which they have a natural affinity during a life or death struggle.

Chapter 7—*Kata* Examples. This chapter uses *kata* from *Goju Ryu* to demonstrate how all of the previous material comes together. Using our examples, you will have a leg up in deciphering the secrets of your own martial art and will be able to analyze your own *kata* in a similar fashion.

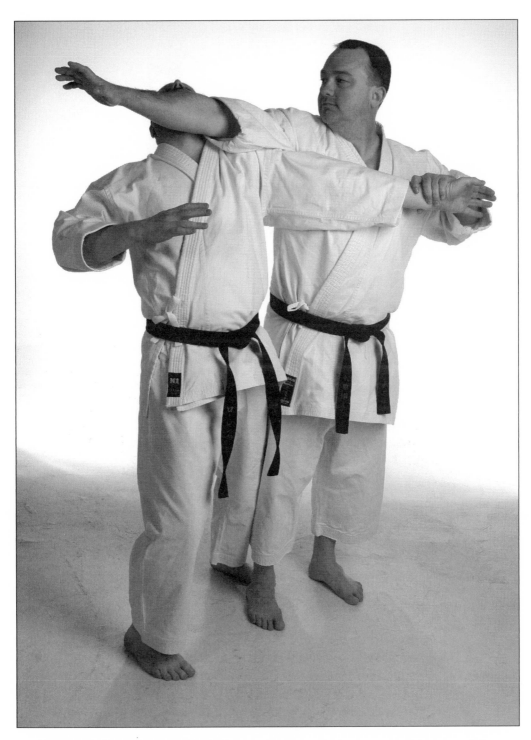

GEKISAI SWEEP, STOMP, *SHUTO*. THIS TECHNIQUE IS A SIGNATURE MOVEMENT OF *GEKISAI KATA*. IN THIS CASE IT IS PERFORMED TO THE OUTSIDE, DISRUPTING THE OPPONENT'S BALANCE WHILE SIMULTANEOUSLY STRIKING THE THROAT WITH A SWORD HAND.

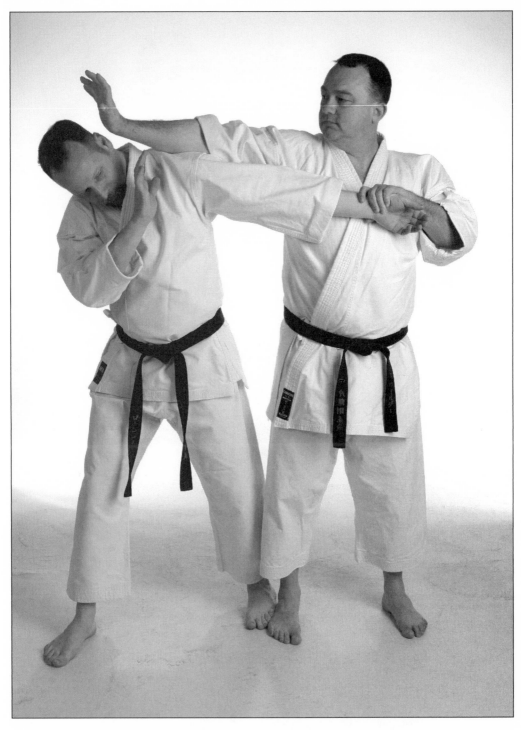

SUPARINPEI PUSH/PULL STRIKE. THIS TECHNIQUE STRETCHES AN OPPONENT BY GRABBING THEIR
ARM, PULLING, AND SIMULTANEOUSLY HITTING THEM WITH A *SHOTEI UCHI* (PALM HEEL) STRIKE.

CHAPTER 1

Background Fundamentals

"We make war that we may live in peace." [3]

– Aristotle

Based on humankind's instinct for self-preservation, combat arts have existed throughout the ages. The highest purse sport in ancient Greece's first Olympic Games was *pankration*, a martial art that translates as "all powers fighting." Alexander the Great's *pankratiasts* spread their fighting form throughout the many regions that his armies conquered (e.g., Egypt, Persia, Syria, Babylonia, Media, and India). Although not widely practiced, the art of *pankration* still exists today.

Over time diverse fighting arts took on unique characteristics of different cultures, especially in Egypt, Turkey, and central Asia. The principles behind Asian martial arts are believed to have spread from Turkey to India, where they were further developed into sophisticated arts. Once codified, these principles spread through the Orient in the form of *kata*. These *kata* proliferated from China to Okinawa and then to Japan, heavily influencing the indigenous fighting arts in those regions.

What is a Kata?

"The word kata comes from the Japanese meaning formal exercise. In Japan kata is not just something that is done in the martial arts. Kata has a deeper and spiritual meaning that is done in almost every aspect of life. There is a formal way for a tea ceremony, to enter a room or to greet a friend. A martial art is a discipline of the mind and body as much as it is a war art. Many different martial arts date back hundreds and even thousands of years. Each generation transmitted their knowledge and secrets to the next generations through kata." [4]

– Joe Talbot

A *kata* is a logical sequence of movements containing practical offensive and defensive techniques that are performed in a particular order. Watching a person perform *kata* is much like observing an exchange of blows between the practitioner and an invisible enemy. The ancient masters embedded their unique fighting systems within their *kata*, which became fault-tolerant methods* for ensuring such techniques could be taught and understood consistently over the generations. Less experienced practitioners could view the forms, imitating the movements of their more knowledgeable brethren.

For centuries oral tradition was used throughout the Orient to pass martial traditions from master to student. Very little was written down, partly because literacy was quite rare outside the nobility and certain privileged merchant classes and partly to keep confidential practices from becoming public knowledge. As students learned the basics and gained their instructor's confidence, they could be initiated into the secrets of his system.

Individuals who understand their art form's strategy and diligently practice its various *kata* learn real-world fighting applications they can use to defend themselves. While each *kata* is always supposed to be performed in exactly the same way, there are a large number of applications, or *bunkai*, from each movement that demonstrate combat techniques. As we watch skilled practitioners go through the movements, it may be possible to visualize joint locks, throws, grappling techniques, and even pressure point applications hidden within the more obvious strikes and punches of each *kata*.

Since these applications are often obscured, intentionally so, we have developed a "secret decoder ring" or modern Rosetta Stone that will teach you how to decipher techniques from your *kata* with real-world utility. Because this information is best understood in a logical progression, we will begin with a bit more history of where all this stuff came from and the strategic concepts within which it is applied.

Chinese Kung Fu

"Anyway, this time I would like to tell you my private opinion regarding, of course, karate-do as follows. I have heard that it is not sure but there is martial arts called 'Three Hand' in India. I don't know the original Indian name. 'Three Hand' is the direct translation of Chinese language from Indian language. I suppose such a martial art was brought to China from India during the Emperor Wu dynasty, and it became the origin of Shaolin Temple."[5]

– Chojun Miyagi

Bodhidharma, founder of the Zen sect of Buddhism, was born in either southern India or Persia, reportedly to a royal family. According to legend, he traveled to the Hunan province in China around 500 A.D., ostensibly to teach Emperor Wu*

---

* Fault tolerant systems are designed to operate successfully regardless of whether or not an error or defect occurs, as opposed to those that can be broken by a single point of failure or even systems that rarely have problems at all. They are highly robust.

the tenets of Zen Buddhism. Hardened by his journey, it is said that he developed great physical and mental prowess. After delivering his teachings to the monarch, he remained in China, spending nine years at the Shaolin Sze so that he could teach Buddhism to the temple monks.

During his stay, he started to teach different breathing techniques and physical exercises to fortify the monks of Shaolin, who were generally weak and unfit in his eyes. He also taught the monks how to develop their mental and spiritual strength, in order to endure the demanding meditation exercises required by their faith. Bodhidharma's teaching is widely considered the birth of kung fu, which means "hard work" in Chinese.

Although there are many similarities between the fighting arts of India and China, there is actually no firm evidence that the Chinese martial systems originated in India. In fact there are several Chinese texts documenting the existence of indigenous fighting forms prior to the sixth century. Regardless, it is known that Buddhism in general and Bodhidharma in particular heavily influenced the Shaolin training. The monks believed that in a weak physical condition they would be unable to perform the rigorous training necessary to attain true enlightenment. Most *Chan Fa* systems are descendants of the 170 hand and foot positions of *Ch'Uen Yuan,* which can be traced back to Bodhidharma's teachings.

The *Shaolin Chan Fa* kung fu was the first codified fighting system in China. As kung fu spread throughout the country, it divided into two main styles—the northern style and the southern style. Linear and hard techniques characterized the northern style, while the southern relied on softer, circular movements. As time progressed, kung fu techniques were often inherited within individual family lines and kept as well-preserved secrets.

Okinawan Martial Arts

"Without doubt, I am sure that the roots of karate-do are in China. I suppose the prototype karate-do might be modified in various ways in my home Okinawa, but I think it is worth enough as we can see the evolution of karate, which was influenced by the uniqueness of Okinawa culture."[6]

– Chojun Miyagi

In Okinawa, the native fighting art of *Te* was practiced long before the introduction of kung fu from China. Once introduced during the 14th century, however, kung fu quickly won popularity and was presented as an art of self-defense under the name *Tote,* which means "Chinese hand." It is widely believed that *Te* was combined with kung fu to form the martial art karate.

* Liang Dynasty

When Japan conquered Okinawa in 1609, an earlier ban on carrying weapons* continued. Fearing insurgency, the Japanese further banned the practice of unarmed martial arts as well. Consequently, the Okinawans had to continue their martial training in great secrecy. No written records were kept. Training was often conducted under cover of darkness at night or in windowless rooms. During the next three centuries, the indigenous martial art took on its own, unique character and was subsequently named *Okinawa-Te*. It was divided into three main styles:

Shuri Te: influenced by the hard techniques of northern kung fu and characterized by offensive attitude.

Naha Te: influenced by the softer techniques of southern kung fu and characterized with grappling, throws, and locking techniques and a more defensive attitude.

Tomari Te: influenced by both the hard and soft techniques of kung fu.

By the end of the 19th century, *Shuri Te* and *Tomari Te* had been subsumed under the name *Shoren Ryu*, which has evolved into several slightly different styles today. Although *Naha Te* still exists in its own right, it is the direct predecessor of modern *Goju Ryu*, which means hard and soft style.† *Goju Ryu* has remained largely unified.

那覇手

naha-te

首里手

syuri-te

泊手

tomari-te

Kanryo Higashionna (Naha Te)

"There are at least three popular versions of his [Kanryo Higashionna's] life story, each one differing in almost every single detail. I present the following version because it appears to be the most logical—which probably makes it the least accurate! Higashionna began his martial arts study in the time-honored tradition: as the result of a beating. This mugging... steeled Higashionna's resolve to learn Okinawa-te, an art which he had practiced occasionally throughout his youth."[7]

– Paul Okami

Kanryo Higashionna *Sensei*,‡ the founder of *Naha Te* was born on March 10, 1853, in the district of Nishimura in the city of Naha, Okinawa. He was the son of Kanryo and Makomado. His father was a merchant who traded food and clothing

---

* First pronounced in 1477 by King Sho Shin, the third king of the second Shô dynasty.
† More precisely, "the hard/gentle way of the infinite fist."
‡ *Sensei* means teacher; literally "one who has come before."

throughout the Ryukyu Islands. At the age of 10, he started to work with his father, because his younger brothers had died very young and his elder brother was physically unable to perform manual labor.

Legend states that in 1867, at the age of 14, Higashionna *Sensei's* father was killed in a fight. Shortly thereafter, he decided to travel to China to learn the deadly martial arts that would permit him to avenge his father's death. A more likely explanation, however, is that he actually left to avoid conscription by the Japanese army.

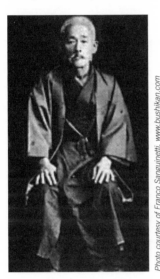

KANRYO HIGASHIONNA

Photo courtesy of Franco Sanguinetti, www.bushikan.com

In 1867 through 1868, the Tokugawa era ended and the Meiji Restoration began. The goal of the Emperor Meiji and his new government was to transform Japan into a democratic state with equality among its entire people. The boundaries between the social classes were gradually broken down. As demonstrated in the movie, *The Last Samurai*, catching up and modernizing the military to bring it up to par with European nations was a high priority for Japan at that time. Universal conscription was introduced to facilitate these ends.

Men on the island nation of Okinawa who fell under this conscription to the Japanese military yet found themselves in an odd position. Not being Japanese, many Okinawans had little interest in joining the military of a nation that had overrun them. Vast cultural and language differences separated the two countries, some of which remain to this day. One option was to leave their island and seek refuge in China, a country with which there had been a long history of friendly relations and trade.

In those days traveling to China was restricted only to merchants, students, or government officials, and permission to travel was granted only by the King of Okinawa himself. The only port of departure was the city of Naha. With the help of the official Udon Yoshimura, Higashionna *Sensei* was able to obtain a permit to travel to Fuchow as a student in 1868.

When he arrived in the city of Fuchow in China, Higashionna *Sensei* was accepted in the *Ryukyu Kan* or lodge where all the Okinawan students lived. He was quickly introduced to the renowned *sensei* Ryu Ryu Ko who had learned the martial arts in the southern Shaolin temple in the mountains of the Fujian Province. Ryu Ryu Ko *Sensei's* family was part of the Novel Court of China before it lost status as result of political turmoil in the country. Ryu Ryu Ko *Sensei* owned a bamboo shop and kept his house on the second floor of the same building. Here he also taught martial arts to a select group of students.

Ryu Ryu Ko tested Higashionna, requiring him to perform menial duties in the yard or shop for over a year before agreeing to teach him the martial arts. Once his actual training began, Higashionna *Sensei* learned *sanchin kata* first. *Sanchin*, which means "three battles," is a moving meditation designed to unify the mind, body, and spirit. *Sanchin kata* is the foundation of many martial systems to this day. While its techniques appear fairly simple and straightforward, it is actually one of the most difficult *kata* for martial artists to truly master. Techniques are performed in slow motion so that practitioners can emphasize precise muscle control, breath control, internal power, and body alignment.

Regardless of the reasons why he commenced his studies, historical records confirm that Higashionna *Sensei* was greatly motivated to learn the martial arts and showed swift progress. He soon moved out of the *Ryukyu Kan* to live and work full-time at Ryu Ryu Ko *Sensei's* bamboo shop. There he was introduced to various traditional training aids such as *chiishi* (weighted stick), *nigiri game* (gripping jars), *tan* (conditioning log), and *makiwara* (striking post).

Although the training was very severe, he excelled at it, learning not only open hand techniques, but also weapons forms such *daito* (long sword), *shuto* (small sword), *sai*, and *bo* (staff) as well. He also learned herbal medicine. In a few short years, Higashionna *Sensei* became Ryu Ryu Ko's top student. He studied for fourteen years in China before returning to Okinawa in 1881.

Upon his return, Higashionna *Sensei* started teaching a select group of students at his own house. Following his instructor's example, his teaching was also very severe. As his fame spread, the King of Okinawa invited Higashionna *Sensei* to personally teach him the martial arts.

In 1905 Higashionna *Sensei* was invited to teach his *Naha Te**[*] in the Naha Commercial School. The school's principal wanted to teach his students the spiritual and moral aspects of the martial arts. This was an important step in the development of *Naha Te*, not only for the recognition of the benefits of the practice but also because, until that time, *Te* had always been taught with a focus on developing skills necessary to kill an adversary in combat.

After his research, Higashionna *Sensei* decided to make an important change in *sanchin kata*, the foundation of *Naha Te*. Although he had learned to perform *sanchin kata* with open hands, he started teaching it with closed hands and slower breathing. He introduced the closed fist to emphasize physical strength more than the ability to kill. The focus on slower breathing promoted its inherent health benefits.[†] Tradition also played an important role in this change because Higashionna *Sensei* noticed that many young Okinawans, without acknowledgement of martial arts, naturally used closed fists when they were going to fight. However, he continued to teach the original way that he learned in China to the select students at his private *dojo*.

---

* *Te* from the city of Naha as it was called then.

† See Principle 13—*don't forget to breathe.*

Until 1905, only a few select individuals practiced *Te*. After that time, karate became more accessible to the general population thanks in large part to the efforts of Kanryo Higashionna *Sensei*. He passed away in October 1915, at the age of sixty-two.

Chojun Miyagi (Goju Ryu)

> *"I remember well my training with Miyagi, in particular the look of his eyes: they were very intimidating. After training he seemed to transform and became gentle and warm… It is very interesting to note that Chojun Miyagi was an exception to kakidameshi. Even though he was very famous, he was held in great respect and awe by all karateka on Okinawa and thus no one dared to test his fighting skill. Of all the teachers I have known, none was respected like Miyagi. This was truly remarkable."*[8]

– Seikichi Toguchi

Chojun Miyagi *Sensei*, the founder of *Goju Ryu*, was born on April 25, 1888, in the city of Naha, Okinawa. He began his practice with Ryuko Aragaki *Sensei* at the age of twelve. Aragaki *Sensei*'s approach was to teach only the fighting itself, with little emphasis on the martial art. After seeing Miyagi's dedication, Ryuko *Sensei* decided to introduce him to Kanryo Higashionna *Sensei*. In 1902, at the age of fourteen, Miyagi began studying *Naha Te* with Higashionna. At twenty, he became Higashionna *Sensei*'s top student.

At the age of twenty-two, he traveled to the main island of Kyushu for his required military service, returning to Okinawa two years later. For the next three years Miyagi studied directly with Higashionna *Sensei*, until his teacher died in 1915.

After the death of his instructor, Chojun Miyagi decided to follow the steps of his *sensei* and travel to Fuchow, China, to learn more about the martial arts. In his first trip in 1915, he went to Fuchow and trained for two months with a student of Ryu Ryu Ko *Sensei*. The old man was very impressed with his skills. Miyagi *Sensei* went to visit the grave of Ryu Ryu Ko *Sensei* as well as the temple where he had trained. In a letter, Miyagi wrote that it was easy to see the footmarks on the patio from the many years of training.

In the early 1920s Miyagi *Sensei* developed the characteristic *Goju Ryu* warm-up exercises or *yunbi undo* with the help of his friend and student Dr. Jinsei Kamiya.* This series of exercises was based not only in martial arts fundaments but also on scientific medical research.

Around this same time, Miyagi *Sensei* developed *tensho kata*, which he began to teach at a high school in Okinawa. *Tensho* translates as "little heaven," or "heaven's

---

* A practicing physician, Kamiya (1894—1964) was also an expert in karate and *kobudo*.

breath." Sometimes called "revolving hands" for its flowing hand techniques, it is a combination of hard dynamic tension with deep breathing and soft flowing hand movements and is very characteristic of the *Goju Ryu* style. This *kata* helps practitioners concentrate strength in their *tanden*.* The *tanden* and hips play a much larger role in Asian martial arts than they do in Western ones. Done a little faster than *sanchin*, *tensho* also emphasizes precise muscle control, breath control, internal power, and body alignment.

Sometime between 1920 and 1930, Miyagi traveled to China for the second time. This was not a productive trip because the relations between China and Japan were not good at the time.

In 1930 Miyagi *Sensei* sent his top student, Jinan Shinsato,[†] to perform a demonstration of *Te* at the Meiji Shrine in Tokyo Japan. This was the year Hirohito was named emperor and there was a huge *taikai* (public demonstration) of martial arts planned as part of the celebration. A *kobudo sensei* (weapons instructor) present at the demonstration asked Shinsato *Sensei* about the name of his art. He found that

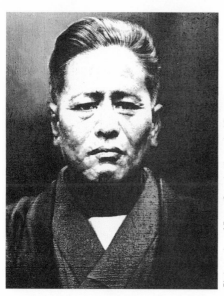

CHOJUN MIYAGI

Photo courtesy of Franco Sanguinetti, www.bushikan.com

he could not answer because until then they only referred to karate as *Te* (hand), *To* (China) or *Bu* (martial art). Upon his return to Okinawa, Shinsato asked his *sensei* about the name of the style that they practiced.

Miyagi *Sensei* decided to call his style *Goju Ryu*.[‡] The meaning was extracted from the *Bubishi*, or book of the poems, where there are references to different subjects including the martial arts. This collection includes a poem entitled the "Eight Precepts of Kempo."[§] Taking a line from that poem, the name *Goju Ryu* identifies the style as the way of the hardness and softness. In this manner *Goju Ryu* became the first style of karate to be named for something other than the city in which it was practiced.

In 1933 *Goju Ryu* was officially recorded and recognized in the *Butotu Kai*[||] in Kyoto, Japan. The official name was recorded as *Goju Ryu Karate Do*, where the meaning of the *kanji* (character) karate was *To* (China) in recognition of the origin of this martial art. In other words, the original translation of "karate" was "Chinese hand" rather than "empty hand" as it is commonly called today.

---

* Considered the center of *ki* energy or center of the body, roughly located at a practitioner's *obi* (belt) knot, two finger widths below their navel.

† A law enforcement professional by trade, Shinsato (1901—1945) was Chojun Miyagi's top student and chosen successor. Unfortunately he died during WWII and was unable to carry on Miyagi *Sensei*'s work.

‡ Though some accounts say that Shinsato *Sensei* may have came up with the name on his own which is certainly possible given the amount of time it took to travel from Kyoto to Naha and back.

§ See Appendix A: *Bubishi* Poem—*Eight Precepts of Kempo*.

|| The institution that groups all the martial arts in Japan.

In 1934 Chojun Miyagi was appointed as the representative of the *Butotu Kai* in Okinawa. Later that same year, Miyagi *Sensei* was invited to travel to Hawaii to teach karate to the Okinawans living on the island. He remained in Hawaii for six months. In his third trip to China, in 1936, he was able to contact the Shanghai Martial Arts Federation. This was instrumental in helping him further his research in the martial arts.

In 1937 Chojun Miyagi was honored to receive the title *kyoshi** from the *Butotu Kai*. This was the first time in the history that somebody in karate received this honor, bringing with it the same status judo and kendo had already achieved.

During World War II, Miyagi *Sensei* lost his top student and chosen successor Jinan Shinsato as well as two of his daughters and a son. After the war, he realized that his martial knowledge could be lost if it was not made available to a larger audience, so he began to teach karate at the Police Academy in Gushikawa, Okinawa, as well as at his home. Among his students were Anichi Miyagi *Sensei*, Shuichi Aragaki *Sensei*,† Seko Higa *Sensei*, Keiyo Matanbashi *Sensei*, Jinsei Kamiya *Sensei*, Genkai Nakaima *Sensei*, and Seikichi Toguchi *Sensei*, among others.

Although Miyagi *Sensei* was adopted into one of the wealthiest families on Okinawa, the war destroyed his assets and wealth. Nevertheless, he devoted his life to karate, which he viewed as sacred like a religion and held in higher esteem than monetary wealth. He structured the system of *Naha Te*, adapted it to the demands of modern society, and made it available to the public as *Goju Ryu* karate. Chojun Miyagi *Sensei* passed away on October 8, 1953 at the age of sixty-five.

Origin of Kata in the West

"Koza city was the home of the United States Air Force base at Kadena and many American soldiers came to the dojo for instruction. At first I had hostile feelings toward Americans so I refused to teach them. Then one day, a student of Higa introduced me to an American soldier and asked me to teach him; this I could not refuse. After teaching him word spread and I was soon teaching about 40 American soldiers… I could not speak English, so I spent countless hours figuring out how to clearly transmit the meanings of kata."[9]

– Seikichi Toguchi

It is widely known that karate was brought to the United States and Europe after World War II. For the most part military men stationed in Okinawa during that period were the first Westerners to learn karate. Returning home after their tours, they were anxious to teach this new fighting system that they had learned in the

---

* Master instructor; equivalent of eighth *dan* black belt.

† Whose grandfather had introduced Miyagi to Higashionna *Sensei*.

mysterious Orient. Sadly, they were passing along knowledge that most had only begun to understand and even fewer came close to mastering.

It stands to reason that the Okinawans who had lost one-eighth of their total population to the war would be somewhat reluctant to teach all of the secrets of karate to their Western occupiers. Culturally, the true secrets of martial arts were passed on only to favored students—often a single one for any given instructor—and only after years of rigorous study and service.

Even if these martial arts masters did want to impart all of their wisdom, the language barrier would have been a significant inhibiter. Trying to explain the philosophy of strategy and tactics in a foreign language is certainly a formula for misunderstanding. Further, it simply takes many, many, many years to truly understand the full depth and subtlety of a martial art.

Many of the early Western karate practitioners were U.S. Marines stationed in Okinawa during the occupation, so let's bring the United States Marine Corps attitude and tradition into the equation. The U.S. Marines are the best at what they do: they kill people, break things, and blow stuff up. They are tough. They never quit and get the job done no matter what the odds. You just do not get that way without a lot of hard, demanding training.

So here's the formula: Take a nearly bankrupt, war-torn county, place it under military rule by occupation forces, add high unemployment, and throw in a means to make a living in U.S. dollars by teaching karate. Add secretive instructors, a language barrier, only a few short years to study, and a bunch of rough-and-tumble soldiers ready to interpret the confusing new art they are learning via the only means they know, their military training.

Furthermore, as karate was opened up to society at large, it was frequently taught to schoolchildren. Many dangerous techniques were hidden from these practitioners simply because they were not mature enough to handle them responsibly.

As a result of all these factors, much of what made it to the outside world was devoid of the principles and rules necessary to understand and utilize hidden techniques. What we got—what showed up on the shores of the United States and Europe—was for the most part, hard, inflexible, intermediate-level karate. There were certainly individual exceptions, of course, but the vast majority of practitioners simply did not learn the finer points of their art. They understood the form, but not the deeper meaning.

Even at *shodan* level,* a practitioner has really only mastered the basic fundamentals of their martial art. *Shodan* most accurately translates as "least of the black belt ranks." Mastery at this level is just the tip of the proverbial iceberg. Not to devalue the accomplishment in any way, but realistically the skill disparity between *shodan* and *nidan** is frequently at least as vast as the difference between an untrained novice and a *shodan* instructor.

* 1st degree black belt.

Karate was never intended to be *only* a "hard" art. Everything in nature is smooth; a cloud has white puffy edges or wispy tailings and a hurricane, as strong as it is, is smooth as well. The hurricane's strength waxes and wanes, yet the wind never comes to a complete standstill and then starts back up again. Just as the wind smooths jagged mountainsides, so too do ocean waves erode jagged shorelines leaving behind a smooth surface.

The only time nature is jagged or has an abrupt edge is when something is rigid and inflexible. Take a stone for instance. If you strike it with another stone to make an edge in the same way our ancestors made flint knives and arrowheads, you will get a sharp surface. Unfortunately it is a brittle one as well. Sharp edges in nature simply do not last. Eventually the sharp edge and the rigid give way to the smooth. It is inevitable. It is the way of nature. We can easily see this in the smooth skipping stones found along any shoreline. It is also demonstrated in the shape of mountains—the older they are, the smoother they become.

Like nature, much of karate (as well as most other martial arts) is smooth and flexible. It is about curves and flow, crashing perhaps, but crashing like ocean waves as opposed to using force in straight, hard, and unnatural ways. Properly performed *kata* have a precise rhythm. Proper pacing is important. Much of the movement is circular.

Subtle nuances make the difference between usable martial application and interesting yet ineffectual dance. Over time, the level of skill and understanding has increased, of course, but even today there are still too many practitioners whose fundamental knowledge of *kata* and application need improvement.

Form precedes speed and both are necessary for power. For example, a properly executed karate punch starts at the ground, from the practitioner's heel. Without a good stance only the upper body is involved and it does not work properly. The elbow must stay pointed at the ground, arm as close to the body as possible. The deltoid muscles in the shoulder must be completely relaxed with tension in the latissimus dorsi and pectoral muscles powering the blow. If the elbow turns outward or the shoulders rise up, the deltoids contract, slowing the punch and reducing the power of the blow.

Everything must be loose to achieve maximum speed with the whole body tensing only at the moment of impact. Hip rotation, if any, is up and down rather than side to side. Practitioners who sway their hips to build power inevitably pull one arm off line, taking much longer than necessary to complete a follow-up blow. A well-trained karate practitioner should be able to throw at least three to five punches per second, any of which have the power to stun or kill an enemy. It takes many, many years of dedicated training to achieve this level of expertise, of course.

When it comes to punching, it does not matter whether you use a traditional *seiken tsuki* (horizontal or fore fist), *ippon ken* (one knuckle), *nukite* (finger strike),

* 2nd degree black belt.

tate tsuki (vertical or standing fist), *shotei uchi* (palm heel strike), or any other type of punch. The underlying principles are the same. Any punch is not solely a hard technique. Speed is built from softness, from relaxation. True power requires excellence in both form and speed.

Kata as a Textbook

"It should be known that the secret principles of Goju Ryu karate exist in the kata."[10]

– Chojun Miyagi

Morio Higaonna *Sensei* wrote, "Karate begins and ends with *kata*. *Kata* is the essence and foundation of karate and it represents the accumulation of more than a thousand years of knowledge. Formed by numerous masters throughout the ages through dedicated training and research, the *kata* are like a map to guide us, and as such must never be changed or tampered with." As Higaonna suggests, it is useful to think of *kata* as a textbook, the essential foundation of any fighting art.

Everything the ancient masters thought their students needed to know was embedded in their *kata*. Copying such *kata* by rote or trying to mimic an instructor was the traditional way to learn. Under such guidance, students gathered the pieces and assembled them, ensured that everything was correct, then repeated the process until it became second nature. This style of learning, called modeling in academia, has persevered because it imparts form and function, transcending language barriers and other inhibitors of communication. Unfortunately it is a poor method of imparting context and deeper meaning.

While many people can breeze through a work of fiction, often seeing movie-like images in their head rather than individual words, textbooks tend to be dry, boring, and about as far from fun as one can get. Although time flies when reading a good novel, it drags when reading a textbook. Take the owner's manual for your vehicle for example. Fascinating read isn't it? Probably not something you look forward to going through.

To make *kata* truly useful, it needs to be interesting. Like a good book, practitioners should look forward to reading it. Repetitive, directed practice and harsh discipline just do not work for most people. Even though it is still fairly common in the Orient, most Westerners are unwilling to spend their first six months mastering a single stance while watching everyone else's training. They ultimately find better things to do with their time.

Learning today has evolved into an interactive art. So too, should martial arts instruction. Students cannot simply be told what to do; at some point they need to understand why. A holistic instructional approach should link history, strategy, technique, and application such that *kata* becomes the living core of the martial art.

Why do the vast majority of us drive modern fuel-injected vehicles with more onboard computing power than the Apollo Lunar Lander? Because they are better, more reliable, and safer than older vehicles, that is why. If we were unfortunate enough to be diagnosed with cancer, we certainly would not want cancer treatments from 1952. We should not be teaching martial arts using methodologies from 1950s either; it simply no longer makes sense.

It is very important to teach and learn *kata* holistically.* Nuance and subtlety are what make the difference between mediocre karate and truly effective fighting art. For example, when Wilder recently returned from Okinawa, he commented on his training there: "The training was all about the basics, the *kihon*, and the subtleness within. The shift of weight, the alignment of the spine, it was about the complexity and the depth of the basics, those fundamental building blocks. It was never about forcing anything; the training was about generating power."

One way to ascertain how powerfully you hit is to have a partner hold a phone book or two against his or her chest. Strike the phonebook(s). If your punch is done correctly, concussive force should transmit through the phone book(s) into your partner, who should feel the blow deep in the chest. Ineffective punches, on the other hand, just make impact on the surface. There is a lot of noise, but little transmission of energy. With minor improvements to the stance that Wilder took back from Okinawa, such as focusing his anchor point on his trailing leg's back heel in *sanchin dachi*, he can easily deliver shock through two phone books, even when he finesses his punches rather than trying for maximum power. The subtlety of body mechanics is extremely important.

So too is concentration. During *kata* practice, practitioners are training to survive in a real fight. In his tome *Fighter's Fact Book*, Loren Christensen† wrote, "As a *kata* judge there is nothing that annoys me more than watching a competitor go through his form as if he were thinking about what he wanted for lunch. You are in a fight for your life, madly defending against attacks from a half a dozen to ten assailants coming at you from every direction. This is not the time to be thinking about lunch."

This mental and physical coordination is an essential component to *kata* practice. It should not be limited simply to competition. As you perform each and every movement of your forms, remember that you are training to keep yourself alive in a real fight. *Kata* is not dance practice nor is it aerobic training. It is the fundamental basis of a fighting art. Like a textbook, it contains all the applications you need to defend yourself in mortal combat.

---

* For more information about teaching and learning martial arts you may wish to refer to Lawrence Kane's book *Martial Arts Instruction: Applying Educational Theory and Communication Techniques in the Dojo* (YMAA Publication Center, 2004).

† Loren Christensen is a prolific author and retired police officer with thirty years of military and civilian law enforcement experience who holds a 7th dan black belt in karate and is proficient in several other fighting arts.

Types of Applications

"In the end a martial artist is training to injure, cripple, or kill another human being. In any drill where students are not regularly hospitalized there is a deliberate flaw, a deliberate break from the needs of reality introduced in the name of safety. In every drill you teach, you must consciously know what the flaw is and make your students aware of it." [11]

– Rory A. Miller

As mentioned previously, there are a plethora of applications for each movement in any *kata*. Although most interpretations are correct, some are better, more useable, than are others. It is important to distinguish between different types of applications so that we can apply them properly. Like tools in a toolbox, we need to use the right one for right situation.

Drills in the *dojo* should not be confused with real violence; they simply help us prepare for it. Treating a real fight like a practice session, on the other hand, can get you killed. Although we do not want to become too hung up on the terminology, there are important differences among the various types of *kata* applications, which can be readily identified through their Japanese nomenclature. A brief description of many common types follows:

Bunkai

Bunkai is the generic name for applications found in *kata*, generally thought of as the most commonly attributed fighting techniques for any given movement. Although any particular set of *kata* movements may have numerous applications any that are performed in exactly the same manner as demonstrated by the *kata* would be considered *bunkai*. If the technique is varied slightly (e.g., performed to the left rather than to the right) but essentially the same, it is more accurately called *henka waza* or "variation technique." Either way, *bunkai* are fighting techniques found in *kata*.

Bunkai Oyo

Bunkai oyo (sometimes simply called *oyo*) are most commonly viewed as the application principles upon which a technique is based. *Oyo* is usually performed as a set of prearranged applications done between partners in a flow drill. While the *bunkai oyo* may exactly mirror what is seen in *kata*, there are many instances where it differs in some way—perhaps performed in a different sequence than the one shown in the *kata*, applied from a different angle, or even transformed in a manner that is only tangentially related to the original *kata* movement. Further, *oyo* may begin with movements from one particular *kata* then add on related techniques that are found in an entirely different *kata*, grouping them together to form a logical progression.

The essential component of *bunkai oyo* is its basis in *kata* principles. It helps explain the essential message of a given *kata*. For example, *saifa kata* translates as "smash and tear." It is of Chinese origin, brought back to Okinawa by Kanryo Higashionna *Sensei*. It incorporates quick whipping movements, hammerfists, and backfist strikes. Although it generally follows the same principles as any other *Goju Ryu kata*, it particularly emphasizes getting off-line (from an opponent's main force) while simultaneously closing distance and exploding through an adversary in ways that can end a fight immediately. *Saifa kata's bunkai oyo* demonstrates these concepts.

Almost every *kata* in *Goju Ryu* karate has a predefined *bunkai oyo*, which practitioners can use to better understand the principles behind its applications. Many other Okinawan and Japanese systems do the same thing. This form of *bunkai* allows the practitioner to do the following:

- Establish flow.
- Exercise the principle of constant attack.
- Explore the unique properties and principles of each individual *kata*.
- Apply dangerous techniques in ways that are not harmful to their training partner.

Okuden Waza

Okuden waza is another name for the secret techniques that have been intentionally concealed in *kata*. *Okuden* refers to the secrets of a school or martial way while *waza* means technique or practical application. Every *kata* contains a significant number of applications, many of which are not obvious to the causal observer. Most of the truly dangerous, advanced techniques are deliberately concealed.

As stated earlier, the ancient masters deliberately camouflaged some of these techniques in order to hide them from practitioners of other styles. Later on, as karate was opened up to society at large, it was frequently taught to schoolchildren. Many dangerous techniques were hidden from these practitioners simply because they were not mature enough to handle them responsibly. In such training discipline, fitness conditioning, and competition aspects of karate where emphasized more than its martial characteristics.

Types of "Fighting"

"The kata are a collection of karate's most brutal and effective fighting techniques, including not only the commonly practiced kicks and punches, but also neck cranks, throws, chokes, strangles, joint locks/dislocations, takedowns and many other grappling techniques." [12]

– Iain Abernethy

One way (among many) in which practitioners can begin to identify practical applications from *kata* is through *kumite* or sparring situations that offer opportunities to practice the *bunkai*. Just as there are various types of *bunkai*, so too are there various types of *kumite*. Once again, it is important to be able to distinguish between the different types:

Kiso Kumite

Kiso kumite is prearranged sparring with an emphasis on technique. It is a set of attack and counterattack sequences designed to teach self-defense skills without the dangers inherent in free sparring. Techniques are pulled from a variety of *kata* and grouped by theme (such as evasion, nerve strikes, short techniques, and so on.). *Ippon kiso kumite* uses only the last attack and defense from each set, followed by an additional set of freeform attacks by the original defender. For safety reasons, practitioners typically start slightly out of range. The attacker makes a long first step, while defender makes a short one to execute techniques at proper fighting distance.

It is important that practitioners give pressure in *kiso kumite*, and that they honor their partner's techniques. Giving pressure means using proper body alignment and good stances such that forward pressure against the opponent is maintained at all times. This approximates realistic conditions where only well-executed movements will be effective. Honoring technique means reacting as if one has been struck with significant force such that practitioners can practice combinations of technique in a reasonably realistic manner.

Because both attacker and defender know exactly what the other partner will do, participants can execute techniques safely while using great quickness and power. As training progresses the patterns are burned into practitioner's muscle memory, facilitating automatic responses in pressure situations. Regardless, it is still not real fighting. We pull the final blow before it lands with full force.

You know it is only a drill when no one goes to the hospital afterward. It would be quite embarrassing to respond to a real-life attack with blazing speed and accuracy only to gently tap your attacker because you pulled the blow. It is very important to understand that *kiso kumite* is not real fighting, only an approximation thereof. You need to be able to mentally shift gears during a real confrontation on the street.

Fuku Shiki Kumite

Fuku shiki kumite is freestyle sparring with *kata* emphasis. Similar to *ippon kiso kumite* advanced practitioners often use it to practice *bunkai oyo* in an unchoreographed manner. Partners may decide to use only techniques for specific *kata* or may select a more freeform manner, but either way the emphasis is on employment of *kata bunkai*.

In traditional schools, padding and other safety devices (e.g., hard cup, head-gear) are generally discouraged as they limit range of movement and ability to perform certain techniques. Further, there are important conditioning aspects to getting hit with a healthy amount of force (in non-vital areas, of course). Being able to absorb a blow is important; a black belt who spends four to six years punching air to achieve his or her rank will often be unable to present an adequate defense in a real fight. In these exercises, the senior partner controls the speed and takes responsibility for safety of both practitioners. While it is a step above *kiso kumite*, this unchoreographed exchange and counter exchange is still only an approximation of real fighting.

Any time practitioners use protective gear or arbitrary safety rules, the will find very different dynamics between sparring practice and actual combat. The same thing happens in other martial arts as well. Olympic-style fencers, for example, use light-weight flexible swords that score with a light touch. Subtle wrist movements and hand quickness are emphasized. If you score a microsecond before your opponent's blade touches you, you win. Intentionally letting a slower opponent stab you is not exactly a viable tactic in a real fight, however, as both combatants would be injured or killed from simultaneous blows.

Further, real dueling swords are much heavier, requiring somewhat different body mechanics and fighting ranges to penetrate and dispatch an opponent. Even in modern times, numerous people are hacked to death by swords or machetes in countries like Rwanda, Sudan, Israel, the Philippines, and even in the United States. Understanding how such implements work in actual combat may be more useful than one might first imagine. Conversely, confusing sporting competition for combat preparation may be more detrimental than one might think.

Sanbon Shobu Kumite

Sanbon shobu kumite is a three-point, tournament style match. Padding and safety gear is more frequently used with this application, though certainly not in every case. Since strict safety rules outlaw anything truly dangerous (e.g., vital point or nerve strikes, joint attacks) tournament matches are far from true combat situations. Weight classes frequently match competitors of similar size/age, and mixed gender competitions are rare occurrences.

Tournaments are great for conditioning. They build reflex action and refine practitioner's timing and reaction skills. It is paramount, however, that tournament fighters do not pick up bad habits and bring them into self-defense situations. For example, we have seen tournaments where contestants were fighting with their backs and sides facing their opponents, since the back was not a legal target for point scoring and would lead to at least a *keikoku* (warning) or *shikkaku* (disqualification) if intentionally struck. Fighting with your back to an attacker is clearly not something you would choose to do in a life-or-death confrontation.

Boxers also follow artificial rules for competitor safety. Kicking techniques are removed entirely. Punches below the waist are illegal. Grappling and throwing techniques, once common in bare knuckles fighting, are no longer allowed. Heavily padded gloves allow straight punches to the chin that might otherwise break a participant's hand. Clearly though the intensity is similar, the strategy and tactics used in a real fight will be markedly different from those employed in boxing competition. Being successful at one application does not necessarily prepare practitioners for success at the other. Once again, rules promulgated to enforce practitioner safety create a barrier between tournament and combat applications. There is nothing inherently wrong with competing in sporting events so long as practitioners understand that they are very different than real-life combat.

Randori

Randori is free style sparring, similar to a practice tournament where points are not counted. This activity is commonly used in grappling arts such as judo or jujitsu and includes high intensity attacks and counter attacks drawn from anywhere within the martial system. The focus is not on any specific *kata* or grouping of techniques.

Once again, freestyle sparring is still not real fighting. The focus is on movement, combinations, timing, and balance. Unlike *kiso kumite*, *randori* can help practitioners enhance their ability to instantaneously react to surprise attacks. Like *sanbon shobu kumite*, however, vital areas are left alone and blows are struck only with sufficient force to score a "victory." In grappling arts, for example, chokes are released when a practitioner taps (the ground, the mat, or a body part), often before he or she loses consciousness. Even if a competitor is rendered unconscious in a match, referees and medical personnel are close at hand to safely revive him or her. Similarly, joint locks do not generally lead to hyperextension or dislocation in a tournament or sparring practice match.

While you never intentionally hurt your training partner, you would certainly never want to pull your punch in a real fight. It is important to avoid building bad habits from *randori*. Practitioners should mentally follow through with the blows that they physically stop short.

Self Defense

All bets are off when it comes to real life self-defense. Real life self-defense is a completely different animal than practice in a *dojo*. Self-defense techniques are a foundation on which to build creativity, spontaneity, and to define multiple applications from any given technique. Size, age, or gender mismatches, unexpected actions by opponents, and other variables need to be considered and compensated for.

There is no magic-bullet technique to fit all situations. In short, once a confrontation begins, practitioners must do whatever works to end it quickly. A fundamental principle of karate, however, is that all techniques should be applied defensively. The famous saying goes, "*karate ni sente nashi*," Which translates as, "there is no first strike in karate." This is outstanding advice. Martial artists should never provoke confrontations. While there certainly are situations in which fighting is the only alternative, it is best to avoid physical altercations altogether whenever possible.

Unlike a sparring match, there are no rules in a real fight. One cannot believe anything an attacker says. If someone is attacking you, he (or she) must be a bad guy (after all, no one reading this book would ever provoke a violent confrontation, right?). While we are not attorneys, hence not offering legal counsel or opinion, our understanding is that the cornerstone of a legitimate claim of self-defense is the innocence of the claimant. A person must be entirely without fault. If a martial artist begins a conflict, he or she cannot claim self-defense. If the practitioner allows a conflict to escalate into a lethal situation when it could have been avoided, he or she shares some degree of culpability and, once again, cannot claim self-defense.

There are countless stories of martial artists picking fights they regret for the rest of their lives because people were maimed or killed and the practitioners are subsequently sued or jailed or both. You cannot afford to let your ego overrule your common sense. In unavoidable combat, however, you must do anything to survive. Never stop until your attacker has been disabled and you can safely get away.

Once a confrontation escalates into combat, adrenaline rushes through your system. This dramatically increases your pain tolerance and helps you survive in fighting mode. This "fight or flight" reaction instantly supercharges your body for a short period of time, increasing pulse rate and blood pressure, while making you faster, meaner, and more impervious to pain than ever before. Embrace your fear in a fight; it can help you win.

In a real fight, martial training can take over automatically. You can literally watch your body perform what it has been trained to do, with your fists and your feet or with a makeshift weapon or even a gun, without really having to think about it that much. That is why we practice repetitiously and realistically. When real danger arises, pre-programmed responses can take over.*

Why Applications are Not Readily Discernable in Kata

> *"Miyagi Sensei asked him to show them his best kata that he mastered in China. Then Machaa Buntoku put on hachimaki (headband) and performed a strange dance in front of them. He danced and danced. Seeing his strange dance, Seiko Higa thought this old man must be crazy or mad because of his old age.*

> *"Jin-an Arazato who was yet young at that time lost his temper to see this dance and told him, "OK. Dance is enough! Show me your fighting technique! I will be your opponent." Arazato delivered a karate-do blow at him, but Arazato was thrown down by the dancing old man and hurt his back. He lost face. Everyone there felt awkward about it, so they bowed to the old man and went home. On the way home no one spoke.*

> *"This anecdote was told to my father by Master Seiko Higa. For the dancing old man, he just showed them his best kata, however, they had never supposed that his dancing was his best fighting technique."* [13]

> – *Kiyohiko Higa*

To the uninitiated, *kata* often looks like dancing, yet to the trained practitioner it can be the key to learning a deadly art. There was an ancient custom in Okinawa called *kakidameshi* where *budoka* routinely tested each other's fighting skills in actual combat. Like the feudal *samurai* before or the old West gunfighters who would follow, the more famous the practitioner, the more often he would be challenged to combat by those seeking fame. These challenges often took the form of sudden ambush or sneak attack. Consequently, while the masters of such arts had to ensure that their forms would work in actual combat, they jealously guarded the secrets of their style. They orally taught the secrets of deciphering their *kata* to a single trusted student, a sole successor who promised to never reveal these secret techniques to the public.

In their book, *Shihan-Te: The Bunkai of Karate Kata*, Darrell Craig and Paul Anderson explain that, "the notion of teaching and practicing in secret was not unique to the Okinawans; the same tradition had existed in ancient China... The

---

* For more about this subject, see Characteristics of Violence in chapter 5.

masters often had what could be viewed as a dual-track system; they taught the same *kata* in two slightly different ways. The outer circle of students, those not yet entitled to the master's secrets, would be taught a *kata* with certain critical details and principles omitted; the inner circle would be taught the same *kata*, but with those details and principles included. To the untrained eye, the difference might be undetectable."

Gichin Funakoshi, the founder of *Shotokan Karate* told an interesting story in his book *Karate-do Nyumon*. An elderly Okinawan karate master contacted Funakoshi expressing the desire to pass on a *kata* before he died. Unable to attend, he received permission to send his son, Gigo, who was shown the secret *kata* in a locked room with shuttered windows. The old man told Gigo that he had only shown that particular *kata* to one person in his life, at that time critically altering it to hide certain techniques.

The average karate practitioner did not always have wide-ranging curricula to learn. Seikichi Toguchi wrote, "Both Higa and Miyagi were very strict and questions were not permitted during training. When we practiced, we were not allowed to perform the *kata* beyond what they had taught us. In essence you were not allowed to learn a new sequence of the *kata* until the initial sections or techniques were approved."

Until the end of WWII most *karateka* typically learned *sanchin* plus one or two other *kata* selected by their master based on their individual strengths, weaknesses, body types, and dispositions. It was not unusual practice a single *kata* for seven to ten years before being given permission to begin another one. Since each *kata* contains a complete, integrated fighting system, the goal was to understand truly all aspects of what they had been given.

After the devastation of the Great War, however, many masters wanted to avoid any further loss of knowledge, so additional curricula were presented. When a practitioner is given a lot more material to digest, it is quite understandable for their level of comprehension to be somewhat less. To confuse matters further, the same *kata* was sporadically taught to different students of the same instructor in different ways, most likely to adapt to body type and other personal characteristics among the various practitioners.

In his fascinating biography of Japan's legendary swordsman, *The Lone Samurai: The Life of Miyamoto Musashi*, William Scott Wilson wrote: "Musashi taught each of his disciples individually at his *dojo*, judging each man for what would be appropriate or inappropriate for him to learn." It is certainly reasonable to assume that many contemporary instructors approached teaching similarly.

It is also possible that the variations were simply due to differences in emphasis among *kata* segments. Instructors frequently emphasize specific sections of a *kata* to

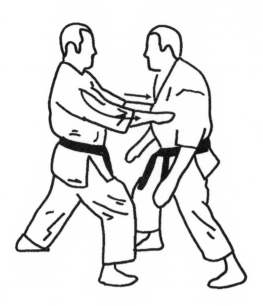

SAIFA KATA: MOROTE KAMA-DE UCHI (DOUBLE BEAR CLAW STRIKE).

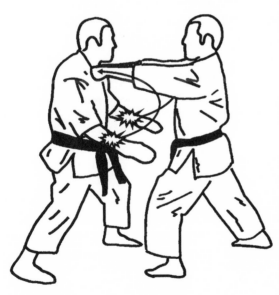

SAIFA KATA: MOROTE SEIKEN TSUKI (DOUBLE PUNCH).

help individual practitioners overcome a particular shortfall in their training. As Taguchi *Sensei* wrote, "No explanation of techniques was given. We simply followed instructions. We were not even permitted to utter a word in response to instructions." If the reason for this emphasis is not explained or rescinded, a *kata* may be forever altered by such changes.

Even when taught exactly the same way, individual students' memories occasionally differed, leading to divergences in the way they performed the techniques. Modern students, even those who learned from direct disciples of the founders of various styles, often find variation between their understandings of certain *kata*. For example, *saifa kata* as taught by Seikichi Toguchi *Sensei*, a direct student of Chojun Miyagi *Sensei* is slightly different than the version taught by Teruo Chinen *Sensei*, another direct student. In the middle of the *kata* one instructor teaches a *morote kama-de uchi* (double bear claw strike) while the other uses a *morote seiken tsuki* (traditional double punch).

Beyond that, everyone has some *kata* they prefer over others. People generally learn better when they like what they are doing. When writing this section, we thought about which *kata* were most important to us and why.

Wilder likes to close with an opponent as much as possible. "I have found that even at 225 pounds, I was frequently the lightest in my judo competition category," he relates. "Closing the gap on my terms was always preferable than having an opponent determine what was going to happen. Although I innately understood this concept, the judo training helped me embrace and analyze the idea of closing, controlling, and ultimately striking my

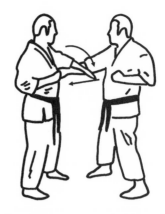

HOOKIYU KATA: CHUDAN UKE (CHEST BLOCK).
THE DEFENDER IS ON THE LEFT.

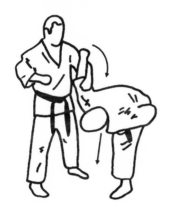

HOOKIYU KATA: GEDAN UKE (DOWN BLOCK)—WHAT LOOKS
LIKE A DOWN BLOCK BECOMES AN ARM BAR).

opponent on my terms and not necessarily having that chosen for me or by the luck of the draw. If told I could take only two or three *kata* to a desert island I would have to say, *sanseiru* and *shisochin* would be two of them because of the way they charge an opponent. It is just a preference built out of body type and psychological make-up."

Kane, on the other hand, says that,

"at 185 pounds, the odds of my being bigger than an opponent really aren't all that great. Rather than crashing through and uprooting someone, I prefer to dance around the edges and break an opponent down with speed and precision. I really like fast whipping techniques such as those found in *saifa* and *saipai*. Those are the *kata* that I'd take to the island." His predilections and Wilder's are different in part due to their divergent body types.

Whatever your individual preferences, you can be successful by focusing

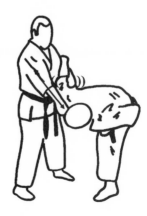

HOOKIYU KATA: GEDAN TSUKI (HEAD PUNCH)—WHAT
LOOKS LIKE A DOWN PUNCH IN KATA BECOMES A HEAD
PUNCH IN APPLICATION BECAUSE THE OPPONENT IS BENT
OVER FROM THE ARM BAR.

on just about any single *kata*, whichever one suits you best, because most every *kata* contains an integrated, holistic fighting system. While it is not obvious to the casual observer, even basic *kata* can demonstrate powerful, hidden techniques if you know how to find them. For example, one interpretation of the *chudan uke* (chest block), *gedan uke* (down block), *gedan tsuki* (down punch) combination from *hookiyu kata** is to block a punch, apply an arm lock to bend your opponent over, and then strike to their temple, a very powerful combination.

Kata demonstrate the angle and direction of attack (either front, back, or side) to which the practitioner is responding. *Kata* also give clues about the type of attack (such as a punch, kick, grab, or push) and what the proper counterattack might be. For example, hand techniques are often delivered to the upper part of the body, while kicks are usually lower. Strikes work against an opponent's force, while throws work with it (using an opponent's force against them).

Though they intentionally hid the secret meanings and techniques within their *kata*, the founders of the modern martial arts did pass along clues for how to uncover them. However, even once we have identified what we think is the ultimate expression of any given technique, it is important to understand that more than one proper application exists for any given movement of any given *kata*.

More Than One Proper Application Exists

"There also is no such a thing as a useless tool. No matter what a teacher says about another style, inherent in any martial art style are the elements to be used for self-defense. However, many instructors have never learned them—and yet they claim to have mastered them. These same people point derisively toward the ignorance of other instructors and the weaknesses of other styles. This is why I say there is no such thing as a bad martial art style, only bad martial arts teachers." [14]

– Marc MacYoung

There is no single, correct interpretation of any particular movement in a *kata*. More than one proper application exists for each movement. Some are better than others, of course, but many exist all the same. Morio Higaonna said, "If you practice the *kata* thoroughly you will come to understand the *bunkai* of the *kata* naturally and completely. However, this will take many years of training, without which you will not gain a true understanding of the *kata*, and will not be able to apply *kata* techniques in real combat. None of the movements is restricted to only one application—in real fight the variations of each application is unlimited." Anyone who says differently simply does not understand what he or she is talking about.

* Hookiyu kata is one of the very first kihon forms taught in many Goju Ryu systems.

We all know the fable of the emperor who had no clothes. The emperor had ordered a special suit for an event but was hoodwinked into thinking that the haberdasher had made him fine clothes when in fact he was actually naked. Of course nobody would admit that the emperor had no clothes since he was, after all, the emperor. That story is an example of consensus reality. While it is amusing in a fairy tale, in real-life consensus thinking can get you hurt. Conventional wisdom is not always correct. It must be evaluated and re-analyzed over time to ensure that it remains meaningful and relevant.

A good example might be the consumption of alcohol. In medieval times there was a commonly accepted practice of imbibing wine, mead,* or similar drinks with meals. The health benefits were frequently extolled in literature and common thought. Over time, however, that changed. In reaction to overindulgence among other things, secular and religious groups began to frown on such practices. Eventually the consumption of alcohol was banned altogether in the United States during the failed experiment of Prohibition.

More recently several medical studies have demonstrated some health benefits from consuming small amounts of alcohol (no more than two glasses) on a daily basis. A medieval physician once wrote that wine "doth quycken a man wyttes; it doth comfort the hert; it doth scowre the lyver, and it doth ingender gode blode. In modern English that translates, "wine quickens a man's wits, comforts the heart, scours the liver, and engenders good blood."

Modern medical research has proven at least some of this statement to be true: the tannins and other phenolic compounds that give wine its flavor and color are also powerful antioxidants, capable of preventing disease. Wine-based antioxidants help prevent unhealthy LDL cholesterol from being oxidized into artery-clogging plaque, as well as helping to decrease the formation of dangerous internal blood clots. Further, a 2004 study by the Fred Hutchinson Cancer Research Center found that men who consumed four or more glasses of red wine per week reduced their risk of prostate cancer by 50 percent, with a 60 percent lower incidence of the more aggressive types of cancer.

The consensus thinking about alcohol has changed over time. The same thing happens in martial arts. There are usually three components to a martial art, the physical, the mental, and the spiritual. These are not mutually exclusive in that they bleed over into onto one another at different times. So when you scrutinize the consensus reality do yourself a favor and look to all of these aspects understanding that at any time one aspect, mental, physical, or spiritual can play a foundational role in supporting the other.

The Buddha taught, "Believe nothing merely because you have been told it. Do not believe what your teacher tells you merely out of respect for the teacher." It is

---

* A variant of wine made from fermented honey, mead was immortalized in Norse mythology as the favorite beverage of gods and heroes. The nectar and ambrosia of the Greek mythos was thought to be made from honey wine as well.

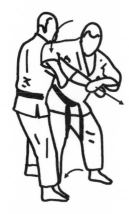

COMMONLY TAUGHT THROW, STEP 1: SPIN, LEAVING
YOURSELF VULNERABLE TO COUNTERATTACK.

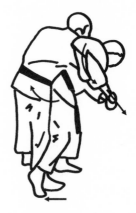

COMMONLY TAUGHT THROW, STEP 2: TURN AND THROW.

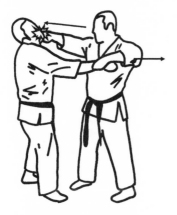

PROPER THROW, STEP 1: STRIKE FIRST,
DISRUPTING THE OPPONENT.

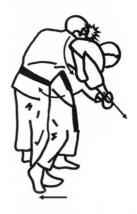

PROPER THROW, STEP 2: STRIKE AGAIN/TURN AND EXECUTE
THE THROW. THIS CAN GET YOU DISQUALIFIED FROM A
JUDO TOURNAMENT BUT IS A MUCH MORE COMBAT-WORTHY
APPLICATION ON THE STREET.

wise to use discernment when you are approaching your training. Just because someone says that something is so, that does not necessarily make it right.

If you are in an instructional role and discover through the study of physiology,
reading this book, or from some other research that what you have been taught is
not correct, be sure to change your own teaching and make sure it is corrected down
the line. Nothing is more foolish that doing what that emperor did, walking around
in ignorance in front of all his subjects.

For example, throws that win sporting competitions can get you hurt or killed
on the street. Compare and contrast a commonly taught throw with a combat
worthy alternative:

Hidden Applications between Kata Movements

"Perception is strong and sight weak. In strategy it is important to see distant things as if they were close and to take a distanced view of close things." [15]

– Miyamoto Musashi

Not only are many secret techniques intentionally obscured in *kata*, but also some are not even shown at all. There are frequently hidden applications (e.g., ear slap, eye rake) *between* movements in *kata*. Watching a skilled practitioner go through a *kata* can be magical. The more you know about the *kata*, the more magical the performance becomes. The key to what the *kata* artists do is often what they are doing when they appear to be doing nothing.

Confusing? Think of it this way—in music, a pause or rest between the notes provides emphasis for the notes that follow, giving these subsequent notes their moment to shine. Without the rhythm and the rests, all the notes would be smashed together creating an unpleasant stream of noise. The same concept applies to *kata*. Mozart said that it is far easier for a musician to play well quickly than to play well slowly. Many people rush through *kata* in a hurry to show power and speed. What Mozart said about music also applies to *kata*. A pause in the *kata* gives the technique that follows a moment to shine.

Look at your own *kata* and ask yourself if it is a blur that is unintelligible or if it is a beautifully composed story of speed, power, technique, and understanding. As you practice, it is important that you take your time. Start with the most basic form you know and slow it down. You will probably find many areas that need improvement and it will take a while to actually complete each form. Remember to look for the forgotten nuances that one cannot always see at full speed.

Do not change the movements, however. Hidden applications between movements should be shown with your mind, not your body. It is all a matter of intent. This is extremely subtle and somewhat difficult to explain. Suffice it to say that watching a very experienced practitioner doing even the most basic of *kata* looks nothing like those who have only been practicing for a few years.

Think of each move of a *kata* as a note of music, and look at the spaces between the notes for hidden techniques that will disrupt your opponent and facilitate your ability to successfully counterattack. For example, between any open-hand chest blocks in *kata*, there can easily be a rake to your opponent's eyes. Expanding on this idea, the return from the block becomes a grab and pull, followed by your next technique. Since head and hands follow the pain,* effective combinations typically move along the body going high-low-high or low-high-low to present openings via

---

* By head following the pain, we mean that your opponent's attention will usually shift to where he has been struck, particularly if he is not a trained fighter who has become sensitized against pain. Further, there is a natural physiological reaction that draws a person's hands toward the body part that hurts. Using this example, if you rake someone's eyes, he is likely to flinch, cover his face with his hands, and momentarily forget about his lower body leaving it vulnerable to your follow-on attack.

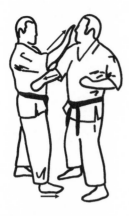

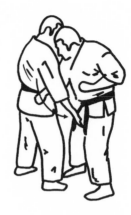

EYE RAKE. ALMOST ANY OPEN-HAND CHEST BLOCK CAN ALSO BE USED TO ATTACK AN OPPONENT'S EYES.

GROIN STRIKE. A GROIN STRIKE WORKS WELL IN CONJUNCTION WITH AN EYE RAKE SINCE HEAD AND HANDS FOLLOW THE PAIN.

disruption. In this manner, you will often see an eye rake followed by a groin strike or an attack to the opponent's knee.

Summary

"Martial arts and self-defense organizations often tend to be extremely cliquish. That is to say that they are often built around a particular way of thinking or more often, one person's persona. In fact, these are indeed cults of personality. These programs often fall into three basic categories. One, because the "founder" of the system, or current grand pooh-bah, is thought by the disciples to walk on water and be the messiah of the martial arts. Two, is the person presents himself as some kind of killer kung fu commando street fighter who has used his devastating fighting system to defeat hordes of attackers in countless combat situations. The third mess is a combination of the first two. Putting it bluntly when you encounter this you have not found an effective self-defense system, you have found a church." [16]

– Marc MacYoung

Violence has existed in one form or another since the first cave man bashed his neighbor over the head with a rock or a stick. Combat arts created to defend oneself from assault have been around nearly as long. As martial forms evolved into sophisticated fighting systems, almost all Asian styles began to utilize *kata*. A Japanese word meaning "formal exercise," *kata* contain logical sequences of movements containing practical offensive and defensive techniques that are done in a particular order. The ancient masters embedded the secrets of their unique fighting systems in their *kata*.

While each *kata* is supposed to be performed in exactly the same way every time, there are almost unlimited combat applications or *bunkai* hidden within each movement. Even more applications can be hidden between the movements of a *kata*. Nevertheless, to the uninitiated, *kata* look very much like complicated dancing. Practical applications and sophisticated techniques remain hidden from the casual observer. There are a couple of important reasons why these mechanisms are not readily apparent.

First, in 1609 when the Japanese conquered Okinawa, the birthplace of karate, they banned the teaching of both armed and unarmed martial arts. Consequently the Okinawans had to conduct their training in great secrecy. Forms were passed between master and disciple through oral tradition with nothing written down. Much of the training was conducted indoors, at night, or otherwise shielded from prying eyes.

A second important reason for the secrecy of *kata* is found in the ancient custom of *kakidameshi*, a tradition where *budoka* in Okinawa routinely tested each other's fighting prowess with actual combat. Techniques not only had to be combat-worthy, but they also had to be held pretty close to the vest. It simply would not do for a competitor to know one's secrets before a fight.

Consequently there was often a two-track system of instruction. The outer circle of students learned basic fundamentals; unknowingly receiving modified *kata* where critical details or principles were omitted. It was a significant honor even to achieve this first level of training, as masters turned away all but the most dedicated of followers. Further, the heads of these martial schools (or martial ways) universally expected instant obedience from students, clarifying little and tolerating no questions.

The inner circle that had gained a master's trust and respect, on the other hand, could be taught *okuden waza*, the secret applications of *kata*. Even within this inner circle, the rules and principles for deciphering all of a system's *kata* were frequently taught only to one student, the master's sole successor, rather than to the group as a whole. Often this instruction was withheld until the master became quite old or very ill, shortly before his death. On occasion the master waited too long to pass along this vital knowledge and it was lost altogether.

In modern times *kata* was spread from Okinawa to the rest of the world, primarily by America GIs and Allied troops who learned karate during the occupation of that country at the end of World War II. Although locally high unemployment drove the many *budo* masters to teach the Westerners as a means to earn a living, most soldiers were not initiated into their inner circles. Further, even when instructors wished to share their secrets, language barriers often inhibited communication.

Later on, as *budo* was opened up to society at large, it was frequently taught to schoolchildren. Many dangerous techniques were hidden from these practitioners simply because they were not mature enough to handle them responsibly. Consequently much of what made it to the outside world was intermediate-level martial arts, devoid of principles and rules necessary to understand and utilize hidden techniques.

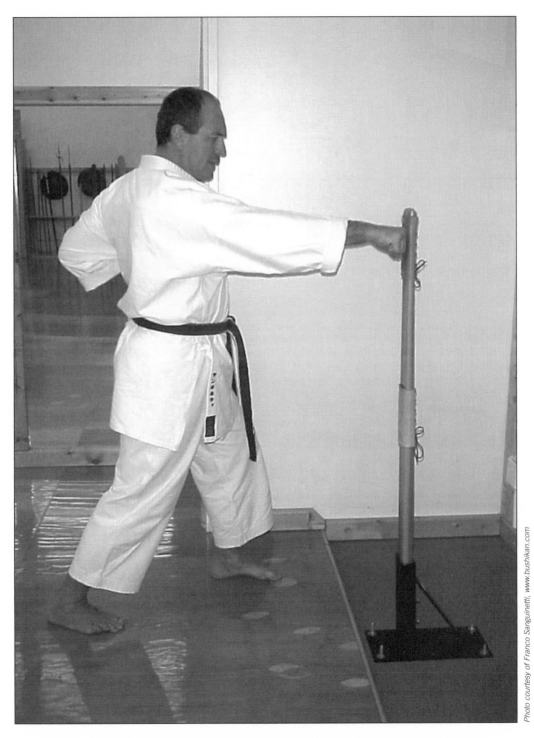

MAKIWARA IS A STRIKING POST WITH A STRAW, CLOTH, LEATHER, OR RUBBER COVERING FOR CONTACT PADDING. IT IS USED FOR PRACTICING STRIKING TECHNIQUES AS WELL AS FOR CONDITIONING THE HANDS, ELBOWS, KNEES, AND FEET. YOUNGER CHILDREN WHOSE HANDS ARE STILL DEVELOPING SHOULD NEVER PUNCH A MAKIWARA. IT IS TOO RIGID AND MAY CAUSE INJURY, SO SUBSTITUTE A MODERN, PUNCHING BAG INSTEAD.

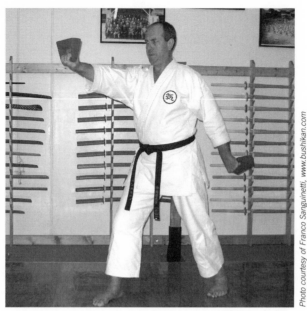

Photo courtesy of Franco Sanguinetti, www.bushikan.com

ISHISASHI IS A STONE PADLOCK RESEMBLING THE SHAPE OF AN OLD-FASHIONED CLOTHES IRON. IT IS USED FOR STRENGTHENING ARMS AND WRISTS.

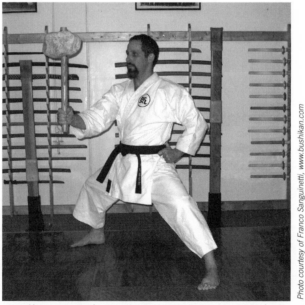

Photo courtesy of Franco Sanguinetti, www.bushikan.com

STONE *CHIISHI. KIGU HOJO UNDO* (SUPPLEMENTARY TRAINING WITH VARIOUS TOOLS) CAN HELP BUDO-KA DEVELOP TREMENDOUS PHYSICAL STRENGTH AND FLEXIBILITY. *CHIISHI* IS A CONCRETE OR STONE WEIGHT AT THE END OF A WOODEN HANDLE USED TO STRENGTHEN THE GRIP, AS WELL AS THE JOINTS OF THE ELBOWS, WRISTS, AND SHOULDERS. *CHIISHI* EXERCISES CONDITION TENDONS AND JOINTS AND HELP DEVELOP THE MUSCLES USED FOR BLOCKING, STRIKING, AND GRAPPLING TECHNIQUES. IF THE *CHIISHI* IS TOO HEAVY TO CONTROL APPROPRIATELY, PRACTITIONERS SHOULD CHOKE UP ON THE HANDLE SO THAT THE WEIGHT IS CLOSER TO THE BODY.

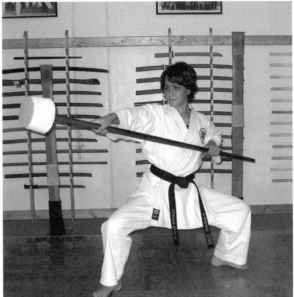

LONG *CHIISHI* (BO EXERCISE). HERE AN EXTRA LONG *CHIISHI* IS USED TO PRACTICE *BO* STAFF WORK, DEVELOPING STRENGTH, SPEED, AND FLEXIBILITY IN *BO* TECHNIQUES.

Photo courtesy of Franco Sanguinetti, www.bushikan.com

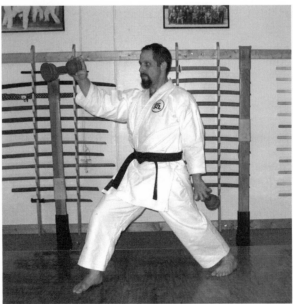

NIGIRI GAME TRAINING. NIGIRI GAME ARE GRIPPING JARS, USUALLY MADE OF CLAY WITH A RIM AROUND THE TOP TO GRIP WITH THE FINGERS. WATER, SAND, OR SMALL STONES ARE OFTEN ADDED TO INCREASE THE WEIGHT. EXERCISES WITH THESE JARS ARE DESIGNED TO STRENGTHEN THE FINGERS FOR GRIPPING AND TEARING APPLICATIONS.

Photo courtesy of Franco Sanguinetti, www.bushikan.com

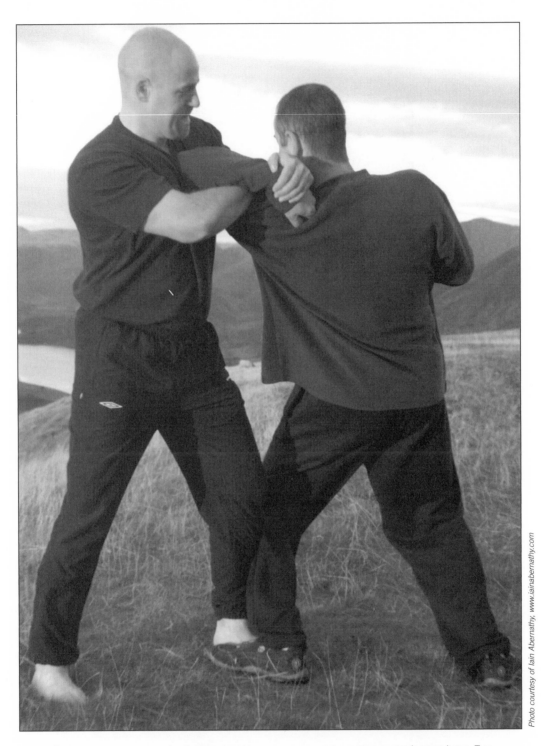

CHINTO ENTANGLED WRISTLOCK. IAIN ABERNETHY APPLIES AN ENTANGLED WRIST-LOCK FROM CHINTO (GANKAKU) KATA. THE RECIPIENT IS MURRAY DENWOOD. THE LOCATION IS THE LAKE DISTRICT IN CUMBRIA, NORTHERN ENGLAND.

Chapter 2

Strategy and Tactics

"A man who does not plan long ahead will find trouble right at his door." [17]

– Confucius

Every martial system contains both a strategy, which may be hidden, as well as tactics that can readily be found in *kata*. Tactics are the applications that you see (or decipher), while strategy is the overarching plan that ties them together into a cohesive whole. Looking at how frequently techniques come up in the various core *kata* of a system can be a good way to ascertain its strategy. Look for patterns that are repeated within and between the various *kata*.

A deep understanding of strategy and tactics is a necessary prerequisite for being able to properly decipher *kata*. To be effective, all martial applications must be grounded in a system's strategy. Picking and choosing individual techniques from a variety of different styles is almost always sub-optimal as there is no strategic concept binding them together. Let's delve into this subject in more detail.

Effective Applications Must Be Grounded in a System's Strategy

"When you truly understand the Way, you can take any form that you want to. It is almost as if you had developed miraculous powers. You can become as light as a feather, as fluid as water, or as stiff as a board. Regardless of the form you take, once you have understood my strategy you cannot be beaten by one man or ten thousand. Once you have understood my strategy you will be a warrior to be reckoned with." [18]

– Miyamoto Musashi

By the height of their empire, Rome's legions (*legio*) had conquered much of the known world. A large reason for their amazing success was a solid strategy on which everything else was built. The core of that strategy was, at its most basic level, based on discipline and unity.

Professional foot soldiers formed the vast majority of the Roman army at that time. These soldiers trained specifically for close-quarters combat. Though the exact formation and structure of the legions varied depending upon the time period one

35

examines, each division of soldiers—century (~80 men), cohort (~480 men), and legion (~5,240 men)—had its own battle standard.

Though used primarily to facilitate command and communication, battle standards also helped to preserve the cohesiveness and pride of each unit, as they represented a concrete symbol of that unit's achievements and were also used in various religious rituals designed to promote unity. The most important standard in each legion was the legionary eagle made of a precious metal (usually silver), a potent symbol of the power of Rome and the honor of the legion. In wartime, officers called standard-bearers (*signifer*) held these battle standards. These individuals stood out from other soldiers by the animal-head skins they wore on their heads.

Just as the military structure of the legion was designed to promote discipline and unity, so too was the equipment the troops were issued and tactics they deployed. Each foot soldier was given a very short thrusting sword (*gladius*), a large shield (*scutum*), a couple of javelins (*pila*), and at least minimal armor (covering much of the head, torso, forearms and shins). When fighting they threw their *pila* to disrupt an enemy, picking off easy targets, then closed ranks to engage in carefully orchestrated hand-to-hand combat. In close-quarters range, they were trained to attack the nearest enemy soldier diagonally across from them, thrusting through the small gaps between their interlocked shields. Roman soldiers almost never aimed for an enemy combatant directly in front of them, relying instead on their fellow warriors to handle that threat.

These short swords and interlocking shields forced the Romans to work together as a unit, each protecting the other. Individual fighting ability counted far less than organization and coordination. They methodically moved forward as a disciplined unit, decimating and trampling their less organized opponents. In this manner everything in the military structure, equipment, training, and tactics all reinforced the Romans' overall strategy.

It works the same way in the martial arts. Everything from stances to breathing, including movement, striking, kicking, grappling, and defensive postures are all directly tied to a system's strategy. It is holistic, self-contained, and unique to every art.

After training for some time, one often hears practitioners claiming that their style is inherently superior to others. This attitude is expected, though not particularly mature. It is part of the growth a person experiences while training. They certainly should have pride in what they do, feeling that they are engaged in a noble pursuit. The challenge at this point in their training is that they are only seeing the *lower part* of the metaphorical mountain.

As a person becomes more skilled they see, like a mountain climber, that there are other routes to the top. The farther a person climbs the closer those routes become until the summit is reached. Willi Unsoeld, a famous mountaineer who in 1963 became one of the first Americans to climb Mt. Everest via a more difficult route, claimed that the reason people climb mountains is for "convergence." Everything slips away to one point and eventually all can be seen from the summit. Clearly the metaphor of a mountain and its many paths is relevant to the martial artist. So what appears to be totally different early in one's training may well prove to be very similar in the long run—even if comparing such divergent art forms as *qigong** and *kali*.†

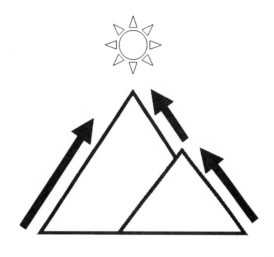

TWO SIDES OF THE MOUNTAIN.

For example, karate metaphorically boils an egg from the outside in, beginning with hard external power then incorporating internal energy with later development. *Taijiquan*‡ boils the egg from the inside out, staring with *qi*§ development and later adding external power as the training progresses. These arts take two different paths, each ultimately leading to the same (metaphorically) boiled egg.

Strategy vs. Tactics

"Strategy is comprehensive planning and conduct for the long-term. Strategy gives us the course of action we take as we attempt to achieve our goals. Tactics are maneuvers we do to carry out strategy. Tactics then only make consistent sense when they are seen as an aspect of strategy, and not an end in themselves—this explains why the way a lot of players approach to the game makes little sense. They make decisions in a vacuum. Many otherwise thoughtful players, when they decide to think and talk about poker strategy, end up focusing and thrashing around various tactical ideas. They end up missing the forest for the trees." [19]

– Steve Badger

---

* A Chinese internal art that is also known as chi kung.

† A Filipino blade art.

‡ Also known as *tai chi chuan*.

§ Internal energy, also known as *chi* or *ki*.

Before we delve more in depth into strategy, it is important to understand the difference between strategy and tactics. Strategy is a plan of action, especially for obtaining a goal. It is high level and philosophical in nature. Tactics, on the other hand, are expedient means of achieving an end. They are low level and immediate. Strategy is what you do to prepare for contact with the enemy while tactics are what you do during contact with the target. This difference is paramount.

The distinction between strategy and tactics is all too often not made clear to martial arts students. The problem becomes one of "what if." Most practitioners engage in similar thinking early in their careers: "if an opponent does this, then I will do that." One simply cannot think of all the "ifs" to cover every conceivable situation. When faced with actual combat in an unexpected encounter, their brain will freeze, if only for a brief moment, rendering the over-thinking practitioner defenseless and vulnerable. If their strategic foundation is strong, on the other hand, appropriate tactics can be employed automatically to instantly react to most any situation.

Ask a salesperson about his or her *strategy* for selling new vehicles and you will more than likely about the features of a given automobile. The conversation may move along to price, available selection, rebates, bonuses, and eventually to how to close the deal. The typical salesperson focuses on the immediate, the tactics of a sale. That is how they earn their commissions, how they are paid.

Ask the same question of a dealership owner, and you will probably get a very different answer. Dealership owners worry more about enticing potential buyers to visit the lot. They talk about the customer/sales "experience," and about marketing, service, referrals and relationships because their job is a *strategic* one. The more vehicles they sell, the better they do, yet they may also earn revenue from service, rentals, marketing relationships, dealer referrals, internet transactions, and other services. It is the dealership owner that comes up with giant inflatable gorillas that market to children whose parents might purchase a minivan, offers free savings bonds to potential customers willing to test drive the latest SUV, or provides a year's worth of complimentary fuel with purchase of a full-size truck.

From a martial combat perspective, a simple *strategy* might be to use only low kicks. There may be several reasons behind adopting such a strategy, including but not limited to the age of the practitioner, his or her physical conditioning and flexibility, the desire to maintain proper balance, and so on. *Tactics* associated with such a strategy might include attacks to the feet, ankles, and knees of an opponent.

Martial artists, salespeople, and a large portion of society either confuse the concepts of *strategy* and *tactics* or, more often than not, make no distinction between them at all. Keeping the discipline of strategy and tactics is essential. *Strategy* is developed while the metaphorical waters are calm, while the mind can work without conflict. *Tactics* work *within* a strategic approach to put out the fire once it is already hot, smoky, and terrifying.

Let's assume for the moment that your strategy is to block an opponent and counterattack. Not necessarily a great strategy, but a simple example. One might logically ask, "When do I decide to close an opponent rather than opening them when they attack?" To close means that you are on the outside of their arms giving inward pressure while opening means being on the inside of their arms giving outward pressure. If you close your opponent, such a maneuver cuts off the attack. If you open the opponent, it facilitates your attack.

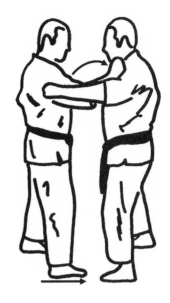

OPENING CHEST BLOCK. THE DEFENDER IS ON THE LEFT.

The right answer is actually that the opponent selects your response; you choose whatever they give you. It is all the same to you. You block and then you strike. Whichever arm they punch with determines whether your movement will to close or to open the attack.

A solid understanding of your chosen style's *strategy* will enable you to make the best use of the various *tactics* that you learn. Without that foundation, you will undoubtedly think too much, practicing a sub-optimized art at best.

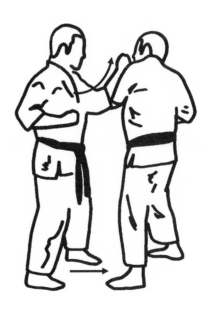

CLOSING CHEST BLOCK. THE DEFENDER IS ON THE LEFT.

Do Not Confuse the Quality of the Strategy with the Skill of the Fighter

---

"What counts is not necessarily the size of the dog in the fight—it's the size of the fight in the dog."[20]

– *Dwight D. Eisenhower*

Morio Higaonna included some interesting historical accounts of Chojun Miyagi, the founder of *Goju Ryu*, in his book *Traditional Karate-Do*. The following episode was discussed in volume 4 of that series: During his stint in the army, Miyagi *Sensei* spent time training at a local judo *dojo* in the city of Miyako while off duty. Though he had never before trained in that particular art, not one of the judo practitioners could successfully throw Miyagi *Sensei* during his two-year stay.

If the skilled *judoka* were unable to defeat this karate practitioner, it might be easy to draw the conclusion that karate is superior to judo or at least that *Goju Ryu* is the better art. Since the almost superhuman physical prowess of Miyagi *Sensei* is well documented, a better conclusion is most likely that a comparison between the two forms is really not relevant in this case. In fact, the judo instructor was quick to notice Miyagi's remarkable physical condition during their first encounter, including the "size of his neck and the extraordinary size and condition of his hands."

Such a remarkable individual would likely have defeated anyone he faced, regardless of his or her martial style. As his fame grew, Miyagi was able to avoid confrontations simply by being recognized, casting doubt and fear into the hearts of potential enemies. In fact, he was one of the few *karateka* for whom of *kakidameshi* was never an issue—no one dared to challenge him. When selecting or evaluating a strategy, therefore, it is important not to confuse the quality of the strategy with the skill of the fighter.

This same concept works in the world of sports as well. There are a couple of ways to advance the ball in a game of American football. You can run or you can pass. Each team determines whether they will focus on the run or on the pass and coaches select players in accordance with that strategy.

During the 1976 National Football League season, the Oakland Raiders under Coach John Madden focused on the pass, using quarterback Ken Stabler and receiver Fred Biletnikoff to secure a Super Bowl victory. The 1972 Miami Dolphins built their team around two world-class running backs, Jim Kick and Larry Csonka. They not only became Super Bowl champions but also the first undefeated team in NFL history. Though the two examples did not occur in the same year, it is nevertheless logical to ask, "So which strategy is better, running or passing?" The key to answering this question is not in the strategy, but in the execution.

Execution of the run or the pass is what makes the difference. An excellent running team can beat a mediocre passing team and vise versa. The same is true in the martial arts. A great kicker can beat an average puncher. A magnificent grappler can defeat a run of the mill striker. It has little to do with style, yet the implementation of a chosen strategy is essential.

Whatever art you choose to practice, you must stick with its strategy to implement it effectively. Anything else will become sub optimal. For example, it does not matter if you hold your fist in a vertical position, or use a twisting punch. It does not matter if you strike with extended fingers, a closed fist, a single knuckle, or an open palm. Unless there are grave points of failure, the type of punch you use is of little consequence because it is a *tactic*. So long as your style of punching (or kicking, or whatever) is supported by a consistent strategy, any version can present a potent formula for victory.

Once You Have a Strategy, Use It

"Wing Chun's origins are in the cramped, tight alleyways of Hong Kong where side-to-side mobility was significantly hampered. This art excels under those conditions. The larger movements and low stances of many northern Chinese styles are designed to work in wide-open, more mountainous areas where movement is not as restricted, but footwork can be treacherous and uneven. Whereas, the low crab-like movements of Hari Mau Silat are extremely effective in the slick, muddy terrain that occurs during Indonesia's monsoon seasons. Each art evolved to operate with radically different environmental conditions and how they fight reflects that. If you are willing to do a little research you will begin to see the wide scope of the factors that affect the art you study. In the same way that a species evolves for existing in particular conditions, so too will a fighting style." [21]

– Marc MacYoung

Once you have a strategy and discover that it is sound, it is absolutely essential that you use it. Never deviate. Since all your tactics will be built around this strategy, failure to follow it will almost certainly lead to an overall failure in combat.

Take the example of Ferdinand Magellan: On March 17, 1521, the famous explorer Magellan was killed in the Philippine Islands. Though he had high-tech (for the time period) weaponry and armor on his side, including warships with heavy guns (cannon), and the finest in swords, knives, and personal protection for both horses and men, he was ultimately beaten to death by a group of nearly naked "savages" armed with bamboo spears and rattan sticks.

How could such a tragedy (from his perspective anyway) have happened? Quite simply, he failed to follow his strategy. Normally, Magellan's men would use their superior shipboard weapons to bombard a target, then swoop in safely ensconced in their armor and mop up any resistance. Because this particular event occurred on a long, shallow beach, the fight took place beyond the range of his standoff naval weaponry. Even worse, he was ambushed in the surf while wearing full armor and heavy, wet clothing.

So there he was without the strength of his long-range weapons, outnumbered, and struggling to stand, let alone fight, in the surf. The defensive value of his armor swiftly became a severe liability. No doubt he put up a valiant struggle as the histories indicate, but truly he was doomed from the start when he threw aside his strategy and chose to face the natives with theirs. Since all his tactics and equipment were built around a strategy he could no longer employ, he was bound to lose. By the time he was engaged with the enemy, it was too late to change anything.

When deciphering *kata* it is a common error to place tactics above strategy. Remember, *strategy* is what is done in preparation of going to war, while *tactics* are what happens on the battlefield. As the example of Magellan points out, if the strategy is no good, it matters little what you do once you get there. Whenever a general looks at an enemy, he or she is searching for weaknesses; looking for an unfair fight that pits his or her side's strengths against the enemy's weaknesses. The Filipino natives used the strength of their mobility and numbers to overwhelm and defeat the encumbered forces of Magellan.

The yardstick of strengths to weaknesses must measure every tactic. To use a military example, an enemy may have a very strong but shallow front line. They are disciplined, aggressive, and fast. Our general has a heavily armored army, yet slow-moving forces. In this instance our general's strategy might be to engage the enemy head on in a manner that limits their mobility and cuts off any reinforcements. The goal is to crush the enemy by weight of armor.

One tactic might be to draw the enemy into a confined space, perhaps a valley, and shell their back lines with heavy armament creating a "no-man's land" behind them so that they cannot retreat. After all, engaging a faster, more mobile, well-disciplined force on an open plain would likely lead to disaster. Heavy artillery can break the ranks, lower the discipline, and allow a head-on engagement that should ultimately crush the enemy.

The strategy is to restrict the enemies' movement thereby taking away their advantage. The tactic is to use standoff artillery to seal the rear and use rolling armament to divide and conquer the front line.

Strategy always supports tactics, *never* the other way around. This applies to evaluating *kata* in the same way. It is essential to understand the ultimate goal, the strategy behind each the movement. Then and only then will the movement's true meaning become decipherable.

The Decision Stick

*"When making a decision of minor importance, I have always found it advanta-
geous to consider all the pros and cons. In vital matters, however, such as the choice of
a mate or a profession, the decision should come from the unconscious, from somewhere
within ourselves. In the important decisions of personal life, we should be governed, I
think, by the deep inner needs of our nature."* [22]

– Sigmund Freud

We have a mutual friend, Rory, who has been personally involved in more violent encounters than most people can conceive of, something over 300 documented
altercations. He leads an Emergency Response Team in a corrections facility, kind
of like a S.W.A.T. team to handle situations where inmates get out of control. When
asked about how he has survived so many encounters unscathed, he talks about having a "decision stick."

So what is a decision stick? Let's start by ascertaining what it is not: Those who
work in the business world are probably familiar with the "decision tree." Decision
trees are excellent tools for making financial or number-based decisions where a lot
of complex information needs to be taken into account. They provide an effective
structure in which alternative decisions and the implications of taking those decisions can be laid down and evaluated. They also help analysts and mangers form
accurate, balanced pictures of the risks and rewards that can result from a particular
choice.

It is a tool that helps map problem resolution processes. Each action one pro-
poses to take follows a different branch of the tree until the problem is resolved.
While it may be a good analytical tool, the decision tree is really not designed for
quick action. A decision tree creates a complex matrix that involves (metaphorically) time, space, height, and width with every branch on the tree. It works only when
you have time to map out decisions before you make them.

In a fight, you do not have that luxury. Decisions—often life or death decisions—must be made in an instant. If you do not have time to use a decision tree,
you must use a decision stick. This "stick" represents a limited set of choices or preferred techniques that you can apply in self-defense situations. Compared to a decision tree, of course, the decision stick offers an extremely narrow set of choices. That
is exactly what you need in the heat of battle. You must be engaged in the moment
of now.

Part of the success of using the decision stick theory is to choose an appropriate
application and let your opponent do what he or she will. That is how our friend

Rory has survived so many violent encounters unscathed.* Proper techniques do not rely on specific actions from your opponent. Techniques do not try to second guess what an enemy will do. They do, however, anticipate expected physiological reactions (e.g., turning the head away from a poke to the eye) as you progress from one technique to another. Stick with your art form's *strategic* framework, selecting applications that naturally fit your style and physical abilities.

Although as we move from an agrarian society to a more service-oriented economy fewer people are involved in using farm machinery; however there is a great lesson about martial arts buried in the common farm tractor. Tractors are the modern horse of today's farm. They haul everything hither and yon and serve as a power source as well. One of the most useful and also most dangerous tools on the tractor is the PTO shaft.

PTO stands for Power Take Off. The PTO shaft sticks out of the back end of the tractor like a short stinger. It is an extension of the drive shaft of the engine, literally connected to the pistons. The faster the tractor engine goes the faster the PTO shaft spins. The PTO shaft is used to provide power for mowers, sprayers and any other piece of farm equipment needed to get the job at hand done.

The PTO shaft is also one of the most dangerous pieces of farm equipment ever created, and a whole lot of people have been accidentally killed or maimed by it. The shaft is easy to step over, bend over, and forget about as the farmer has other things on his or her mind. Such inattention, however, can be a fatal mistake because the PTO shaft does what it does with no thought or consideration. It spins—quickly and with great power. It doesn't know about the coming birthdays, the plans that a person has or anything of the sort, it only does what it does and it does it very well, mindlessly.

The PTO shaft as designed by the engineers has only one focus: to turn. The machinery does not discern between pants, gloves, or even a loose branch. Regardless of what gets caught in the shaft, it does exactly what it is designed to do, turn over and over again.

Similarly, you're only thought during combat struggle should be to strike down your opponent. *Budo* techniques need to be similar to this mindless piece of farm machinery. The response to a movement by an opponent needs to be instantaneous, deliberate yet with no real thought. An action equals a response, instantly. A karate technique, or any martial arts technique for that matter, needs to be clear of any cluttering thoughts.

The only concern that a martial art practitioner should have at that moment is… none. The response and the technique once enacted needs to be as mindless as the spinning metal PTO shaft on the back of a tractor. Your response follows a decision stick. It must be straight, simple, and to the point. In combat, everything else is meaningless.

---

* While Kane has witnessed, interceded in, and stopped or prevented hundreds of fights, tangling with drunken football fans pales in comparison to battling hardened criminals as Rory does on a regular basis. That's the difference between fighting someone who really wants to hurt you and someone who truly wants to kill you. While Kane has room for error, Rory does not. Keep this in mind while training; your first mistake could be your last.

Strategy of Goju Ryu

"I believe that in the beginning of 1953, he [Miyagi] felt death was near. His blood pressure was very high and I noticed that his strength and stamina were low. Looking back, I see now that with the approach of his death he felt that the time was right to impart his secret theories of karate to me. These theories included kaisai no genri (the theory on karate kata), how to create hookiyu (unified) kata and the concept of creating and developing a teaching system for karate. These were all fundamental to create a legacy for future generations.

"I cannot stress enough how puzzled I was that he discussed these things. Until this time he never taught theory. As I previously mentioned Miyagi never explained what we did or the reason behind it…"[23]

– Seikichi Toguchi

Traditional instruction in Asian martial arts relies heavily upon modeling relationships where students observe and attempt to imitate their *senseis'* techniques, transcending potential language barriers and other inhibitors of communication. While this is a particularly powerful method of introducing students to the gross physical movements of an art form, lecturing is required to communicate essential strategic frameworks as well as important nuances of individual tactics or techniques. Without a teacher's counseling and assistance, it could literally take a lifetime of practice to truly understand an art form's strategy and figure out how to apply it. Most Westerners are simply not prepared to wait that long.

In order to help you identify and understand the strategy of whatever art form you study, we have selected our own style, *Goju Ryu* karate, to cover in depth. After all, it is what we know best. All styles will have a similar strategic foundation upon which their applications are built. In fact, many other styles have strategic and/or tactical elements in common with *Goju Ryu* simply because there are only a limited number of ways in which the human body can move as well as a finite set of vital points where it can be broken easily.

For example, both a "horse" stance and a "cat" stance are found in almost all martial arts. They may not be performed in *exactly* the same way for every art form, but the essential body mechanics hold true. While the cat stance in Japanese martial arts is generally performed with the ball of the lead foot on the ground, it is usually done with only the toes touching the ground in the Chinese arts. Kobudo practitioners perform this stance a bit more flat-footed than karate practitioners do. Regardless, all martial forms use the same stance for similar applications.* Due to

---

* For an illustration of this technique you can look up neko ashi dachi (cat stance) in the glossary of techniques at the end of this book or see it in the next section of this chapter where we demonstrate various stances to addresses the concept of imbalance.

this commonality, we believe that by understanding our style a little better, you will gain important insight into your own martial art.

In *Goju Ryu* karate, the fundamental strategy is to (1) close distance, (2) imbalance, and (3) use physiological damage to incapacitate an opponent. A detailed description of each strategic element follows:

(1) Close Distance

Closing distance is a brilliant strategy for unarmed combat. It allows the practitioner to bring all his or her "weapons" on-line, leaving nothing out. In striking range, practitioners are able to punch, kick, or grab. When they move just slightly closer, they can perform a throw, choke, arm bar, or hold. Further, closing distance invades an opponent's personal space, a strategy that can be quite disruptive.

People of all nations have a concept of personal space, an invisible barrier through which only intimate associates cross. In America, it is fairly large, extending perhaps a couple of feet from one's body in all directions—especially directly in front. We are socially conditioned to maintain that space.

Try this drill to understand the concept. Choose someone you know, but only as a casual friend, acquaintance, or business associate.* Walk up to the person that you have selected, stopping only a couple inches away and try to have a conversation. Your violation of that person's personal space likely will be unnerving, and they will instinctively move back, sometimes even without consciously knowing it.

There are several black belts from other styles who practice at our *dojo* from time to time. Many, especially those who achieved rank through styles that emphasize kicking, have a difficult time acclimating to the *Goju Ryu* fighting distances. As you probably experienced in the aforementioned drill, these black belts unconsciously want to step back. Our mere presence inside their comfort zones can disrupt their techniques, giving us immediate advantage.

Everything in *Goju Ryu* is built around this strategy. The stances are designed to either fight at close range, to close distance quickly, or to recover and control the fighting range. All techniques, even kicks, can be utilized up close. In *saifa kata*, for example, we find a close-quarters knee strike, a brief pause that lets the adversary double over, and then an immediate front kick.† The emphasis of that particular movement is on the knee strike, a tactic that supports the strategy of closing distance and fighting in short range.

Closing distance puts your opponent at a tactical disadvantage. Loren Christensen reinforced this point when he wrote, "Far too many martial artists scramble backwards in response to a straight charge by an attacker. This works for a step or two, but when an attacker explodes forward driving you back more than three or four steps, the chance of entangling your legs increases to about 100 percent."

* Be a little bit careful about whom you select, however, so that you are not accused of sexual harassment or something worse.
† It's actually slightly more complicated than that but we'll save further explanation for later.

Closing the distance is effective because it has a propensity to imbalance an attacker, disrupting his or her plans.

(2) Imbalance

Happo no kuzushi, the eight directions of imbalance:

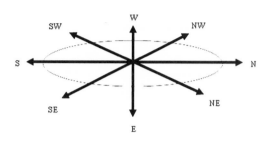

EIGHT DIRECTIONS OF IMBALANCE.

It has been said that nature kills a horse from the ground up. A horse that cannot walk or run properly is unable to search for food or escape from predators. Similarly, a martial artist whose body is out of position will surely be defeated. Strength of technique and ability to move to attack or defend rely on proper footwork and good balance.*

The most commonly used stances in *Goju Ryu*, as with many other martial styles, include *sanchin dachi* (hourglass stance), *zenkutsu dachi* (front forward stance), *shiko dachi* (*sumo* or straddle stance), and *neko ashi dachi* (cat stance). Each stance has a different purpose with different dynamics. Similarly the directions of strength and imbalance vary as well.

Sanchin dachi (hourglass stance) is a well-balanced stance used for close-quarters fighting. It is performed with feet shoulder-width apart; weight distributed about 55/45 front to back. The forward foot is about one step ahead of the rear foot. Toes are pointed slightly inward, especially on the front foot, where it is more pronounced. The knees track straight ahead, aligned with the hips. Back is straight, spine aligned, with the pelvis pulled forwards and upwards to straighten the lower back as well. Shoulders sit straight above the back with head centered above that such that a straight line goes from the top of the head straight down through the center of the body.

---

* For more information about this and other vignettes of martial wisdom, you may wish to refer to Kris Wilder's book, *Lessons from the Dojo Floor* (Xlibris 2003).

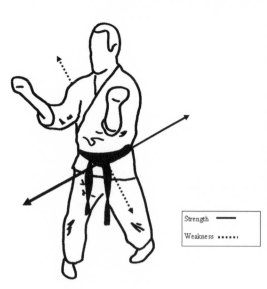

SANCHIN DACHI (HOURGLASS STANCE): LINES OF
STRENGTH AND IMBALANCE.

Zenkutsu dachi (front forward stance) is a strong forward stance designed for deep distance-covering lunges or to receive driving attacks such as tackles by an opponent. It looks a lot like a hurdler stretch and is performed with the feet shoulder-width apart, forward leg bent 90 degrees at the knee, rear leg straight and extended approximately two shoulder-widths behind lead foot; the torso is erect. If you drop to a kneeling position from this stance, you will discover that your back knee aligns with your front heel (assuming that you are doing it correctly, of course). Weight is distributed approximately 75 percent on the front leg and 25 percent on the back leg.

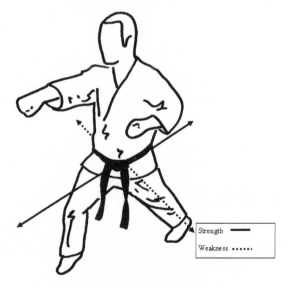

ZENKUTSU DACHI (FRONT STANCE): LINES
OF STRENGTH AND IMBALANCE.

Shiko dachi (*sumo* or straddle stance) is used to uproot an attacker from beneath his center and is commonly used in Japanese *sumo* wrestling (hence the nickname). To execute it correctly you must be touching an opponent's body with yours. This stance is too immobile to be used successfully at any distance. It is performed with feet spread approximately two shoulder-widths apart, toes pointed outward at 45 degrees. Weight is distributed evenly over both legs so it is a fairly stable stance. Knees are bent deeply and pulled back as far as possible with the torso erect. Lower legs/shins are approximately vertical. If you lean forward and put your hands on your knees, you'll look like a baseball umpire. Don't do that! Instead, pull your shoulder blades together, keeping your upper body vertical.

Neko ashi dachi (cat stance) is almost always a defensive response designed to regain advantage. It works off the natural flinch reaction. Rear knee is bent, with foot flat on ground, and toes facing to the outside. The front foot rests lightly (~10 percent) on the ground approximately one shoulder-width forward of the rear leg. Toes face forward, flat on ground, with the heel of foot raised.* Crouch slightly, with front leg in center of body, bent a little at the knee. If you slide

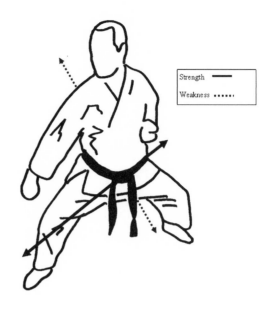

SHIKO DACHI (SUMO STANCE): LINES OF STRENGTH AND IMBALANCE.

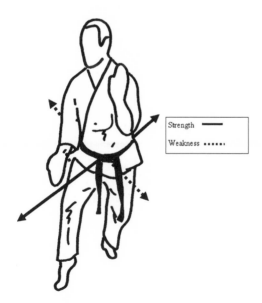

NEKO ASHI DACHI (CAT STANCE): LINES OF STRENGTH AND IMBALANCE.

the front foot behind you, it should clear the back foot rather than entangling it. Keep your torso erect while thrusting backwards with your buttocks.

Imbalance goes beyond just the stance, however. Vision, breathing, and movement can be attacked as well. In fact, if any two of the three can be incapacitated the fight is already won. *Kata* from a variety of different styles demonstrate techniques designed to attack vision, breathing, and/or movement.

Further, imbalance can also apply to any of the five senses. Strikes to the eyes, nose, and ears are fairly common. It is very challenging to fight what you cannot

* As mentioned earlier, if you practice a Chinese martial art, you'll probably rest the tips of your toes on the ground in a slight variation from the Japanese/Okinawan method.

see. And anyone who has experienced a severe ear infection (or even a really bad head cold) knows how hard it is to maintain one's equilibrium when your ears do not work correctly.

A solid shot to a limb can cause numbness, temporarily blocking sensation as well as the ability to defend or attack properly. Kane's son Joey recently attended a birthday party at an indoor skateboarding park in Tukwila, Washington. One of the teenage semi-pro skates who was practicing at the time lost his balance at the crest of a large half-pipe and fell off, landing heavily on his arm. Although he appeared to have nothing broken, only a severe contusion, the arm immediately began to swell and go numb. Even a teenage adrenaline junky can be stopped by enough pain. He was in no condition to do anything other than nurse his wound, to which Kane proceeded to examine and apply first aid.

Goju Ryu attempts to imbalance from both the outside as well as the inside of the attacker. For example, *kiai* (spirit shout) is often a psychological tool (e.g., distract or frighten opponent) as much as it is a physiological one (e.g., increase practitioner's focus and power). Just gazing upon an adversary with intense concentration can be unnerving. Further, in *budo,* properly delivered strikes can cause hydrostatic shock that damages internal organs, because blunt force trauma from a blow to a vital area can initiate shock waves that cause significant internal damage beyond the surface impact of the strike.

(3) Use Physiological Damage to Control

Adrenaline rushes through your system in combat, supercharging the body for a short period of time. Interestingly for men, it's almost instantaneous yet of short duration while in women the adrenaline rush builds slower and lasts longer. Either way, adrenaline increases pulse rate and blood pressure while simultaneously making a person faster, meaner, and more impervious to pain than ever before.

Unfortunately it works the same way for an attacker as well. As a consequence, strikes to non-vital areas generally have very little effect. As a law enforcement officer, Loren Christensen has had to fight criminals even after they have been shot. "And they still fought like maniacs," he relates. "I know of two occasions where suspects had been shot in their hearts and they fought the officers for several seconds before they crumpled dead to the ground... I saw two cases of people shot in the head—one person took five rounds—and they were still running around screaming and putting up a fuss." In the heat of battle it is very difficult to stop a determined opponent.

The creators of *kata* certainly understood this challenge. They developed techniques to defend themselves through physiologically damaging an opponent. Strikes or grabs to an attacker's vital (anatomically weak) areas can elicit pain, temporary paralysis, and dislocation of a joint, knockout, or even death. Every movement in *kata* in *Goju Ryu* as well as any other martial art has practical self-defense applications, most of which attack vital areas.

Without a long-range weapon or total surprise, it is virtually impossible to simply walk up to someone and damage a vital area. Even in untrained individuals, the natural flinch reaction helps protect their vulnerable cores. A close examination of *kata* generally reveals that it uses strikes to set up imbalance and imbalance to set up strikes.*

A simple example is the *mae geri* (front kick), *hiji ate* (elbow strike), *uraken uchi* (backfist) combination in *gekisai kata*. The kick is executed from *sanchin dachi* but lands in *zenkutsu dachi*, allowing the practitioner to rapidly close distance. Furthermore, after striking an opponent's midsection or groin with your extended foot, you pull it back down 90 degrees to land in the proper stance.† In practical application, your landing will be aimed at your opponent's knee, ankle, or foot. When properly executed, this kick not only strikes while closing distance, but it imbalances your adversary as well.

If done correctly the kick component of this combination strikes a vital area (the groin), imbalances (pain/loss of stance integrity), and strikes again (knee, ankle, or foot). Since head and hands follow the pain, the victim will hunch over and bend down (imbalance) meeting the rising elbow (strike) to the solar plexus that immediately follows your kick. This will cause your opponent to raise back up again (imbalance), opening for the backfist (strike) to his or her face. In total this simple combination attacks several vital areas—groin, ankle/foot, solar plexus, head—increasing the likelihood of physiological damage.

All *kata* work this way. Simply put, if you can incapacitate the opponent's vision, breathing, or movement, you are in an excellent position to defeat an enemy. Any two out of three will pretty much guarantee success.

Principles of Enforcement

"Failure comes only when we forget our ideals and objectives and principles." [24]

– *Jawaharal Nehru*

The strategy of *Goju Ryu* can be expanded into a set of principles that help practitioners better understand and apply the style. The list covered here is a subset, as principles necessary for deciphering *kata* are discussed in more detail later. Practitioners of other arts should recognize many of these philosophies as well. Topics we will cover here include the following:

---

* See Principle 3—*strike to disrupt; disrupt to strike.*

† This also provides a nice counter/evade application should an opponent capture your kicking leg via *sukui uke* (scoop block) or similar technique. In this fashion you increase your odds of maintaining your balance long enough to use the mechanical leverage of your entire body weight to escape your opponent's grab.

1. If you move, better your position.
2. Always move at an angle.
3. Do not use two steps.
4. Do not kick above the waist.
5. Fight the whole body.
6. See everything.
7. Blocks are an opportunity to disadvantage an opponent.
8. Avoid going to the ground.
9. The only secret of *Goju Ryu* is to say the name backwards.

1) If You Move, Better Your Position

This point expands on the strategy of closing distance. Economy of motion is very important in a real fight. It conserves energy, always an important consideration. Moreover, it maximizes your chances of landing a blow while minimizing the openings through which an opponent might successfully assault you. While it is possible to overwhelm an average person with an all-out assault, wild uncoordinated blows or erratic movement will doom you in an encounter with an opponent who has learned to take advantage of such errors.

Ensure that you better your position with each move. Do not simply close distance to meet an opponent, do so strategically. Utilize the best technique you can deliver at each fighting range. For example, you may wish to begin with a kick that helps to close to striking distance. From there you punch and shift, moving in to grappling range. From there you execute a foot sweep or a throw, knocking your opponent to the ground. From there you shift in closer to deliver a joint lock or a stranglehold. Each movement ratchets the opponent further into your control. It becomes progressively more and more difficult for your adversary to escape.

While various martial art forms will have divergent strategies or preferences for fighting range, they all have techniques that can be effectively applied at various distances from an opponent, such as grappling, striking, and kicking. The next two principles, moving at an angle and not using two steps expand upon this concept.

2) Always Move At an Angle

We've already discussed the most common stances along with their strengths and weaknesses. It is important to use your strength against an opponent's weakness. This principle supports the strategy of closing distance. When doing so, it is always best to avoid force to force. Force to force encounters put your strengths against an opponent's strengths. Unless you are built like a pro linebacker,* that's probably not a good idea.

---

* For those unfamiliar with the game of American football, linebackers are defensive players who rush the passer (quarterback) or cover wide receivers during pass plays, and defend against the run. They have to be big, fast, and strong. The average professional player in this position stands a little over 6 feet tall and weighs upward of 250 pounds. Most defensive sets have between three and five linebackers.

Get off-line. Being off-line means attacking from any direction other than the main strength of your opponent's stance. If he is in *shiko dachi*, for example, you might go straight up the middle. If he is in *zenkutsu dachi* you will certainly not want to meet her head on. The angle you choose always avoids the main strength of your opponent's stance and/or his direction of movement.

Moving to the outside is safer; inside is faster but less safe. If you are outside, an opponent can only reach you with one arm and/or one leg. The other limbs must cross his or her body to strike you. While safer, it also limits your targeting opportunities as the person's vital core is relatively inaccessible. If you are on the inside, both arms and both legs may target you directly. Conversely, you have free access to the opponent's vital areas as well. In such an encounter, the first one to strike usually wins. For this reason, less experienced practitioners are almost always taught to go outside if they are able to do so, closing an adversary down. Advanced practitioners with more experience to draw from may choose to attack to the inside, opening an opponent for the attack. Obviously unexpected actions by an attacker may supersede your preferred choice, but

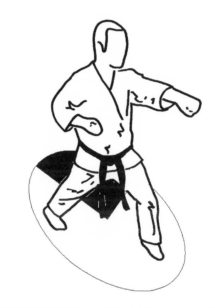

ZENKUTSU DACHI (FRONT STANCE): THE CIRCLE SHOWS THE MAIN STRENGTH OF THIS TECHNIQUE, WHILE THE SHADED PORTION IS WEAK.

either way you have only two options—inside (open) or outside (close).

Similarly punches and kicks are generally are performed at an angle. A straight jab in boxing is fairly easy to see and avoid, while an uppercut is more difficult to stop. The same concept holds true in karate. For example, only the most basic *kihon kata* (e.g., *hookiyu, gekisai*) in *Goju Ryu* demonstrate linear (straight in toward the chin) head punches.

To be clear, there is nothing wrong with a linear punch so long as it comes from an off angle rather than straight in where it is easy to see and block. Effective head punches rise from below (e.g., elbow strike, uppercut), drop from above (e.g., hammerfist, swing strike), or come in at an angle (e.g., knife hand strike, backfist).

Kicks frequently avoid straight lines, coming in at angles as well. Examples include *mikazuki geri* (hook kick), *mawashe geri* (wheel kick), and *kensetsu geri* (joint kick). In *Goju Ryu*, even *mae geri* (front kick), which looks straight actually rises in an arc from below, making it more difficult to block.* Virtually any angle of attack that makes a technique more difficult to block and thus more likely to connect can be found in *kata*.

3) Do Not Use Two Steps

New martial arts students typically learn by conjunction—block *and* strike, step *and* kick, block *then* shift, turn *and* throw, and so on.† Conjunctions are examples of cognitive thought, the concept of joining two ideas together. Because students need to learn complex concepts in small, manageable pieces, such terms are a great way to introducing new skills, and very necessary. Outside the *dojo*, however, conjunctions get you hurt. Why? Precisely because conjunctions require cognitive thought, something we cannot afford in a real fight.

Two of the most animal-like characters in literature and cinema are Frankenstein's Monster and Tarzan. Animal-like in that they understand violence as a means to meet a need and in that they both speak in language that is very basic yet understood. There are few barriers between their perceived needs or desires and their actions.

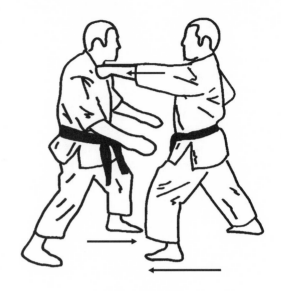

ZENKUTSU PUNCH: EVEN IF YOU BLOCK THE FIRST STRIKE, REMAINING INSIDE AN ATTACK LEAVES YOU VULNERABLE TO FOLLOW-ON TECHNIQUES (E.G., PUNCH, KICK).

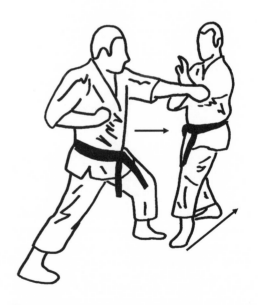

ZENKUTSU PUNCH: SHIFTING OUTSIDE NOT ONLY EVADES THE PUNCH BUT ALSO CLOSES THE OPPONENT, MAKING IT HARDER FOR HIM TO STRIKE AT YOU WITH A FOLLOW-ON TECHNIQUE (E.G., PUNCH, KICK).

---

* Much like an uppercut, which is much harder to block than a straight punch.

† Even advanced practitioners show each *kata* movement discretely and separately as they perform the form.

Both Frankenstein's Monster and Tarzan are unencumbered by the two beats formed with a conjunction. It is a straight shot—stimulation action, rather than stimulation *and* action. Clearly civilized individuals cannot walk around in a feral state responding at our most basic level with whatever is needed to get the necessary results as fast as possible. However, in a life or death situation on the street, that is exactly what is required to survive.

The pacing in which most *kata* are performed is slow enough that every individual technique is shown discretely with a conjunction between. In a fight we need to move to a world of block/strike rather than block *and* strike, eliminating that conjunction. Once practitioners understand that these conjunctions are artificial, they must work to remove them when actually applying concepts from their *kata*. This does not change the *kata*, only its applications.*

4) Do Not Kick above Your Waist

This tenet reinforces the entire strategy of *Goju Ryu*—closing distance, unbalancing, and controlling with physiological damage. Some styles, particularly Korean ones that emphasize leg techniques, include a lot of flashy kicks to the head and upper body. Such moves look really cool and are used a lot in tournaments, *kata* competitions, and movies. Unfortunately, many of these techniques are not practical in a self-defense situation.

While Wilder also has a black belt in tae kwon do and still retains a fair amount of flexibility, he has never even attempted to kick someone's head in a real fight. "No matter how fast you are, it simply takes way too long to cover the distance required to execute such maneuvers efficiently. They are relatively easy to anticipate, block, and counter. And they leave you off balance far too long. Kicking below the waist, on the other hand, covers a lot less ground and is, therefore, much faster for me to use. If someone trains for that high kind of kicking that's fine. They just have to know the risks…," he explains.

In *Goju Ryu*, kicks above the waist are rare (only shown in a single *kata*, *suparinpei*) and usually executed when an attacker is already lying on the ground. In addition to the benefits of more speed and less distance, low kicks are considerably better at helping practitioners maintain their balance. Whenever a person's foot leaves the ground, he or she becomes vulnerable and is temporarily rooted to the spot where the support foot rests. That is why practitioners of Asian martial arts tend to glide-step across the floor when moving in stance rather than lifting their feet clear off the ground as Westerners traditionally walk.

Further, fighting in *Goju Ryu* is extremely close. Kicking range for us is often punching range for other arts. Consequently, there is frequently not enough room to do anything more than a knee strike against an opponent, at least initially. Of

---

* See Rule 12—*there is no pause,* for more information.

course when they bend over or fall back from the pain, then we can follow through with a traditional kick. That is why the initial knee lift is emphasized as the basis of all *Goju Ryu* kicks.

Real fights are sloppy affairs. They are close, fast, and furious. A great kicking tactic in such encounters is to chop away at your opponent's knees, shins, ankles and/or feet. Such attacks are quick and vicious. They are difficult to see, even harder to avoid, and cause significant physiological damage with minimal effort. Kane has had arthroscopic surgery to repair cartilage tears in both knees.* He will be the first to tell you that damage to a knee is quite debilitating. Once practitioners have entangled an opponent's feet with their kicks, they have a much better chance of landing upper body blows with their hand strikes.

When was the last time you had time to stretch out before a real fight? No matter how flexible you are, it is fairly difficult to execute a high kick at full speed and power with cold muscles. Even if you can snap off a few high kicks, you'll almost certainly pay for them later (e.g., pain from pulled or strained muscles). Yet you simply cannot say, "Excuse me, Mr. Bad Guy. I need to take a time out to stretch my legs so that I can kick you in the head. Could you please wait a minute before you punch me in the mouth?"

Further, you are probably not going to be wearing a loose-fitting *gi* the next time you find yourself in a real-world life or death encounter. The constrictive street clothes that most people wear are simply not conducive to the extreme leg movements necessary to kick above someone's waist. While that may be pretty obvious with dresses or long skirts, it often holds true for jeans and slacks as well.

High kicks are just not effective in a real fight. Loren Christensen sums it up quite well: "I was in dozens of street brawls as a police officer, and not once did I do a leaping, spinning kick like Jean-Claude Van Damme." While they look spectacular in movies and on TV shows, kicks above the waist are neither practical nor desirable in actual combat.

5) Fight the Whole Body

This principle is mostly about imbalance. *Goju Ryu* tends to attack arms to arms and legs to legs. As described previously, if you can entangle an opponent's feet with your kicks, it is much easier to land an upper body blow from your hands and vice versa. Once your opponent's knee has been blown out from a *kensetsu geri* (joint kick) or his foot or ankle crushed from a *kakato geri* (stomping heel kick), the likelihood of his paying attention to anything else is greatly diminished. If nothing else, pain will weaken your opponent's concentration, put him on the defensive, and lesson his resolve. The desire to escape may overwhelm any aspiration to continue the attack.

The old joke is that kung fu was invented by two monks, "Hilo-hi" and "Lohi-

---

* Thankfully not at the same time! One surgery resulted from a skiing accident, while the other was from a tournament injury.

lo." Expanding on this idea, we tend to ride the body high-low-high or low-high-low, changing up and down between techniques to disrupt an opponent as much as possible. The more you can keep an opponent off balance and on the defensive, the better your chances of surviving a violent encounter unscathed.

6) See Everything

Sun Tzu in his famous book *The Art of War* wrote, "It does not take sharp eyes to see the sun and the moon, nor does it take sharp ears to hear the thunderclap. Wisdom is not obvious. You must see the subtle and notice the hidden to be victorious." In *Goju Ryu*, the principle of seeing everything has to do with not focusing too much on one part of an opponent's body (e.g., hands, feet).

As we attempt to disrupt an attacker by working his or her whole body, so too will a skilled opponent try to work us. If a practitioner pays too much attention to any one part of the opponent's body, he or she increases the risk of falling for a feint or otherwise being struck by an unanticipated blow.

There are a lot of theories about where to look at an opponent during combat. These include the hips, pelvic girdle, hands, neck, or eyes. While all of these have their pros and cons, the essential principle is to focus on *everything and nothing simultaneously*. For the sake of argument, let's say that you prefer to look at the triangle formed by the opponent's chin and shoulders, a popular approach. Since many practitioners tense their neck muscles, flex their shoulders, or even pull their arm back before striking this seems like a reasonable place to look.

If you choose to concentrate on a specific location, you must be able to detect movement everywhere, including movement in your peripheral vision. You do not necessarily have to move your eyes much. You simply cannot afford, however, to be taken by surprise if an adversary tries to stomp your foot or kick your ankle while you are focusing on his neck.

Further, you must be aware of your surroundings in combat. Unlike the safe, wide-open environment in the *dojo*, real fights typically take place in and around obstacles. You need to be aware of loose rocks, patches of mud, spilled drinks, broken bottles, overturned chairs, moving vehicles, and any other dangers that surround you as you tangle with your adversary. Dogfighter pilots in WWI attacked with the sun at their back to temporarily blind or disorient an opponent. The same tactic was used by gunfighters in the old west, knights in medieval Europe, and *samurai* in ancient Japan. If they could not get their backs to the sun, *Shinobi* ninja in feudal Japan used to flash sunlight off of their sword blades to temporarily blind their opponents. You must constantly be aware of your environment and use it to your advantage.

Another environmental consideration is people in the immediate vicinity. Bystanders may be innocent witnesses, potential sources of aid, or friends waiting to back up your opponent. While karate is primarily a striking art, it does feature groundwork (e.g., locks, chokes) as well. Before going to the ground in a fight, you must be absolutely certain that your attacker does not have friends waiting for an opportunity to kick your head in once your have become entangled and vulnerable.*

7) Blocks Are an Opportunity to Disadvantage an Opponent

Blocks are an opportunity to disadvantage an opponent. Do not miss the chance to do so. As stated in the introduction, the word *uke* in Japanese really translates better as "receive" than it does "block." When you receive someone's attack you make it your own, controlling it in a fashion designed to expeditiously end the fight.†

This concept reinforces the strategy elements of closing distance, as well as unbalancing, and (hopefully) physiological incapacitation as well. Aggressively meeting an attack places you at an advantage. The greater the level of pain or injury your defense causes, the better your strategic position.

If someone has the audacity to strike at you, make him or her regret it each and every time you touch the person. The more aggressive your defensive response, the less likely an adversary is to continue his or her attack. Further, if your attacker's friends are watching your response may convince them that they would be foolish to join their buddy in the conflict. Either way, if your opponent is disadvantaged by your defense, he or she is far less likely to be able hurt you.

8) Avoid Going to the Ground

Marc MacYoung‡ wrote, "It's not that I am against ground fighting. Through some brutally earned experiences I have some seriously controversial views on the subject of grappling and submission fighting in the streets. While it is a good sport system, the commonly held and wildly misguided belief that it is the ultimate fighting system is a dangerous delusion. While grappling has its time and place, trying to use it in a serious altercation can and will result in grave injury."

The primary problem with ground fighting, as we see it, is the vulnerability of being on the ground. In one-on-one encounters, grappling techniques work quite well. It is very comforting to be able to incapacitate an attacker without seriously injuring him or her (e.g., chokes, submission holds). Unfortunately a large number of fights involve more than one person. If your attacker has friends and you go to the ground, you lose the mobility necessary to handle multiple opponents.

Remember the story of Magellan? The manner of his death reinforces the fact that a practitioner must fight his own fight on his own terms; not someone else's. A martial artist must utilize the strengths of his or her own system. In the case of karate, that system relies on primarily striking techniques (e.g., punches and kicks). Even though they share certain tactics, grappling arts such as judo and jujitsu utilize

---

* See item number 8, Avoid Going to the Ground, for more information.

† See Rule 8—*there is no block,* for more information on this topic.

‡ A former bouncer and street fighter, Marc "Animal" MacYoung teaches experience-based self-defense to police, military, civilians, and martial artists around the world.

totally different strategies than striking arts employ. It is important for martial artists to have at least a passing familiarity with the strategies of other styles, but in a life or death situation, you should rely on at the methods you know best. That is why we do not go to the ground in *Goju Ryu*. Groundfighting is simply not the strength of our style. Further, it is inherently dangerous to the practitioner to utilize grappling applications in actual combat.

The bottom line is that going to the ground in a real fight is very dangerous and best avoided if at all possible. Kelly Worden* agrees, writing "In reality, whether in the streets of our inner cities or on the battlefield in a war zone, it takes nothing more than a simple boot knife or folding pocketknife to kill or maim a grappling strategist during a physical engagement."

Working stadium security, Kane has helped break-up hundreds of fights. He relates that "combatants went to the ground perhaps 30 percent of the time, not counting situations where one person fell and the other stood over him or her while continuing an attack. The most severe injuries I have seen happened when two guys, yes it was always guys, became enjoined in a wrestling contest and then one or the other's friends weighed into the battle. Kicks to the head are brutal. They are vicious, bloody, and extremely dangerous. Believe me; you really do not want to be the recipient of one."

9) The Only Secret in Goju Ryu is to Use/Say the Name Backwards.

The name *Goju Ryu* means hard/soft style, literally the "hard/gentle way of the infinite fist." The famous Chinese philosopher Lao Tzu said, "The softest things in the world overcome the hardest things in the world." Similarly, an ancient Japanese proverb states that, "*ju* (soft) many times controls *go* (hard)."

Judo and aikido could be considered the ultimate embodiments of these axioms, as their strategy is to use an opponent's power against him. Although there is a common misconception that karate is a totally hard-style martial art, most of *Goju Ryu* is soft and flowing with exploding instances of hardness (e.g., at the moment of impact from a strike).

To use or say the name backwards is, perhaps, a better explanation of the *Goju Ryu* strategy. It is soft/hard. Loose, relaxed muscles move much more swiftly than hard, rigid ones. Since force equals mass times acceleration, the faster you move the harder you hit, regardless of the distance you cover. Even when touching an opponent before initiating your attack you can generate more power by ensuring that your muscles are relaxed until the moment of the strike (e.g., sticking hands or bouncing *ki* applications).

---

* The first American *Datu* and Senior Blademaster of modern arnis.

Tactics of Goju Ryu

"In Okinawa, karate is not practiced primarily as a sport or even as an exercise for health. The Okinawans consider karate a life long pursuit to be practiced as training for both the body and mind." [25]

— *Morio Higaonna*

Looking at how frequently techniques come up in the various core *kata* of a system can be a good way to ascertain its strategy. These individual techniques are, of course, the tactics that support that strategy. In the twelve core *kata* of *Goju Ryu*, *te waza* (hand techniques) appear about 70 percent of the time. This reinforces the idea that *Goju Ryu* is fundamentally a striking art. Here is how the techniques break out:

- Hands (*te waza*) ~ 70 percent
- Feet (*ashi waza*) ~ 20 percent
- Throws (*tachi waza*) ~ 5 percent
- Groundwork (*ne waza*) ~ 5 percent

Forms of Compliance

"Victorious warriors win first and then go to war, while defeated warriors go to war first then seek to win." [26]

— *Sun Tzu*

If you drill down through the tactics of *Goju Ryu* as demonstrated by its *kata*, you will find strikes from hands or feet to anatomical weak points, attacks to joints (e.g., locks, separations), throws, nerve attacks, and chokes. Each of these tactics supports the fundamental *Goju Ryu* strategy of closing distance, unbalancing, and using physiological damage to incapacitate an opponent. While predilections regarding usage vary widely, almost all martial arts use these same tactics.

Striking Anatomical Weak Areas

Striking anatomical weak areas such as the temple, eyes, throat, solar plexus, groin, and knees, and ankles is an efficient way to dispatch an enemy. The shorter the fight, the less likely you are to get hurt. There are three forms of strikes in the martial arts: (1) vascular, (2) neurological, and (3) structural.

Vascular strikes damage the circulatory system and the flow of blood throughout the body. Neurological strikes affect nerves and the nervous system. Structural strikes affect the mechanical structure of the body: bones, tendons and muscles. These three types of strikes are not mutually exclusive. In other words, a vascular strike may have neurological and/or structural impact as well. For example, a hard blow to the temple can initiate structural, neurological, and vascular damage all at once, cracking the skull, shocking the brain, and causing internal hemorrhaging.*

Blows generally contour the body, aligning the striking surface to the target hit.† For example, *Goju Ryu* utilizes several different parts of the hand to punch various targets along a person's body, including the *seiken tsuki* (traditional fore fist punch), *ippon ken tsuki* (one knuckle fist),‡ *shuto uchi* (ridge or knife hand), and *tetsui uchi* (hammerfist). Kicks contour the body as well striking with the ball, heel, or edge of the foot to align with a target in a manner that will cause maximum damage.

Regardless of the type of strike employed, crashing techniques that send energy toward the center of the body and neurological strikes that cross energy from one side of the body to the other are most effective.§

Attacking the Joints

Locks can be directed against an opponent's joints, which are twisted, stretched, or bent with the practitioner's hands, arms, legs, or body. This can cause dislocation or hyperextension of the entangled limb. Each attack is a little different:

- Hyperextension—to move a joint in a direction past its normal range of motion.
- Dislocation—to displace a bone from its normal connection to another bone at a joint.
- Lock—to make fast by interlocking parts of your body and your opponent's body.
- Separation—the act of pulling or twisting a joint apart.

The joints can be attacked with the arms or the legs using both entanglement procedures and strikes. For example, a powerful *kensetsu geri* (joint kick) to the knee can easily hyperextend or dislocate that joint (depending on what angle is struck). It works best when an opponent's weight is posted onto his leg that is then kicked from the side. You can facilitate such situations by pulling downward on the attacker's arm and shifting slightly outside commensurate with the kick.

An arm lock, on the other hand, is usually performed by entangling an opponent's limb with your own. To be successful, this type of attack must be performed at extremely close range where your body touches that of your opponent so that he does not have enough space to twist or turn away. Your shoulders, chest, or upper body often facilitate such techniques, providing more leverage than your arms are capable of alone.

* A really good reason to avoid getting kicked in the head.
† See Rule 11—contour the body.
‡ Using either the first or second finger depending upon whether you strike upward or downward.
§ See Kyushu (vital points) in chapter 5 for more information.

Throws

Throws cause injury to your opponent when you hurtle them onto the ground with impetus. We both have trained with a world renowned judo instructor named Kenji who likes to say that, "the concrete hits much harder than the fist." While throws are not a primary tactic of karate, they are an excellent disrupting technique; one that frequently also causes physiological damage. As with joint locks, this type of attack must be performed at extremely close range where the body touches that of the opponent so there is not enough space for the opponent to twist or turn away. Further, if you allow too much space, your adversary can turn inside your attempted throw to execute a counter-throw or disruptive strike against you.

It is important for practitioners of striking arts to be familiar with the primary tactics of other forms. When you know the strengths and limitations of other forms, it becomes more difficult for you to be caught off-guard in a confrontation with someone whose training is different from yours. Although throws performed by karate practitioners tend to be a bit more violent (e.g., punch first, then throw) than similar techniques judged acceptable in judo competition, the movements are essentially the same.

Another advantage of familiarity with throws is learning how to fall properly without becoming injured. The Japanese term for breakfall techniques is *ukemi waza*. There are four basic types of falls: front, back, side, and rolling. Properly executed *ukemi* cushions vital areas, absorbs shock, and allows you to be thrown to the ground without injury.

Unlike judo, which is practiced on *tatami* mats, karate is typically practiced on a hardwood floor, so proper breakfall techniques are essential. With enough practice it becomes so automatic that you can even roll on concrete without injury. A judo practitioner we know had a bit too much to drink, fell into an empty pool, and bounced back up—completely unhurt.

Nerve Attacks

Nerve attacks are not considered stand-alone applications in *Goju Ryu*. They are used in conjunction with other techniques. Nerve knockout or pain compliance* in and of itself is a dangerous thing to use—not so much for your opponent, but for you. *Dim mak*, *kyushu jitsu*, pressure point fighting, or whatever you want to call it is very, very sexy. The idea of just being able to tap an opponent into submission like a Vulcan nerve pinch[†]—to have such power at your grasp—is a dangerous and very enticing path to follow. The problem is that such techniques do not always work.

A logical audit of *dim mak* will tell you just how a skilled practitioner uses it. First the practitioner becomes skilled in other aspects of his or her chosen art; very capable of operating on a mechanical level (e.g., kicking, punching). He or she also

---

* The strategic application of painful techniques designed to control an opponent.

† As seen in the science fiction movie/television series *Star Trek*.

learns submission techniques such as locks, pins, or other mechanical leverage applications that will cause an opponent to surrender. Only then are pressure point manipulations added to the skill set.

To fight using pressure points alone is risky because they do not work on everyone.* Further, what works on one person may not work on another. Law enforcement and corrections officers apply mechanical force (e.g., locks, holds, strikes) when a situation becomes physical because such techniques always work (assuming, of course, you do them properly).

A critical analysis of *Goju Ryu kata*, as with those found in most martial arts, shows that a large number of the strikes, rubs, and other techniques take advantage of commonly accessible pressure points. If, for example, you strike the forearm in the exact right location (e.g., Lung 6) you can deaden the nerves and render it temporarily unusable. Even if you miss that vital spot, a strong enough strike will have much the same result (especially if you break the bone). *Goju Ryu* relies on mechanical force to cause damage, treating the nerve attack as an added bonus.

Chokes

There are two types of choking techniques. First, by applying pressure to the trachea of an opponent, you can cut off the oxygen supply to his or her lungs. The second method applies pressure to the carotid arteries, denying a blood supply to the brain. While both are effective, the latter is somewhat less painful for the recipient. In the same manner as throws and locks, chokes must be performed at very close proximity to an opponent so there is little room for escape or counterattack.

Applying a choke in a real fight causes most people to freak out. Loss of breath is very frightening. Practitioners who choose to utilize this technique must use proper body mechanics to overcome a frenzied opponent. A lot of practitioners believe that chokes are a good way to incapacitate an opponent without permanently injuring him or her. If applied too long or incorrectly, however, chokes become deadly, so exercise appropriate caution when using these techniques. Practitioners who learn how to perform chokes are generally taught resuscitation techniques as well. We wholeheartedly agree with this practice.

Summary

"When confronted by a would-be assailant, you have three choices. You can: (a) run away, (b) give him what he wants, or (c) defend yourself. You will have to evaluate the situation—sometimes in a matter of seconds—and decide which course you will take. If you feel that your attacker intends to harm you, then obviously you must defend yourself. Generally, however, if you can get away or end the confrontation

---
* See Principle *4—nerve strikes are extra credit* for more information.

without physical force you should do so. This has nothing to do with the morals of using physical force...it's just that the chances of being hurt are much greater if you engage in combat." [27]

– *Paul McCallum*

A deep understanding of strategy and tactics is a necessary prerequisite for being able to properly decipher *kata*. Strategy is a plan of action. In martial arts as in war, it is what you do to prepare for engagement with an enemy long before the fight begins. Tactics, on the other hand, are expedient means of achieving an end, in this case defeating an adversary. Tactics are selected during the heat of battle. Like a house without a solid foundation, tactics without strategy will ultimately fail. The tactics of every combat art have been developed within a strategic framework that allows them to work effectively.

Tactical thinking is based around the concept of "if"—"if he does this, I will do that." The challenge is that you simply cannot think of enough "ifs" to anticipate every conceivable situation. When faced with an unexpected movement during actual combat, your brain will freeze, if only for a brief moment, rendering you temporarily defenseless and vulnerable. If the strategic foundation is strong, on the other hand, appropriate tactics can be employed automatically without conscious thought, letting you react appropriately to most any situation without hesitating.

In *Goju Ryu*, for example, the strategy at its simplest form is to close distance, imbalance, and use physiological damage to incapacitate an opponent. The tactics of *Goju Ryu* support this strategy, reinforcing the fact that karate is fundamentally a striking art. Looking at its core *kata*, you will find about 70 percent hand techniques, 20 percent foot techniques, 5 percent throws, and 5 percent groundwork.

It is important to avoid confusing the quality of the strategy with the skill of the fighter. During his military service Chojun Miyagi *Sensei*, the founder of *Goju Ryu* karate, spent time training at a judo *dojo* while off duty. During his two-year stay, not one of the judo practitioners was able to successfully throw him. Reading this story, one could easily infer that karate is better than judo. Realistically, however, Miyagi's remarkable physical conditioning probably had much more to do with his success than any differences between the two arts.

Once a practitioner understands his or her chosen art's strategy and discovers that it is sound, it is imperative that it be followed. Since all the tactics are built around this strategy, failure to follow it will almost certainly lead to failure in combat, a regrettable situation. In a fight, life or death decisions must be made in an instant. To survive a practitioner must be engaged in the moment. There is no more time to plan. Responses must follow a "decision stick." They must be straightforward, simple, and immediate. In combat, everything else is meaningless.

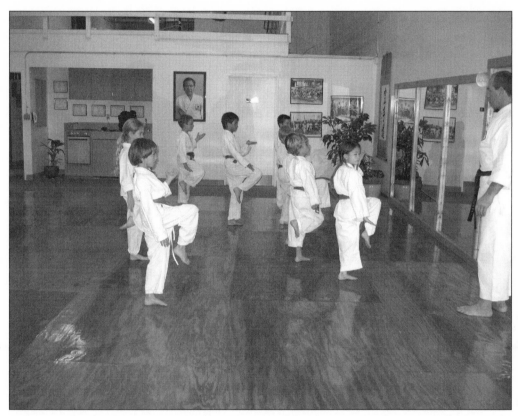

Kids *saifa: hiza ate*. Here, Franco Sanguinetti's kid's class practices *saifa kata*. This movement is a knee strike.

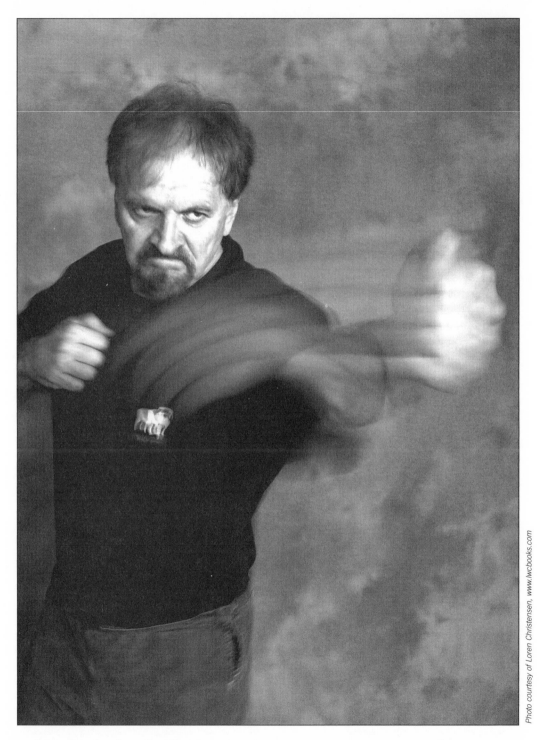

SPEED BACKFIST. LOREN'S BOOK SPEED TRAINING IS ONE OF OUR REFERENCE SOURCES AND AN OUTSTANDING READ. THIS PHOTO IS ON THE COVER OF THE VIDEO THAT GOES WITH HIS BOOK. LOREN IS A RETIRED POLICEMAN, VIETNAM VETERAN, HIGH-RANKING MARTIAL ARTIST AND PROLIFIC WRITER. HE HAS EARNED A TOTAL OF 10 BLACK BELTS: SEVEN IN KARATE, TWO IN JUJITSU AND ONE IN ARNIS.

CHAPTER 3

Principles

"One must learn how to apply the principles of the kata and how to bend with the winds of adversity." [28]

– Choki Motobu

Principles outlined in this chapter form the philosophical context within which valid *kata* applications can be identified. They apply to most any martial art form that uses *kata*, particularly striking arts such as karate. These principles differ from the rules that follow in chapter 4 in that they apply broadly to all techniques rather than to deciphering an individual movement.

The rules of *kaisai no genri* (discussed in chapter 4) are tactical in nature, deciphering practical applications from the specific movements of any particular *kata*. The principles we'll delve into in this chapter, on the other hand, form a strategic context within which practitioners can identify what types of applications work and thus weed out invalid interpretations of *bunkai* from any *kata*. In order to make full use the rules, one must first understand the principles, the foundation upon which they are built.

We will discuss the following principles in detail:

1. There is more than one proper interpretation of any movement.
2. Every technique should be able to end the fight immediately.
3. Strike to disrupt; disrupt to strike.
4. Nerve strikes are "extra credit."
5. Work with the adrenaline rush, not against it.
6. Techniques must work at full speed and power.
7. Techniques must work on an "unwilling" partner (e.g., opponent).
8. Strive to understand why it works.
9. Deception is not real.
10. If you are not there, you cannot get hit.
11. Cross the T to escape.

12. Stances aren't just for *kata*.
13. Don't forget to breathe.
14. Use both hands.
15. A lock or hold is not a primary fighting technique.

1) There is More Than One Proper Interpretation of Any Movement

"In actual combat it will not do to be hampered or shackled by the rituals of kata. Instead, the practitioner should transcend kata, moving freely according to the opponent's strengths and weaknesses." [29]

– *Gichin Funakoshi*

There is more than one proper interpretation for any movement in *kata*. As Morio Higaonna wrote, "None of the movements of the *kata* is restricted to one application—in a real fight the variations of each application are unlimited." Of course there are some interpretations that are better than others. Practitioners are frequently taught only *bunkai* and/or *oyo* or *kumite*. With a little creativity most can figure out *henka waza* on their own. *Okuden waza*, on the other hand, requires a "secret decoder ring." Its applications are rarely obvious.

The principle of more than one proper interpretation is really about creativity, thinking outside the box. We bring it up to spur your experimentation. According to Iain Abernethy, "it is a grave error to insist that a *kata* movement has only one single application. Each *kata* movement has many possibilities. To limit oneself to a single *bunkai* for a single movement is limiting to both the individual and the art of karate." He is right, of course. In fact the death of each master during ancient times held the risk of irrevocable knowledge loss. *Tomari Te*, for example, is pretty much a lost art today.

When a practitioner learns to apply various principles and rules to decipher *kata*, such knowledge should be passed along, at least within that practitioner's school. While we acknowledge that newer students should not be overwhelmed with esoteric knowledge, nor should immature practitioners be taught lethal applications before they are responsible enough to handle them, there are very few truly valid reasons for instructors to withhold "secret" techniques from their advanced students.

Experiment! Have fun with your *kata*. Learn what works and what does not. Look for the best application for any given technique as it applies to you—your unique physical characteristics and body type, your mentality and emotional approach to combat, and your other predilections. Decipher and share secret techniques amongst other practitioners of your style. What works best for you may not be best for them. On the other hand, you might just find a new interpretation that works even better than whatever you came up with on your own. Keep an open mind.

2) Every Technique Should Be Able to End the Fight Immediately

"Bombs do not choose. They will hit everything." [30]

– *Nikita S. Khrushchev*

The art of striking an opponent, whether it is in hand-to-hand combat or a technological warfare, is always based on two principles: accuracy and energy. Accuracy is simply hitting your target. Energy is the amount of power you can project into that target.

The most classic example of the trade-off of accuracy versus energy was found in the cold war between the United States and the former Soviet Union. The United States decided that it could strike multiple targets with just enough warheads to totally obliterate each one. The country's leaders spurred the developed of precision guidance mechanisms that could deliver lethal cargo within inches of an intended target. Today's ubiquitous global positioning satellite (GPS) systems are an offshoot of that military technology.

The USSR, on the other hand, had less technical skill, albeit substantially higher than most other countries in the world. They chose to simply strike with as much mega tonnage as they could get into the air, destroying the target and everything for miles and miles around. A deficiency in accuracy for the Soviet military was solved through the development of bigger bombs. It was a trade off.

Hand-to-hand fighting works in much the same way. The more accurate you are, the less energy you need with each blow. Most members of the martial arts community have met an elderly practitioner or someone of small stature who can shatter bricks, boards, or bodies with effortless grace. As accuracy and energy converge, the results can be devastating. Each movement of a *kata* is designed to cause serious bodily harm to your opponent in the shortest amount of time possible. This is most obvious with strikes, but that is not the whole story.

Most times that you "block" an aggressive motion you are actually striking your opponent.* At the very least, a good defensive movement should make your opponent think twice about continuing to attack you. Any time you touch an opponent you should use that opportunity to damage them. Kane has witnessed more than one real fight where a martial artist broke, hyperextended, or dislocated their attacker's arm with a blocking technique. Defensive movements that stop or redirect an attack are just as likely as strikes to put the opponent out of the fight.

* See Rule 8—*there is no block.*

Offensively or defensively, if you have accurately attacked an aggressor's vital area you can elicit pain, temporary paralysis, dislocation of a joint, knockout, or even death. Eye, ear, throat, solar plexus, knee, and ankle blows can cripple or kill someone. Punching a person in the stomach, on the other hand, may just piss him off. All useful applications cause physiological damage to vital areas. It is critically important to understand where these areas are and how your *kata* techniques target them.*

Acupuncture requires a high degree of precision as you are using a tiny needle to stimulate the nerve. A karate strike, on the other hand, does not need to be nearly as precise. In general the harder you hit, the larger the area you affect. Every movement in *kata* is designed to hurt someone. If you aim at a vital point, strike vigorously, and miss slightly, it really doesn't matter all that much. To go back to our opening analogy, you do not necessarily need the pinpoint precision of a U.S. nuclear missile if you hit hard enough like a larger Soviet bomb.

All blows should be full speed and full power every time. Realistically, it's only a feint if an opponent blocks it.† We have seen many tournament fighters throw halfhearted fakes that would have connected had they put sufficient zip on their first strike. Instead, they were focusing on the follow-throughs that were ultimately blocked—laughable faux pas in a sparring competition; deadly mistake in a real fight.

The proper defensive mindset is "him, down, now!" You simply cannot mess around in a real fight and walk away unscathed. The ancient masters understood this all too well. They could not rely on modern medicine to repair damaged cartilage, stop internal hemorrhaging, or stave off infection. They intentionally designed every offensive movement (and many defensive ones as well) in every *kata* to immediately end the fight. Perceived applications that do not do this are simply wrong. In such cases there is a better, more realistic application still waiting to be uncovered. You just have to find it. Every technique should be able to end a fight immediately.

---

3) Strike to Disrupt; Disrupt to Strike

"Whether fighting an enemy armed or unarmed, keep him on the defensive. Chase the enemy with your body and your sprit. This is excellent strategy. You can easily open targets for yourself with a little effort, but then you must have the courage to go in and kill the enemy without delay. You must be totally resolved when you are fighting; otherwise you will easily lose. By constantly creating difficulties for the enemy, you will force him to deal with more than one thing, giving you the advantage in killing him swiftly." [31]

– Miyamoto Musashi

* See "Vital Points" in chapter 5 for a complete, detailed description of each vital area.
† See Principle 9—*deception is not real.*

Your attacker is rarely going to stand there like a *makiwara* (striking post) and let you apply your techniques unopposed. You need to disrupt him or her in order to be able to strike and strike to disrupt. Get the opponent off balance, upset his design, and move in for the kill.

This sounds ruthless, but it has to be. Remember, if there were any way to avoid a confrontation, we assume that you would have already taken it. The Chinese sage Lao Tzu wrote, "There is no glory in victory, and to glorify it despite this is to exult in the killing of men." As a trained martial artist, the only fights you get into are those that are completely unavoidable. That means that the aggressor really wants to hurt you. Your life is on the line!

There are several philosophies about how to attack the body. The two fundamental versions are multiple attacks versus one hit, one kill. Multiple fast attacks from many angles can overwhelm an opponent to the point that his defenses can no longer function. One strike delivered to a vital area with sufficient power, on the other hand, is all that is needed for a victory. Both philosophies are valid and built into the strategic foundation of various arts.

When placed in a defensive situation the human body reacts by covering its vital areas. Those vitals can be best described as the centerline of the front of the body, or the conception vessel. The conception vessel runs down the exact center of the body from just underneath the lower lip to the area in front to the anus. Damage to the conception vessel rocks a person to his or her core, physically.

Today much emphasis is placed on core body strength. Whether in the National Football League, the Canadian Football League, Major League Baseball, Premier League Soccer, competitive weight lifting, professional ice skating or even Pilates, core body strength is pushed because it provides the foundation for most physical actions. In attacking the conception vessel, or "cracking the conceptor" as it is sometimes called, you are attacking with intent to destroy your opponent, to render him or her unable to respond with further attack. There are several means to crack the conception vessel; however, we will focus on striking since it is the most common.

As kids, our most common defense against attacks by older siblings or unruly classmates was to turn away, bend over at the waist, hunch our back, and cover our head with our arms. Occasionally we might move our hands around hoping to swat away a blow. This response is rooted in a natural reaction. These vital points, or soft bits, need to be protected and the very structure of the human body predetermines the way in which it protects itself. We get small and cover up. The mind then uses this natural pattern to fire off assisting signals to accomplish the goal of defense and, ultimately, survival.

People block, defend, or cover with their arms in the same way in which they eat, from outside to in. Again, this inward motion uses the body's natural response of getting small and covering up. That is why inward blocks are faster than outward ones.

Try this drill with a partner: One person will attack (*tori*) while the other defends (*uke*). At first you will work outside-in, and then repeat the exercise inside-out. In both drills, *tori* pokes *uke*'s chest gently yet swiftly with his finger (almost like trying to tickle the *uke*). At first *uke* will start with his arms up and out to the sides, like the classic stance of surrendering to the police. With each poke, the *uke* drops his hand down and in to block. From this starting position *uke* should be able to stop or deflect every attack fairly easily, especially if he reaches forward and intercepts *tori*'s attacks very close to *tori*'s body.

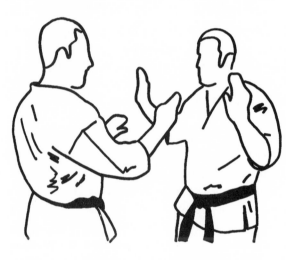

TAP DRILL: STARTING POSITION.

From this benchmark, *tori* will change his attack and aim for *uke*'s shoulder. Once again *uke* will try to block the attacks. Rather than down and in, his arms will move up and out. This should be significantly harder. Movements outward away from the core are always slower and less natural than movements in to protect it.

Now, let's get back to the philosophy of overwhelming assault versus a single killing strike. If you need to hurt someone severely, putting them out of a fight, you need to attack his or her core, the best defended area. Whether you use a single attack or a million, you must disrupt the opponent's natural reaction in order to reach a vital area. Practically, it is always best to assume that you will need more than one successful strike to end a fight. After all, there are several documented cases of criminals continuing to attack police officers after being shot multiple times. Bullets tend to hit a bit harder and sink a bit deeper than fists. If it takes less strikes to put down an attacker than expected so much the better.

Either way, "strike to disrupt/disrupt to strike" is a very effective methodology for breaking through an opponent's defenses. If you try to punch someone in the face, for example, odds are good that he or she will block it. Even untrained individuals are instinctively good at protecting their heads. Stamping on a person's foot or kicking his or her ankle first, however, causes the head and hands to follow the pain. The person involuntarily looks down and flinches inward. This usually opens up a shot to the head. You strike the foot, disrupting the stance and concentration. This disruption affords you an instant of opportunity to attack the head.

Most *kata* work the body: striking to disrupt, and then using the temporary disruption for an even better strike. Attacks to the feet, knees, or ankles, slaps to the ears, and assaults to the hands, wrists or elbows are all obvious disruptive strikes that are much easier to achieve than attacking the core directly.

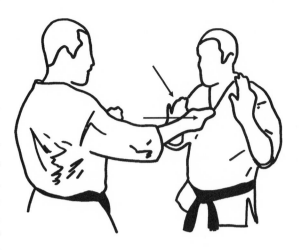

TAP DRILL: INSIDE WITH BLOCK.

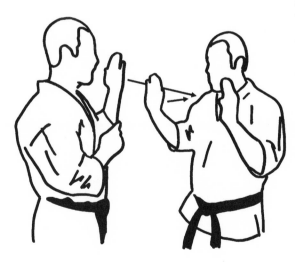

TAP DRILL: VARIATION TO OUTSIDE TO SHOULDER.

The idea is to work your way in, and then crack the conception vessel. To ensure clarity, it is important to understand that such actions can and usually should be simultaneous rather than consecutive. For example, the aforementioned ankle kick/head strike can be performed with a simultaneous right to left kick and left to right strike, a kind of scissor movement. Furthermore, good stances allow a practitioner to assault an opponent's legs with his or her own feet and/or knees simply by moving forward while simultaneously attacking with hands or arms.

4) Nerve Strikes are "Extra Credit"

"When you attempt to execute a throw, joint lock, or some type of submission hold, size and strength can play a major role in its effectiveness. If prior to applying the technique you are able to strike or press a vital point, you can cause your opponent to lose the use of his limbs or become unconscious. It would seem self-evident how valuable this would be in self-defense situations. Once you have been able to incorporate vital points into your particular martial art, you will be surprised how effective their addition will be." [32]

– Rick Clark

According to acupuncture theory, there is a definite flow of energy in the human body. The energy starts in the lung meridian and flows to the large intestine, stomach, spleen, heart, small intestine, bladder, kidney, pericardium, triple warmer, and gall bladder, ending with the liver. The process is then started again and continually makes this circuit through the body over a twenty-four-hour period. Techniques from various *kata* strike, rub, or press these points to help disable an opponent.

Traditional Chinese Medicine divides the world into five elements that interact with each other: wood (liver and gall bladder), fire (heart and small intestine), earth (stomach and spleen), metal (lung and large intestine), and water (bladder and kidney). Although acupuncture and acupressure work on the so-called "cycle of creation," martial arts are more focused on the "cycle of destruction," hence studying how to cause damage using these same principles.* In the cycle of destruction wood destroys earth, earth destroys water, water destroys fire, fire destroys metal, and metal destroys wood.

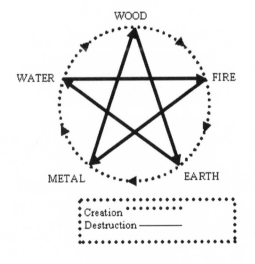

CYCLE OF DESTRUCTION.

To elaborate further, wood destroys earth as a tree's roots burrow into the ground. Earth controls water as a clay pot can contain liquids. Water self-evidently extinguishes fire. Fire destroys metal as

---

* Though we do learn how to heal/reverse damage caused by these strikes, of course.

in a forge. Metal destroys wood as a saw cuts through a board.

Although *atemi waza* (pressure point techniques) do not work against everyone, practitioners can usually cause maximum damage using the least amount of force to an adversary using this method. For example, the lung meridian is considered metal, while the gall bladder meridian is considered wood. Since metal destroys wood, you would want to strike a metal point first, then a wood point. Grabbing Lung 8 (metal) on an opponent's wrist followed immediately by striking Gall bladder 20 (wood) at the side of the neck can result in a knockout. Crossing the sides of the body is especially powerful.

Pressure points are rarely manipulated with a straight motion. In most cases practitioners will attack pressure points at a 45-degree angle. As a general rule, the larger the person or the larger the bone, the larger the vital point will be. When done properly, most people (more than 80 percent) will react strongly to pressure point techniques. Some, perhaps 15 percent, will react to some, but not all pressure points. There are also a small number of individuals who do not respond to most points at all, so practitioners cannot rely solely on this method to stop an attacker. It is best to think of it as an extra bonus.

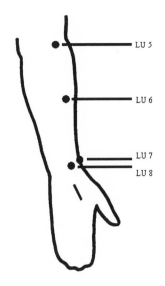

LUNG MERIDIAN ALONG THE ARM (CLOSE-UP) VIEW.
LUNG 8 IS AT THE WRIST.

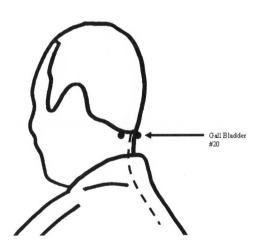

GALL BLADDER 20 CLOSE-UP VIEW.

In his article *Pressure Points*, acupuncturist/martial artist Bruce Everett Miller wrote, "While the medical effects of acupuncture are very real, they are not usually of such magnitude that a single point can stop a person who is attacking. The proof of this is not only in the observed effects but also by the fact that professional practitioners of acupuncture use a combination of points to create a healing effect. In almost all cases, a series of 3 to 5 points or more are used and the points have to be stimulated for 3 to 30 minutes to obtain the desired effects. So, if professional practitioners of acupuncture need several points and sometimes several treatments at these points to cause their effects, how do you expect to stop an attacking person with a single (or even a couple) of acupuncture point strikes?"

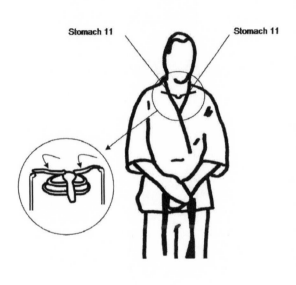

STOMACH 11.

For example, there is an excellent nerve bundle (Stomach 11) under the collarbone that causes extreme pain and buckles the knees of most people. To access this point, curl your fingers around the clavicle so that your fingertips dig in behind it. For even greater effect, you can dig your thumb into the end of the collarbone where it meets the suprasternal notch at the base of your opponent's throat. While this point is generally not used in combat, it makes an excellent demonstration example. When discussing nerve techniques in class, we typically show this particular application since it is easy to perform, gets an extreme reaction on almost everyone, and can easily (and almost always safely) be emulated by our students.

Over the years, this technique has always worked successfully on every student in our kid's class without exception. Not so with the adults. We have one student named John for whom perhaps one in eight nerve techniques are ever effective. Perhaps it is a high threshold of pain or perhaps he was simply born with less sensitivity than other people, but although a few techniques really light him up the vast majority do absolutely nothing. This particular example does not work on him at all. Another student, Jason, seems to have had his nerves surgically removed. On him, literally nothing works.

As you can see, nerve strikes simply do not work on everyone. They also become much less effective if the recipient has trained to "seal up" certain points, has certain mental disorders, or is in an altered state of consciousness due to drugs and/or alcohol. As a much younger, somewhat reckless man, Wilder had an interesting experience that reinforces this point. He recalls being under age at a keg party, which at the time seemed like an attractive idea. "We all piled into our friend's car and set off for the kegger. Soon the cold beer flowed on the warm summer night. The hits of the seventies popped out of a set of small speakers pulling in an AM radio station. Life was good—until being at the wrong place turned into the wrong time as well," he recalled.

As with most cases of violent activity there were precursors to what Kris was about to witness. "Bob was an older kid. He wrestled, played football and was as strong as an ox. Just about as smart too. He had been at the party earlier, left and then came back. During his absence he took what we later discovered was mescaline, a psychotropic drug. By the time Bob returned to the party he was quite agitated and aggressive. Psychotropic drugs have can have different effects on different people and in this case, they brought out the worst in Bob. Unfortunately everyone else was pretty drunk by that time too. So we had the volatile combination of various drugs, youth and testosterone all looking for a reason to get ugly. The spark was a disagreement over a pool game."

Kris recalls that he quickly realized that his adventure had led him to both the wrong place and the wrong time when a plea for the confrontational parties to cool down was answered with a one-sided fistfight with Bob dishing out the fists. "Bob had dispatched at least three people that I saw, perhaps more that I didn't, before the violence exploded out the sliding glass door and onto the lawn. People scattered, but in a flash Bob knocked his next victim down with a double leg tackle. The poor guy was unable to fend off Bob's explosive punches. I just stood there watching as his face became a mass of bruises, swelling, and blood.

"Another guy finally took action. Using a rock the size of a small watermelon he lifted it over his head and smashed it down onto Bob's hunched and muscular back. I stood slack-jawed watching Bob stand up and declare, 'Who the @#*|@ did that?' His reaction, or lack thereof, finally snapped me out of my lethargy. The guy who threw the rock and I both charged at once. I don't know what happed to the other guy because all I saw was a blinding sheet of blue light and the flower bed coming at my face. I was out for a moment then got up and ran without wiping the dirt from myself. My jaw sat on my face awkwardly. Everything began to hurt all at once.

"I shot back through the house and locked myself in the bathroom, hoping to escape through the window. Alas, I found out too late that it was too small. Changing plans, I opened the bathroom door, planning to make dash through the house and escape out the front. As I bolted for the main entrance, I stopped long enough to see Bob with a shotgun pointed up the stairs. Kelly, another guy, was the only person between me and the business end of twelve-gauge shotgun. Kelly begged Bob not to shoot. He leveled the gun anyway and pulled the trigger. Click—misfire! I ran for the door, shocked at my stupidity for standing there so long.

"As I reached the driveway a car was pulling out toward the exit kicking up dirt and loose gravel. Still running, I yelled at the driver to slow down then dove into the open back window, making it only half way in. The driver didn't stop but I managed to hang on." Later that evening," Kris says, "the County Sheriff's department was able to track Bob down using a couple of dogs, making an arrest as he had fled through some nearby brush."

There are many points in this incident where blunders and stupidity reigned supreme. Mistakes were certainly made, compounded by alcohol and youth. Those you can discern for yourself. "The main lesson that I took away (other than to drink in moderation and to avoid psychotropic drugs) was that nerve strikes simply do not work on a chemically altered person," Kris relates The rock that was slammed into Bob's back should have broken it or at the least knocked the wind out of him, yet it did absolutely nothing to alter his aggression. Simply put, nerve strikes would have not worked in such a situation. They certainly have their place, but the application window is pretty narrow.

Similarly, Kane recalls an instance where an out of control football fan was arrested, broke a pair of handcuffs trying to escape, and was subsequently re-subdued by no less than ten police officers. "It was the only time I've seen a group of officers resort to using their batons at the stadium. That's just not something you want to do where it can be overseen by thousands of witnesses and might even be captured by one of the many television crews working the game. For the most part they applied extra mechanical leverage rather than striking the guy to bring him back in line but it was no easy task. He simply felt no pain no matter what they did—pretty clear evidence that in certain situations you can only obtain control through mechanical force."

In acupuncture you have to find an exact spot to place your needle to properly affect a nerve. In acupressure, your fingertips have a slightly larger area to work with. As stated earlier, hit a general area hard enough with a karate strike and you will have a good chance of affecting the surrounding nerves, assuming that your opponent has some propensity to react to pressure point techniques, of course. Regardless, as previously mentioned, you simply cannot count on getting the reaction you desire every time solely from the pressure point.

Some nerves are manipulated via strikes. Others take a rubbing or grinding movement. Others still, take pressure to stimulate. Regardless, these techniques require a lot of study and research to fully understand. Rick Clark wrote an excellent book about pressure point fighting titled, originally enough, *Pressure Point Fighting* (Tuttle Publishing, 2001). If you are interested in knowing more about this aspect of the martial arts, his book is a very good place to start. Pressure point techniques are an excellent addition to your martial repertoire, but as you can tell from our previous experiences, you should not rely on them as single techniques alone.

5) Work with the Adrenaline Rush, Not Against It

"As someone who has worked with thousands of soldiers, I venture to say I am the only man on earth who was given a paratroop brigade to train single-handedly, I have come to the firm conclusion that a rule I live by called the principle of uniformity is valid and critical for survival in conflict. I am convinced it can only help you under the stress of conflict; it certainly cannot get you killed. The principle of uniformity is actually only a practical off-shoot of the time-honored concept that, 'what you train is what you do under stress.' Under stress, we tend to do what we have been trained to do." 33

– Eugene Sockut

Once a confrontation escalates into combat, adrenaline rushes through your system. This dramatically increases your pain tolerance and helps you survive in fighting mode. This "fight or flight" reaction instantly supercharges your body for a short period of time, increasing pulse rate and blood pressure, while making you faster, meaner, and more impervious to pain than ever before. On the upside, embracing your fear in a fight can help you survive, channeling your adrenaline rush into productive energy.

On the downside, the adrenaline rush severely limits your fine motor skills and higher thought processes. It also supercharges your opponent who will have an equal adrenaline rush! The techniques you employ in real combat, therefore, must be straightforward and simple to execute—requiring neither fine coordination nor complicated thought. They also must cause incapacitating physiological damage to stop a determined aggressor who is hyped up on the natural stimulant of adrenaline.*

Proper techniques must take advantage of natural physiological reactions such as the flinch. Imagine a time when you were driving down the highway and a rock hit your windshield, or, if you do not drive, a time when a hornet buzzed past your ear. That natural flinch reaction sends your hands racing toward the threat while your body tries to get smaller or get out of the way. As we have previously noted: hands rise, body drops.

---

* And possibly some unnatural ones as well—remember Mescaline Bob?

This natural response is triggered in the lowest level of the brain. The primitive "lizard brain," or (to be more scientific-like) the archipallium, is the center of self-preservation and aggression. When a person feels threatened, the archipallium takes over. If it could talk, the lizard brain would articulate its function with this simple statement: "Stay out of the way, I'll handle this!" At this point you become a non-thinking reptile. You no longer think; you simply act.

While the ancient masters may not have understood brain chemistry as well as scientists do today, they were certainly very familiar with the effects of adrenaline. None of their *kata* had applications that relied on fine motor skills to work properly. Further, they trained realistically and repeatedly such that high-level cognition was no longer necessary. They reacted instinctively, utilizing preprogrammed techniques in a strategic and systematic manner.

For example, as most practitioners know, there are a lot of grabs and pulls in karate *kata*. Most do not require (nor do they show) wrapping the practitioner's thumb around an opponent's limb as a conventional grip might imply. Not only can it be difficult to get a solid grip in the heat of battle that way, but your fingers may not find adequate purchase on a fast moving, sweaty or bloody limb. Latching on high up on the arm (toward the elbow) then sliding your hand forcefully along it toward the opponent's wrist while progressively tightening your hold is a reasonably good way to secure a grip. Even so, it does not always work.

Rather than grabbing with the fingers, we often use a hooking technique with the whole hand or execute a similar pressing technique with the palm. Either way this controls the opponent through downward pressure called *muchimi* or "sticky" hands. By pressing against an attacker's limb and simultaneously dropping your body weight, you can drive an opponent toward the ground whether or not you wrap your fingers around his or her arm. This type of pull is generally much more effective than a traditional grabbing technique that requires a successful wrap with your thumb.

Applications like *muchimi* work with the adrenaline rush, enhancing its benefits and minimizing its detractors. Trying to grab an opponent's little finger to perform a lock in the heat of battle, on the other hand, would be just plain silly. Simple, straightforward techniques that can be executed using gross motor movements with minimal thought are ideal. A great example would be cutting down a punch with *muchimi* to temporarily post an opponent's weight while simultaneously blowing out his or her knee with a joint kick. Shift/block/strike/incapacitate—it really is as simple as that.

6) Full Speed and Power

"Hopefully we can build techniques that are fault tolerant and allow for some margin of error. Kata does take this into account by the use of multiple attacks or continuation of attacks to your opponent. While it is nice to think in terms of 'one strike, one kill,' the reality of self-defense is that we may be forced to use multiple techniques to achieve our goal." [34]

– *Rick Clark*

Kata practice is about perfection. Applications are often broken down into multiple parts so that practitioners can understand each component and get it just right. We practice our forms over and over again striving for perfection. Why? Because in the fury of battle things get sloppy. The better trained we are, the better we will be able to perform at full speed and power in the midst of an adrenaline rush. Under such conditions much of our control vanishes. Our perfect *kata* form degrades markedly. With proper training, it can be fully effective nevertheless.

There is an old television clip of a running back on an NFL football team looking into the camera and saying, "Just give me eighteen inches of daylight." For those of you without a working knowledge of American football, what he meant was that if his linemen (blockers) could give him a small opening to run through, he could accomplish great things—he had enough foot speed that once he broke clear, the pursuing players had little chance of catching him. As a martial arts practitioner, you need only change the size of the opening, but not the philosophy. We only need a few inches of "daylight" through which to execute a technique.

Real fights are sloppy affairs. Everything happens at full speed and power. They are fast, sweaty, bloody, and brutal. There is no time for perfection. All that matters is survival. If your technique did not work exactly the way you meant it to, you cannot stop the action and redo it. It has to be good enough, timed well enough, and have just enough space to work the first time.

If it is ugly yet effective, that's just fine. Nothing more is required. Unlike *kumite* in the *dojo*, there is no "time out" or "redo" in mortal combat. Self-defense is about ending aggression quickly. That changes everything. We have all heard the phrase, "The best laid plans of mice and men often go awry." Similarly, a military general might say, "No plan survives contact with the enemy." That's okay. Do not look for perfection; just get the job done.

Recalling an incident where a martial arts instructor was in the wrong part of town at the wrong time, Wilder related the following. "I didn't see the fight, but I did see the results after the guy got beat down pretty good. It shook his *dojo* and the majority of the students' foundation. In fact it took great effort to prevent their organization from flying apart. Knowing this guy's method of practice and ideas regarding fighting, I believe that he sought perfection in the situation when it called instead for whatever it took to get the job done. You just can't do that and expect to prevail."

Heed this lesson: In *kata* practice, your form might call for eighteen inches of daylight, but all that you are going to get, and maybe all that you really need in a real fight, is one inch. Take your techniques and test them with this in mind, "Can I do this with far less perfection than what the *dojo* calls for?" Ask yourself, "Can I do this with only one inch and one eighth of a second, rather than eighteen inches and a full second to react?"

One way to safely approximate real fighting in *dojo* practice is to go full speed and power with proper padding and protective gear. The problem is that such equipment takes away many of your weapons. For example, you cannot grab successfully with padded gloves nor can you apply most pressure point techniques.* Further, some techniques are simply too dangerous to apply even with padding. Examples may include eye gouges or rakes, ear slaps, and joint strikes.†

Rather than training full speed and power with a partner where someone might get seriously hurt, we recommend that you practice your *kata* in combat-like conditions instead. Wait until the end of a particularly hard training session or simply go out and run hill sprints to near exhaustion before working your favorite form. Then do it as fast and powerfully as you can. Imagine a real opponent receiving every blow. Try to show every technique, but change the pacing where necessary to remove pauses shown solely for emphasis. Unlike normal *kata* practice, it is okay to get a little sloppy, to lose a little control. Strive for as good as you can do, but do not be concerned if you do not achieve perfection. In fact, if you are doing it perfectly, you are definitely not tired enough.

Although Kane has had hundreds of punches thrown his way and has even had knives pulled on him a couple of times, in most dangerous situations he has had a radio to quickly summon backup or law enforcement support. He recalls, "It's really not all that hard to outsmart a drunken football fan when you're stone cold sober and relatively crafty. Very few precarious affairs escalated into real fights. I was able to talk, laugh, or threaten my aggressors into submission, staying out of harm's way until help arrived. A few times, however, I was not so lucky. Not only have I had to fight my way out of ugly situations, but I have had to intervene to stop others from seriously hurting each other as well."

In almost all of the fights Kane has seen, both participants went all out—full speed and full power. By the time things escalated to violence, very little if anything was held back. The first blow, for example, virtually always went toward the face. Just about any blow to the head can cause serious damage to the victim.

* Though most of us cannot perform pressure point techniques safely at full speed on a training partner anyway.

† Some forms of protective gear are better than others, but virtually nothing will stop a full power kick to the side of the knee from causing significant damage or a full power shot to the eye from causing injury.

Untrained individuals often have a propensity for hurting themselves as much as they do their opponents; however, in the heat of battle they do not notice the pulled muscles, strained joints, and other hazards. Kane recalls, "One guy accidentally broke his own hand punching a metal stair rail, and then proceeded to pummel his opponent without regard to his injury. He didn't even notice that he was bleeding until after the handcuffs were snapped into place." Even in short conflicts, combatants generally emerge exhausted, shaky, and hurting once the adrenaline wears off.

It is hard to recreate such conditions in training without injuring yourself, but it is important to come as close as you can. Doing *kata* when you are totally exhausted and buzzing with adrenaline is a very good approximation of a real fight. You can mentally force yourself to perform even while you body is screaming at you to quit. It is very good training, so long as you do not overdo it to the point of serious injury. This ought to be a once a week activity at most. We feel that it is definitely worth pulling a few muscles in practice if it helps you survive during a real fight.

The bottom line is that practitioners need to know what is necessary for success and not let perfection become the enemy of the good enough. In a real fight at full speed and power, good enough is plenty.

7) It Must Work on an "Unwilling" Partner

"Not to be the bearer of bad tidings, but the reason someone uses a weapon on another human being is to stack the deck in their favor. People don't use weapons to fight, they use weapons to win. The absolute last thing any attacker wants to do is to fight you with equal weapons. If he was looking for a fight he wouldn't have attacked you with a weapon in the first place. And if he knows you have a knife, he is going to attack you with a bigger and better weapon to keep you from winning. You pull a knife and he gets a club. You pull a club and he pulls a gun. There is no fighting involved, you use the superior weapon to disable your opponent. And you do it before he does it to you." [35]

– *Marc MacYoung*

Let's face it, only "bad guys" begin confrontations. They only do so when they are pretty sure that they are going to win. Your attacker is not interested in a fair fight, if he or she can get an assassination instead. Sneak attacks, ambushes, and dirty tricks are tools of the trade. As the old saying goes, "all's fair in war."

If you are going to train well, you must perform realistically. Even though opponents in a real fight will be as uncooperative as possible, in *dojo* practice many practitioners have a tendency to "help" their training partners too much. For example, in tandem sparring drills, many junior practitioners do not really aim their blows. They just put out a punch or kick near their partner who easily blocks it.

Punches work against an opponent's force while throws work with it. If there is no force, you cannot really tell whether or not the technique would have been effective. Further, when practicing sweeps or throws some practitioners tend to drop easily, never really making their partners struggle to perform the techniques properly. In reality, such practice can be very detrimental. There is a big difference between "honoring" your partner's technique and simply letting him do what he wants unhindered. A little pain in practice goes a long way to avoiding real hurt in a fight.

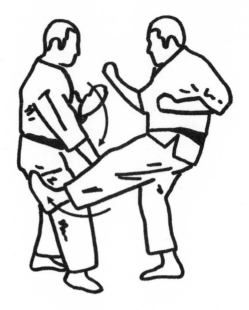

Gekisai oyo (TANDEM APPLICATION DRILL): SWEEP BLOCK TO RE-DIRECT THE KICK.

When Kane first began training in karate, he was frequently matched up with another practitioner named Mike. They took their training very seriously, often practicing after class and/or on weekends. Working toward their green belt tests, they frequently performed *gekisai kata dai ichi bunkai oyo*, a prearranged tandem drill using techniques from *gekisai kata*. One of the sequences calls for a *mae geri* (front kick) from one partner, while the other partner turns his body and sweeps aside the kick with his arm. Lawrence and Mike soon reached a point where they could perform this *oyo* swiftly and well.

One day in class, they had the opportunity to perform this drill with Scott, a visiting *yudansha* (black belt). The first time Scott threw the *mae geri*, Lawrence took a solid blow to the groin, a very painful and quite embarrassing situation. Nevertheless, it was also a very good learning experience.

During their friendly practice sessions, Lawrence and Mike had subconsciously aimed their kicks away from each other's private parts, eliminating the need to seriously block the attacks. Turning their bodies a little was all it took to avoid getting hit by the un-aimed blows. Since the blocks were relatively unnecessary, they had not been training realistically, although they were not aware of it. The first properly aimed, full-speed blow clearly pointed out that shortcoming, however.

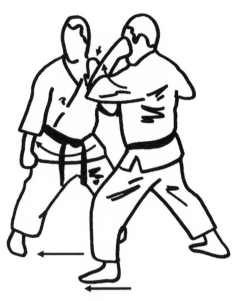

GEKISAI OYO (TANDEM APPLICATION DRILL): FOLLOW-ON PIVOT/ELBOW BLOCK. DEFENDER IS ON THE LEFT.

Fortunately it happened on the practice floor rather than in real combat.

Similarly, at the end of one version of the *saifa kata bunkai oyo*, there is a foot sweep takedown followed by a strike.* If a practitioner leaves too much space between himself and his opponent and/or fails to break the opponent's balance, he sets himself up for an easy counter throw. Once again, when Lawrence and Mike worked together, one partner just fell down whenever the sweep was applied. Scott, on the other hand, threw a vicious counter throw the first time Lawrence tried the technique improperly, giving Scott enough space to turn in. Fortunately, Lawrence knew how to fall properly, an essential skill if you are unexpectedly slammed onto a hardwood floor.

Honoring a partner's technique means behaving as if the movement had been performed at full speed and power. It should never imply letting a partner get away with sloppy or ineffective technique.† The attacking partner learns best when the receiver makes progressive, but realistic, resistance in proper proportion to skill level. In this fashion, a practitioner can identify and correct weaknesses in technique or interpretation thereof in the relative safety of the *dojo*.

When deciphering *kata* applications, you cannot rely on unpredictable movements by an attacker. In other words, assuming that the opponent will attack or respond with a specific technique (e.g., uppercut, elbow strike) is simply not realistic. There are far too many possibilities to account for every one. Even if you could plan for every tactical contingency in advance, you should not count on having the emotional wherewithal in the heat of battle to logically pick responses off a mental list. You must train your body to react without conscious thought.

On the other hand, your applications should anticipate predictable responses by your opponent. Examples of predictable responses include a second punch from the opponent, your groin strike bending the opponent over, or your arm whip causing his head to snap up and back. Training, therefore, must work similarly. It is essen-

---

* The other main version uses a similar movement to show a knee strike that drops the opponent followed immediately by a standing choke.
† Except when first learning the basic movements of a sequence, of course.

tial that the applications you practice have a very good chance of being effective in a real fight.

To help your training partners figure out where that may be the case, you must honor their techniques with predictable and realistic responses as appropriate. You must not, on the other hand, reinforce bad behavior and unrealistic technique. It benefits no one to do so.

---

8) Strive to Understand *Why* It Works

> *"Sepai contains many hidden techniques and combinations of movements that are designed to confuse the opponent in combat. A simple example of this is feinting a strike to gedan (down) then striking jodan (high) or vice versa. By simply watching the kata, it is impossible to determine the true meaning of the techniques. For example, in the case of striking naka daka ippon ken (sepai double punch using 'one-knuckle' fist), the real meaning is in the foot stamp and not the punch."* [36]

> — *Morio Higaonna*

Bunkai are like tools in a toolbox. Practitioners need to use the proper one for any given situation. While you *can* use a hand drill to pound nails, it is inefficient and hard on the drill. You are far better off with a hammer. Understanding why an application works can help ensure that you use it in the proper situation.

In Japanese martial arts understanding can be classified in two ways, *omote* and *ura waza*. *Omote* signifies the outer or surface training; while *ura waza* can be translated to denote the inner or subtle way. *Omote* is the most common and easiest to understand and communicate to others. *Ura waza*, on the other hand, are the subtle details that make the obvious succeed.

Practitioners develop confidence by not only being able to execute a technique in a variety of situations, but also by understanding why it works and where it is best applied. Ed Parker, the founder of American Kenpo Karate, summed it up perfectly when he said, "I would rather have one technique work for me than a hundred work against me."

Karate, for the most part, is *not* composed of complicated variations of techniques; it is about directness of the application and the *ura waza* or the understanding of the technique. Having some understanding of the inner workings of a simple movement sets a practitioner up for success in properly applying it. The secret of martial arts can be found in the basics. In Japanese these basics are called *kihon*.

Repetition is essential. However, at some point, the law of diminishing returns takes effect. You can have twenty years of experience or one year of experience twenty times. Without the *ura waza*, or inside understanding of an application, the repetitions become as exciting as running on a treadmill at the local gym. Some people are told the inner applications while others discover them through diligence. Whatever your path, seek the inner teachings as a desert nomad seeks water.

Without the *ura waza,* you might never understand how to actually apply the techniques you practice in your *kata*. For example, when Wilder first learned *seiyunchin kata* many years ago, his *sensei* explained the various *bunkai* associated with that form. Being new he accepted most of the explanations at face value.

One in particular troubled him, though. There is a segment in the *kata* where the practitioner holds his right arm up vertically, covers his right elbow with his left hand (held horizontally below the joint), shifts forward, and performs a vertical backfist. The explanation provided suggested that the practitioner was protecting his right elbow with his left hand. Wilder recalls, "I spent a lot of time trying to figure that one out. Why would I use some of the more delicate bones in my body to protect an elbow that is just plain hard? It didn't make sense on many levels."

As he surmised, the explanation he received did not make a whole lot of sense. Logically speaking, why *would* you protect one of the toughest bones in your body with a collection of the weakest? If the technique were done on the inside of the elbow, perhaps to protect against hyperextension, that explanation would absolutely add up. But to the outside as shown in the *kata*, it seems ridiculous. Another instructor Wilder talked to thought that movement might represent an augmented block, *henka waza* with the hand actually on the side of the elbow rather than below it.

That explanation did not make a lot of sense either. Let's face it; the most likely attack to the center of the body is a punch. If you need to use a supported block to stop someone's punch, you had best take off running. The concept of using both of your arms to block one of someone else's just does not fly. If you plan to stop a kick with your arms following this scenario, then your body is way out of position. Arms can readily be used to deflect or catch a leg, but force-on-force encounters between arms and legs are best avoided, unless *you* are the person doing the kicking.

Finally when Wilder was working with a *Shito Ryu* practitioner, he discovered a more logical application for the movement that had been bothering him. This practitioner explained that in practical application, the *kata* was showing a defense against a double grab or similar attack, something you want to cut off *before* the opponent makes contact. You use the left arm to horizontally pin the attacker's hands, dropping your body weight to really lock it in. He went on to explain the concept of *muchimi*, showing Wilder how to do it. When Wilder asked about the idea of an augmented block, he said, "If you have to block like that, you should be going that way as fast as you can," as he pointed behind himself and grinned. The technique was actually a lock—not a block where someone was so strong that both hands would be needed for defense.

In this optimized application, when the pin and both strikes happen at the same time as the weight drops, a devastating counterattack hidden within this simple movement is uncovered. This explanation is much more realistic than either of the others. It is also straightforward and exactly what is shown in the *kata*, actually a pretty basic *bunkai* (technically *henka waza*) rather than some obscure *okuden waza* (hidden technique). The only difference between this application and the one shown in the *kata* is that our palm faces down rather than up.

What makes it powerful is a thorough understanding of why it works. For example, Rule 10 tells us that touching our body in *kata* indicates touching an opponent. In the case of this *kata*, the "touch" is really a pin (much like a grab), using *muchimi* to hold the arms in place, which obviously is much more efficient and effective than a one-handed grab against two arms.

Muchimi is the concept of controlling an opponent's limbs without actually grabbing them. It is sometimes called "sticky" hands because the point is to stick to an opponent without wrapping your thumb around his or her limb, which is both slower and more dangerous (for you). Often times a hooked hand is used. *Muchimi* is used in many *kata* from many different martial arts styles.

This same sort of misinterpretation could be made from another application in *seiyunchin* where it appears to show a reinforced block yet is better interpreted as follows:

Once you understand why a technique works and understand its limitations, you can apply it correctly. No technique works in all situations. Like stances, they all have strengths and weaknesses. The key is choosing a technique that exploits an opponent's momentary weakness in order to overcome him or her.

For example, the *Shito Ryu* practitioner explained that the weakness of the aforementioned double grab is that it takes both limbs to apply. The optimized counterattack that he helped Wilder discover requires only one limb to entangle two, freeing the second for attack. This one-on-two application exploits the aggressor's weakness beautifully.

9) Deception Is Not Real

"They attack with one purpose and one purpose only—to destroy the enemy. They do not take false postures when they prepare for attack. They simply attack with all their heart and soul." [37]

– Miyamoto Musashi

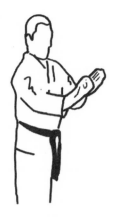

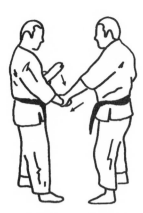

SEIYUNCHIN KATA: THIS MOVEMENT LOOKS LIKE AN AUG-
MENTED BLOCK IN PERFORMANCE OF THE *KATA*. IN PRACTI-
CAL APPLICATION, THE TECHNIQUE IS REALLY A GRAPPLING
TECHNIQUE.

SEIYUNCHIN KATA APPLICATION: GRAB.
DEFENDER IS ON THE LEFT.

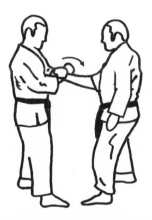

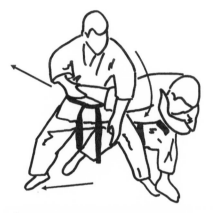

SEIYUNCHIN KATA APPLICATION: COUNTER WITH WRISTLOCK.

SEIYUNCHIN KATA APPLICATION: FOLLOW-ON ARM BAR.

While deception can help you avoid violence, it is not terribly practical once a
fight has already begun. Karate was created by civilians to defend themselves against
civilian aggressors in real life self-defense situations. Because of this origin, karate
kata do not presuppose a trained response that can somehow be manipulated or confused. Consequently holding back some secret technique to deceive an adversary is
not very realistic. Unfortunately some practitioners explain *kata* movements that
way straight-faced and earnestly! Such explanations are uneducated at best.

Ask any boxer if he or she has a secret punch that will be held back for the tenth
round and you'll probably get laughed at. The answer is clearly no. Every boxer wants
to end a fight as soon as possible. Boxers like any sane individuals prefer to hit rather

than be hit. The longer the fight, the more punches the boxer will have to take.

In a real fight, shorter is always better, safer, and more preferable. The longer you wait to deploy your best applications, the lower your chances of actually succeeding when you try to do so if you've already taken damage from an opponent. Miyamoto Musashi reinforced this point when he wrote, "I must say, to die with one's sword still sheathed is most regrettable." Karate (or most any other martial art for that matter) is the same when it comes to fighting. It is about application, immediate, fast, and unrelenting. Once combat begins, nothing is held back.

Now you might be thinking to yourself, "What about honor and the code of *Bushido*?" What we are describing is not about the precursor to violence, it is about the *actual* engagement, immediate and dire conflict. We are talking about ending the confrontation instantaneously—not after an exchange of blocks and punches, or after sizing one another up, or after playing the escalato dance.* It happens now and it ends now. The idea that one is going to use a lure to entrap an enemy or hold back a secret technique is ludicrous.

This does not, however, mean that trickery cannot be used in a fight, or better still, to avoid getting into one in the first place. It simply must be done in the proper context—before contact with the enemy. Once the battle begins, it is too late.

Dave Lowry shared a fantastic example of this concept in his article *The Karate Way*: "Once an Okinawan karate expert was challenged to fight a bull. On the sly, for several days before the match, he went to the paddock where the bull was kept and jabbed its nose with a sharp prod. By the time of the fight, the bull was so terrified of the karate man that when the beast was led into the ring and saw its tormentor, it bellowed and ran away in fear… What about the fellow who was plotting to challenge the karate expert? He must have had some serious second thoughts, watching that bull run in apparent fear of the very presence of the expert. That was one less challenge the expert would have to meet in the future. It was a trick, but it was also smart strategy."

Practitioners cannot count on deception during a fight; it is simply not effective. It must be used *before* a confrontation spirals upward into violence, preferably to de-escalate and avoid the conflict altogether. Once engaged in combat, deception is not real.

---

10) If You Are Not There, You Cannot Get Hit

"Speed in fighting depends not just on your hands and feet in swiftness, but other attributes such as non-telegraphic moves and awareness. Speed in fighting is to hit your foe without yourself being hit." [38]

– Bruce Lee

---

* The upward spiral of one-upmanship that almost invariably leads to violence.

On his web site fightingarts.com, Christopher Caile wrote, "Several cardinal rules or options have already been breached if you are about to be attacked. Rule one is don't be there. Rule two is run, evade or escape. There is also the option of talking your way out of the situation." This is of course, sage advice. If you are not there, you certainly cannot get hit.

In fact, we'd go so far as to say the only way to guarantee survival in a fight is not to engage in combat in the first place. Sometimes, however, you have no choice. In these cases the only escape is to physically fight your way out of a bad situation. Even (or perhaps especially) when engaged in the heat of battle this rule still applies: "If you are not there, you cannot get hit."

In his book, *A Connecticut Yankee in King Arthur's Court*, Mark Twain wrote about a battle between his mythical hero, Sir Boss, and the famous Arthurian Knights of the Round Table. Sir Boss refused the heavy horse, strong armor, obscuring helmet, stout shield, and heavy lance of his opponents and instead mounted a lightweight steed in his court dress, using a rope lasso as his weapon. With their bulk, weight and poor vision, the knights had no possibility of catching him. He was easily able to ride circles around them, slapping them on their backs before he finally lassoed them into submission. This is a great example of not being there, hence not getting hit. By the time the Knights were ready to strike, Sir Boss was no longer there.

But when the enemy does get the "jump" on you, there are several strategies to make you faster and harder to hit. One of the most important is being aware of the "tell." Poker players coined this term, which refers to some movement or gesture that lets them ascertain that an opponent is bluffing. In the martial arts, the tell has been called by many names including the adrenal dump, the twitch, and so on. All of these refer to the final signal of impending attack; the immediate precursor of violence.

Violence almost never happens in a vacuum. There is always some escalation process—even a really short one—that precedes it. If you do not see the tell you are bound to lose. Even if you are really, really fast, action is always faster than reaction. Missing the tell is what gets you "sucker" punched. It could be drop of the shoulder, a tensing of the neck, a puckering of the lips, or any other small movement that precedes an attack.

Because it is subtle and small, it is difficult to detect. Consequently, the best way to find the tell is to look for a change; the physical manifestation of an adrenal response implies a person is about to attack you. Looking for the tell is a not the same as looking for a change in the person, however. You actually look for a change in the person's energy. Here are some examples of where changes of energy constitute a tell:

- A person who was standing still moves slightly. A weight shift is far subtler than a step, but the change is very possibly preparation for attack nonetheless.
- A person who was looking at you suddenly looks away or, conversely, a person who was looking away suddenly makes eye contact.
- A person who is shouting becomes suddenly quiet or, conversely, one who has been quiet begins raising his or her voice.

Once you see the tell, you can react. You can be defensive or offensive as the situation warrants. Either way, if you are not there when your opponent strikes, you cannot get hit. When you counterattack, you must strike and move, hit and move on. Be elusive.

In his famous *Book of Five Rings*, Miyamoto Musashi wrote, "You must constantly move around the fighting area and make sure to befuddle the 'gang' by constantly moving into them and keeping them to one side. You must constantly chase them and not permit them to surround you. They are generally not prepared for this type of retaliation and you will have them under your control. Practice with the idea of moving from one technique directly into the rest without hesitation." This is outstanding advice.

The term *mushin* or "no-mind" is frequently used in the martial arts world. Japanese and Okinawan forms of both armed and unarmed combat use it often. The concept of *mushin* refers to the absence of thought. In *mushin* the mind is open and not fixed on anything in particular. It is the opposite of daydreaming. When all extraneous thoughts are brushed aside, practitioners can react instantly to any threat as it appears.

Let's use the example of a combination technique. Any combination will do, but for example we'll use punch and chop and punch. If you plan to use this triple threat, what is your intent in delivering the combination? Is the goal to knock down the opponent, break his arm, or some other specific end? If so, you have taken a great leap down the path to failure. Why? Because such a goal is too specific. It assumes participation on the part of an enemy who will do his or her level best to disrupt you. Your goal needs simply to be to make them stop.

Once you have thrown the first punch, forget about it. It should no longer have relevance in your mind. Strike and move on. Your mind should immediately move to the next place you'll be. There should be no punch and move and chop and move and punch again. If there is, you have afforded your attacker time and space. It should be punch—chop—punch, all the time moving. In effect never being where you are—either with your mind or your body. By the time the attacker realizes where you are, you're already gone. Like Twain's Sir Boss, if you are not there, you cannot get hit.

11) Cross the T to Escape

"Raking fire was particularly devastating. Ships of this era were weakest at the bow and the stern, if an attacking ship could maneuver to cross the enemy in front or behind then they could fire directly down the length of the ship as the guns came to bear. The round shot bursting through the timbers resulted in a storm of splinters through the deck, in many ways similar to the effect of modern shellfire… The commander aimed to 'cross the T', maximizing his firepower at the expense of his opponent." [39]

— Broadside

Those who have watched *Mutiny on the Bounty*, *Pirates of the Caribbean*, or *Master and Commander*, or toured a real-life historic ship like the U.S.S. Constitution* have seen how the majority of offensive weaponry in old naval sailing vessels was arranged along the sides. Typically there might be a small chase gun or two at the stern (back) and similar small armament in bow (front), but the overwhelming majority of weaponry was stowed along the sides. This was due to architectural constraints of ship design.

Simultaneous firing of all guns along one or both sides of the ship was called a "broadside." Based on the sheer number of weapons alone, if one ship could unleash its broadside against either end of an opponent vessel,† the attacking ship could do devastating damage while being virtually unscathed by return fire. Broadside to broadside engagements, on the other hand, often led to the sinking of both ships. The naval maneuver that applied broadside to bow or stern was called "crossing the T," since the two vessels were aligned in a T formation to each other.

Crossing the T is a good way to think about escapes from holds and throws. In other words, if the attacker is at 90 degrees, escape 45 degrees. Similarly, if they are at 45 degrees, escape 90 degrees. To understand better what this means, try this simple exercise. Have a partner stand face to face with you and grab you around the throat with both of his hands. Your opponent should grip as tightly as you can stand. Now, simply turn sideways. Use your hips to spin your body forcefully so that you end up facing 90 degrees to your partner. Unless there is a huge disparity of strength between you and your partner or you fail to use your hips to turn your entire body at once, your partner should be unable to continue to hold on to your neck.

When blocking an opponent you can force him open or force him closed. Opening allows you access to his centerline while closing lets you cross him up and attack from his side. Closing an opponent is another great example of crossing the T. In other words, by blocking and simultaneously shifting to the outside a person you can cross the T. This movement is a staple of almost all striking arts. It is advan-

---

* Nicknamed "Old Ironsides" for her survivability in combat, she is the oldest commissioned sailing ship in the world that is still afloat (The HMS Victory is about thirty years older, but is permanently dry-docked). A wooden-hulled, three-masted frigate, she was larger and more heavily armed than the standard frigates of the time, very formidable in combat.

† Sometimes called a "down the throat" or "up the kilt" shot.

tageous because it provides maximum firepower for you and places you at the least risk of receiving damage from your opponent.

When you have closed an opponent, you control the limb you just blocked. For example, you block a head punch then control his arm with forward pressure using *hiki uke*. Because you now know exactly where the attacker's arm and hand are, you can readily avoid any further attack for as long as you maintain controlling pressure. That leaves only one limb, the opponent's leg that can reach you directly. He will have to realign his body in order to assault you with either of his other two weapons (arm or leg). During that moment of advantage, you can counterstrike with impunity using any of your unencumbered weapons.

Crossing the T is a nautical way of seeing a martial strategy. This battleship strategy transfers seamlessly to a hand-to-hand martial art because it is solid. It is rooted in efficiency and practicality. These two items—efficiency and practicality—are the hallmarks of solid strategy. By crossing the T practitioners have a strategy to escape from throws, holds, chokes, and most any entanglement attack. Specific tactics for escape will vary, of course, depending on the martial style you practice.

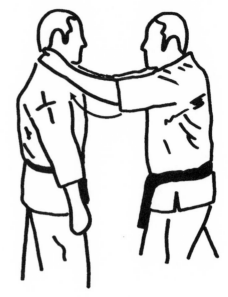

DOUBLE THROAT GRAB.

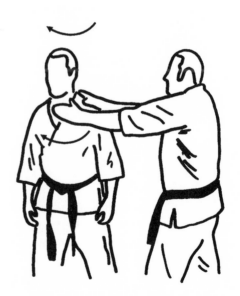

TWIST/ESCAPE.

12) Stances Aren't Just for Kata

"Stance training builds the physical foundation essential for the techniques of Northern Chinese kung fu, including tai chi chuan. In all martial arts, except for those involving grappling, the feet and legs must support the body, providing a stable foundation for defensive and offensive techniques using the arms or legs. The legs are also used to kick, control the opponent and change the body's orientation. In tai chi chuan, power is delivered through a highly disciplined twisting action around the spine, which classically begins with the foot and continues twisting through the ankles, knees, hips, buttocks, torso, shoulders and arms. Or, as the Chinese say "The whole body is the fist." The techniques often require using the torso, hips, shoulders, knees and elbows in addition to the hands and feet common in other martial arts. Strong, disciplined legs (meaning the entire structure of feet, ankles, legs, knees and hips) are essential to the success of such whole body techniques." [40]

– Rita Burns

Although Wilder grew up on a farm, he never owned horses. He found it fascinating, therefore when a blacksmith came to shoe some horses that his employer owned. Taking time out to watch the blacksmith at his craft, Wilder learned an important lesson; one we both agree is one of the most fundamental principles of martial arts.

As Wilder watched the shoeing process, he noticed that the blacksmith was extra particular about ensuring that each shoe fit perfectly. Explaining his diligence the man said, "Nature kills a horse from the ground up." Though it may take a moment to realize it, the blacksmith was absolutely right. If a horse cannot walk properly, it cannot find food, shelter, or escape from predators. If the feet do not work properly, everything else will surely fail.

The same concept applies to martial artists. Poor footwork can certainly cause us to lose a match, or become seriously injured or even die in combat situation. An ill-timed slip may put even the best warrior out of position to defend himself thereby ensuring his swift demise. Strength of technique and ability to move to attack or defend rely on proper footwork and good balance. Taking this cue from the blacksmith, learn your footwork and understand it, so that you can secure your success in matches or combat if necessary.

Here's a good analogy: Pretend for a moment that you have gone camping and upon setting up your tent discover that you have placed it over a large rock. If you want to get a good night's sleep, you will have to move the tent. The process you use to move and reset the tent is very important to this theme of footwork. To move the tent you will first have to lift the stakes to loosen it, and then remove a pole or two. After moving the tent to a better spot, you replace the poles then use the stakes to make the tent taut again, proceeding in that order.

It is the same in martial arts. It is important that the bones be in place first. Like tent poles, bones are the structures over which the muscles are going to be stretched. They must be in order first. If they are not, to continue the camping analogy, the tent will be distorted and weak. This distortion can be seen in *kata* when the architecture, that is, the bones, are misaligned and the practitioner uses muscle strength to put power into a technique. When the bones are aligned in conjunction with the use of the right muscles, this combination becomes much stronger than either could be alone.

Imagine a poorly staked tent in a strong windstorm. It will have less structural integrity to withstand the storm than an identical unit that has been properly staked. Any *budo* technique is much the same, as a simple shove can demonstrate. Unaligned bones and improper muscle tension in martial arts are as detrimental to success as a poorly staked tent in a windstorm.

A common misconception is the widespread belief that stances are just for *kata*. We have seen literally hundreds of e-mails and blog postings along the lines of, "Stances? Oh that's just for *kata*. In real life it doesn't work that way." People tend to disregard the importance of stances in combat. Bad idea!

Proper body alignment is critical in a fight. Lose your balance and you likely lose your life (or at least your well being). Further, much of the *okuden waza* in karate *kata* use stances and movement to unbalance an opponent. Practitioners can attack their opponent's feet, ankles, and knees simply by engaging with proper stance, balance, and body alignment. Combining leg and hand techniques into one swift attack can be devastating. Further, proper stance facilitates maximum power for your strike. Without it, you are at a serious disadvantage.

This does not mean that you must always use the *exact* same stances in combat as you would in *kata*. *Zenkutsu dachi* (front forward stance), for example, is often performed as *shozenkutsu* (half-front stance), a shortened, more mobile version of the longer form seen in many *kata*. You must, however, exercise great caution in doing so, ensuring that changes are strategically supportable and consistent with proper stance dynamics.

For example, *zenkutsu dachi* is commonly used to close distance much like a lunge-thrust in fencing. Shortening the stance to *shozenkutsu* in this application may require two steps when only one should have been necessary, ceding valuable momentum to an opponent. This stance is also used to receive strong forward attacks such as a tackle while counterattacking with movements like a clavicle strike and hammerfist to the head. If your stance is not deep and strong enough in such situations you will be bowled over whether your counterstrike is successful or not.

Similarly, some stances such as *shiko dachi* (*sumo* or straddle stance) are very difficult to perform in certain types of street clothes. To off-balance an opponent, however, you must get below his or her center of gravity. Inability to perform this stance correctly limits the scope of your tactical response. If your clothing selection limits the stances you are able to perform, you must choose applications that can be properly executed with what you are wearing.*

Such issues notwithstanding, practitioners must have proper body alignment and good stance in order to optimize their techniques in battle. Similarly, high kicks generally do not work in actual combat.† Self-defense engagements are fast, furious, and typically happen at very close range. Balance and movement are paramount. Often there is not even enough room to leg strike at all, except with the knee.

Of course, once your opponent bends over from your knee strike, you can follow through with a kick from the foot, but that is a secondary movement. Regardless, even if there is enough room, when you raise your foot high into the air, you take more time to strike your opponent, weaken your balance, and very likely open yourself to counterattack and disaster.

Loren Christensen reminds practitioners to know the difference between kicks for self-defense and kicks for show: "How about a sidekick that thrusts straight up overhead into a vertical line? Where in the heck would you use that in the street? What would it do to your pants? And let's not even talk about doing a vertical sidekick while wearing a dress. OK, the kick will work when you are lying on the ground and kicking up in the face of an attacker. But standing?"

Low kicks to vital areas such as feet, ankles, or knees are much harder to see and avoid, are less damaging to your balance and stance integrity, and are much more likely to connect with your opponent. And, you can perform then in regular street clothes, an important consideration. Most importantly, they do not disrupt your balance or stance integrity. Stances aren't just for *kata*; they are an essential component of effective self-defense too.

13) Don't Forget to Breathe

"Proper breathing is of utmost importance whether one trains in martial arts, the performing arts, or athletics. Its value can be seen most clearly in a martial arts struggle where the ramifications of improper breathing can cost a fighter the match." [41]

– Seikichi Toguchi

Most *dojo* training sessions begin and end with *mokuso* (meditation), the process of emptying your mind and focusing on your breathing. This brief meditation helps

---

* Better yet, change your clothing selection instead.

† Unless you are vastly more skilled and much, much quicker than your opponent.

to set an appropriate mood and allows practitioners to focus on training without outside distraction. It is an emotional barrier that separates *budo* training from the rest of the day. Further, it affords an opportunity to practice proper breathing.

Correct breathing is a vital component of energy management. Try this: pick your favorite *kata* and perform it ten straight times without pausing. Do your preparatory bow only at the beginning of the first set. Similarly, perform the ending bow only after the last one so that you get good aerobic stimulation. Once you get done, are you winded or could you do it another ten times?

If this simple exercise leaves you gasping for breath, odds are good that you are not breathing properly during your routine. The biggest mistake most beginning and intermediate *budoka* make is forgetting to breathe. Some students literally hold their breaths throughout most if not all of their *kata*. This holds true not only for *kata* practice, of course, but *kumite*, tournament, and self-defense applications as well.

Proper breathing is critical for all types of athletes. Boxers, weight lifters, cyclists, and marathon runners all must learn proper breath control to succeed. Avid football fans have probably noticed their favorite players have started wearing a small band across their noses to help force open the airway to boost performance. In the martial arts arena, how many of us have been scored upon in a tournament match during that moment of defenselessness where we think about nothing but sucking in more air? A good fighter looks for such openings in his or her opponent.

"I remember how fascinated I was by the fact that even such a simple thing as breathing was subject to being relearned and mastered as part of martial arts training. I had no awareness then that there would come a day when the controlled-breathing technique I had learned would save my life," Joe Hyams wrote in his famous book *Zen in the Martial Arts*.

Hyams then went on to describe how he survived a case of Weill's disease, a rare and usually fatal illness that he had contracted from tainted water. By slowly controlling his inhalations and exhalations via deep abdominal breathing he was able handle the excruciating pain of his illness and fever. In the hospital he was even able to use breath control to regulate his heart rate, staving off a near heart attack.

Proper breathing significantly increases a person's ability to handle pain, illness, or injury. Pregnant women, for example, are taught special breathing techniques in order to handle the pain of natural childbirth. *Budoka* often focus on their breathing during meditation to take their minds off distractions such as the discomfort of sitting in *seiza* (kneeling) on a hardwood floor* for long periods of time.

Most martial practitioners, those who study karate, aikido, kendo, *kobudo*, *qigong*, *tai chi*, and so on, are taught to breathe in through their noses and exhale through their mouths using their diaphragms to move the maximum amount of air possible through the lungs. Practitioners breathe in through their noses rather than

---

* We don't get to use padded mats like the yoga folks do.

through their mouths partially because the paranasal sinuses* produce nitrous oxide, which becomes part of the gas intake in nasally derived air.

Dentists sometimes use nitrous oxide to relax their patients before oral surgery. It works by relaxing and opening the air passages so that more air flows through the lungs,† which allows more oxygen to be absorbed in the alveoli. This nitrous oxide also helps sterilize the sinuses as well as the nasal air passageways strengthening the body's immune system.

This process is reinforced via *ibuki* breathing techniques found in such *kata* as *sanchin* and *tensho*. *Ibuki* breathing is a strong form of breath control typified by audible inhalation and exhalation, which exaggerates the type of breathing that *budoka* should be doing automatically all of the time. Proper breathing has a calming effect on the mind and body. It can be used to overcome fear and anxiety preceding and during violent conflict. Psychologists use similar breath control techniques to help their patients relax during therapy.

Michael Brown, a *sandan* and nationally ranked karate competitor wrote, "Proper breathing can be learned, but only through years of constant practice can it be mastered. If we wait until we are on the *dojo* floor to think about and practice our breathing, we might as well wait until we are about to crash our car before finding out if the brakes work. Like *kata*, proper breathing is an exercise that should be practiced daily outside the *dojo* so that when we come in to the *dojo*, it is automatic."

Competitive swimmers must carefully coordinate their stroke with their breathing. So too must *budoka*. Proper breathing facilitates *kata* movement. Practitioners typically breathe out strongly during hard techniques and breathe in during soft techniques or movement. In other words, they breathe out and tense for power and breathe in and relax for speed.‡

There are technically two types of breath control utilized in *kata*. The first, *ibuki*, can be thought of as quick energy breath. It is used during kicks, punches, and blocks. The second is known as *nogare*, or slow breathing. *Nogare* breathing is usually done when moving from one position to the next or where there is a pause for emphasis during the *kata*.

Weight lifters often grunt forcefully to lift that last bit of weight. A forced exhalation, grunt, or shout can focus concentration and increase power. It can also disrupt an enemy. Anyone who has ever been through boot camp can remember flinching away from a drill instructor's shout.

Similarly, most martial systems incorporate the concept of a *kiai* or spirit shout, a strong exhalation of breath that adds power to technique, disrupts an enemy, and reduces shock to the practitioner's body. Done properly, it comes from the abdomen rather than the lungs. Almost all *kata* have movements where a simultaneous *kiai* is

---

* Cavities in the frontal section of the skull that are connected to the nasal passage.

† The bronchial tree.

‡ Since tense muscles cannot move quickly.

required.* Most schools encourage practitioners to let additional *kiai* fly whenever they feel so compelled, personalizing their *kata* to a small degree. You must be judicious in this application, however, as it is impossible to maintain good breath control if you are constantly shouting with every technique. And, frankly, too many *kiai* can make your *kata* look more like a circus act rather than a show of technique.

14) Use Both Hands

> *"Always return your weapon along the same path it traveled out on. In this way you can use it again without having to relocate and rethink your attitude. The same applies to bringing the opposite hand back to the hip when you execute a punching strike. You must do this with authority and not in a haphazard manner. To fire a powerful punch requires that you fire straight and true while at the same time bringing the other hand back into firing mode. Otherwise both movements will be weak."* [42]
>
> – *Miyamoto Musashi*

Both hands are utilized simultaneously in almost all techniques. Whenever you throw a basic punch with one hand, the other invariably returns to chamber at your side. In a *kata*'s application, there is often something in that returning hand, especially when it is closed.† For example, as one hand deflects an attack, the other secures a grip for a joint lock or counter-throw; or you may be striking an attacking limb and also your opponent's body with a block and counterstrike combination.

In his book, *Pressure Point Fighting*, Rick Clark wrote that "two hands are utilized in self-defense techniques. If someone throws a basketball aimed at the center of your chest, do you attempt to catch the ball with one hand or two? My guess is that you would use both hands. It is a natural reflex of the body to use both hands when catching the basketball. Likewise, when someone is punching or kicking at you, your natural tendency will be to use both hands for a defensive maneuver."

Proper martial techniques are built from natural instinctive responses. Since reflex actions typically cause us to bring up both hands in response to a threat, it seems reasonable that a large number of defensive techniques utilize both hands. *Yama uke* (mountain block) and *wa uke* (valley block) are good examples of this. Because the proper application of defensive postures is actually *offensive* in most cases, one hand does the majority of checking or deflection necessary to keep you from getting hit, while the other does a controlling or attacking movement. *Yama uke*, for example, could be a simultaneous block and elbow strike.

Using both hands is important for offensive techniques as well. *Hikite* is a push/pull concept that ensures proper body mechanics for maximum power in each

---

* Almost always with a strike.

† Also see Rule 5—*a hand returning to chamber usually has something in it.*

technique. This concept works both with empty hands as well as with weapons and is a fundamental concept for properly executing many martial techniques.

To understand how it works, start with a basic chest punch. Now, imagine a large rubber band stretching from your left hand around your back to your right hand. As one hand punches, the other returns to chamber at your waist pulled by the rubber band. If you put your mind in the chambering hand while visualizing this imaginary rubber band launching your punch, you will find your attacks are both faster and more powerful. Adding a body drop (lowering your weight and center of gravity) to this push/pull from your hands amplifies this effect.

To add yet another layer, do the chest punch again, but from a *zenkutsu dachi* stance this time. As you step into the stance, one hand goes to chamber, while the other punches using the previous visualization technique. As you sink into the stance, put your mind in your back heel, ensuring it is anchored to the ground, then to your lower buttocks to sink into the stance and lower your center of gravity. Finally move your mind to your waist to drive forward, giving pressure. Combining the push/pull from the movement and the punch together gives you the maximum impact. This is all done simultaneously, of course.

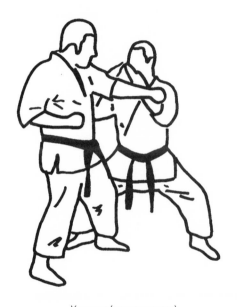

YAMA UKE (MOUNTAIN BLOCK).

When examining your *kata*, pay particular attention to the off-hand, the one that is not executing an obvious technique. There are often *okuden waza* associated with the apparently unused hand. The most obvious example is a grab or pull associated with a defensive posture (check/control) anchoring an opponent's weight for a *kensetsu geri* (joint kick), or pulling the opponent off balance for a lock or a throw.

Similarly there may be an eye rake or ear slap associated with the hand returning to chamber. In many cases the disruption necessary to set up your obvious strike comes from hidden techniques executed by the off-hand.* As we have stated before, every movement of every *kata* is there for a reason.† This applies to both hands, not just the one executing an obvious technique.

* Also see Principle 3—*strike to disrupt; disrupt to strike.*
† Also see Rule 4—*every movement in every kata has martial significance.*

15) A Lock or Hold is Not a Primary Fighting Technique

"In my own dojo we use the phrase, 'blow before throw,' to remind us of the importance of striking and weakening the opponent before throwing. It is important to clarify that the aim of the initial blow is to drop the opponent. Only if they remain standing do we make use of the blow's distracting effect in order to set them up for the throw." [43]

– Iain Abernethy

A lock or a hold is never a primary fighting technique in the striking arts. Even in grappling arts, such as judo or *jujitsu*, you simply cannot just walk up and apply a lock or a hold to an unwilling opponent. Throws work the same way—you must maneuver your attacker into a position from which you can imbalance him or her and then apply the technique. The concept of striking to disrupt and disrupting to strike* is critical to the successful execution of such techniques.

In fact, the goal is actually to drop the opponent with the initial strike, applying the lock or hold only when further control is required (e.g., restraining a criminal until police arrive). Although many locks and holds can be applied standing up, the majority are most effective when applied to an opponent on the ground. It is simply easier to control the person's movement or immobilize him that way. The problem is that if you go to the ground in a self-defense situation and your attacker has any friends around, you have put yourself in an extremely vulnerable position.

It is essential to have complete control of your opponent if you wish to become engaged in the act of throwing. The trick to successfully applying locks, holds, and throws was expressed best by Oleg Taktarov, an expert in *sambo*† and Ultimate Fighting competitor. He said that the trick is "no space, no space, no space, and no space."

He's right: The most fundamental requirements for a successful throw include no space for the opponent to escape, no space for the opponent to turn, no space for counterattack, and no space to disrupt your technique in any fashion.

The same holds true for locks and holds. The more you limit an opponent's movement and choices, the more successful you will be. The attacker can use any space you give to counter your technique. Grappling range is the closest fighting distance imaginable: to the extent possible, your whole body must be touching your opponent's. The rule of thumb is get close quickly and execute swiftly. Take control and give the opponent no space.

The bottom line is that a lock or a hold is never a primary fighting technique in the striking arts. Disruption is a critical component of successfully applying such

---

* See Principle 3—*strike to disrupt; disrupt to strike.*

† A Russian military martial art.

techniques. When analyzing your *kata*, it is important to remember that the goal is actually to drop an opponent with your initial strike, applying the lock or hold only when further control is required.

Summary

"When analyzing kata we will be reverse-engineering techniques. We are given traditional kata, yet the creator of this kata is no longer living. At best, we can give an educated guess to various bunkai in the kata. We may not be able to tell with a high degree of certainty what the defensive movements are that the kata may involve. I do believe we can have some confidence in what type of attacks the various kata would be defending against. I strongly believe physical attacks remain constant across generation and culture.

"If our bunkai for kata is based on the types of attacks we're likely to encounter, it is irrelevant if these techniques were not the intended bunkai of the creator of the particular kata we are analyzing. The important factor here is that we have techniques in the kata we practice to defend against attacks we suspect we will most likely encounter. It does not matter if the bunkai we use was not first envisioned by the creator of the kata—just so long as we have workable techniques that will be applicable to our particular needs." [44]

– Rick Clark

The principles described in this chapter create a strategic framework within which practitioners can identify valid interpretations of *bunkai*, *henka waza*, and even *okuden waza* from the *kata* they practice. These principles can be summarized as follows:

1. **There is more than one proper interpretation of any movement.**
   In actual combat, practitioners transcend the artificial limitations of *kata*, finding near limitless interpretations for any given technique. Look for the best applications that work for your unique physical characteristics, mindset, and other predilections. What works best for you may not be the best interpretation for other practitioners.

2. **Every technique should be able to end the fight immediately.**
   Every movement in every *kata* is designed to cause serious bodily harm to an opponent in the shortest amount of time possible. You simply cannot mess around in a real fight and walk away unscathed. *Kata* were developed before the advent of modern medicine, which cures injuries that would have been fatal a century ago. Consequently the ancient masters designed every offensive technique and most defensive ones to immediately end a fight.

3. **Strike to disrupt; disrupt to strike.**
   Your attacker is rarely going to stand there like a *makiwara* and let you hit them. You need to disrupt his or her designs, get the attacker off balance, and then move in for the kill. Simultaneous attacks to the feet, ankles, or knees, slaps to the ears, and assaults to the wrists or elbows are all obvious disruptive strikes that make attacking the vital core of the body possible.

4. **Nerve strikes are "extra credit."**
   While nerve strikes can be useful, they do not work on everyone. They also become much less effective if the recipient has trained to "seal up" certain points, has certain mental disorders, or is in an altered state of consciousness due to drugs and/or alcohol. Rather than relying solely on such techniques to stop a determined attacker, practitioners should consider them extra credit, to be combined with other types of strikes.

5. **Work with the adrenaline rush, not against it.**
   In actual combat the adrenaline rush supercharges your body for a short period of time, making you faster, meaner, and more impervious to pain than ever before. Unfortunately it severely limits your fine motor skills and higher thought processes. *And* it has the same effect on your attacker. Consequently applications must be straightforward and simple to execute while causing incapacitating physiological damage sufficient to stop a resolute aggressor.

6. **Techniques must work at full speed and power.**
   Kata practice is about perfection. Real fights, on the other hand, are messy affairs. They are fast, sloppy, and brutal. There is no time for perfection. All that matters is survival. Self-defense applications must be good enough to end aggression quickly. Practitioners must know what is necessary for success and not let perfection be the enemy of good enough.

7. **It must work on an "unwilling" partner.**
   Assuming that an adversary will attack or respond with a specific technique is simply not realistic; fights are too unpredictable. *Kata* applications do, however, anticipate predictable anatomical responses.

8. **Strive to understand why it works.**
   In Japanese martial arts, understanding can be classified in two ways, *omote* and *ura waza*. The former means surface training, while the latter can be translated as inner or subtle way. *Ura waza* are the subtle details that make the more obvious *omote* succeed. Like stances, all techniques have strengths and weaknesses. Understanding why an application works can help practitioners ensure that they will use it in the proper situation.

9. **Deception is not real.**
   Karate was developed for civilians to defend themselves against aggressors in a real-life environment. *Kata*, therefore, do not presuppose a trained response that can somehow be manipulated or confused. Practitioners cannot count

on deception during a fight. It must be used before a confrontation escalates to violence, preferably to avoid conflict altogether.

10. **If you are not there, you cannot get hit.**
The only way to guarantee success in a fight is not to engage in combat in the first place. Violence almost never happens in a vacuum. There is always some escalation process that precedes it; identify that escalation and it can be avoided. When forced to fight practitioners should be constantly moving, striking, and moving on. By the time an opponent reacts to your strike you, should already have moved to another place and launched another attack.

11. **Cross the T to escape.**
Crossing the T is a nautical analogy for martial strategy specifically related to holds and throws. It describes a broadside cannon attack against the unprotected bow or stern of a historical sailing ship. This concept transfers seamlessly because it is soundly rooted in efficiency and practicality, two hallmarks of sound strategy.

12 **Stances aren't just for *kata*.**
Proper body alignment is critical in a fight. Lose your balance and you cede valuable, often fatal, leverage to your opponent. Much *okuden waza* in karate *kata* uses stances and movement to unbalance and weaken an opponent. Combining simultaneous leg and hand techniques in one swift attack can be devastating.

13. **Don't forget to breathe.**
For athletes in all types of sports, correct breathing is a vital component of energy management. *Ibuki*, or quick energy breathing, is used during kicks, punches, and blocks. *Nogare*, or slow breathing, is done when moving from one position to the next. *Budoka* (martial artists) are taught to breathe in through their noses and exhale through their mouths using their diaphragms to move the maximum amount of air possible through the lungs.

14. **Use both hands.**
Both hands are used simultaneously in almost all techniques. *Hikite* is a push/pull concept that ensures proper body mechanics and maximum power in both offensive and defensive applications. Furthermore, when examining *kata* for *okuden waza* pay particular attention to the off hand, the one that is not executing an obvious technique.

15. **A lock or hold is not a primary fighting technique.**
A lock or a hold is never a primary fighting technique in the striking arts. Even practitioners of grappling arts cannot simply walk up and apply a lock or a hold on an unwilling opponent. Disruption is a critical component of successfully applying such techniques. In fact, the goal is actually to drop the opponent with the initial strike, applying the lock or hold only when further control is required.

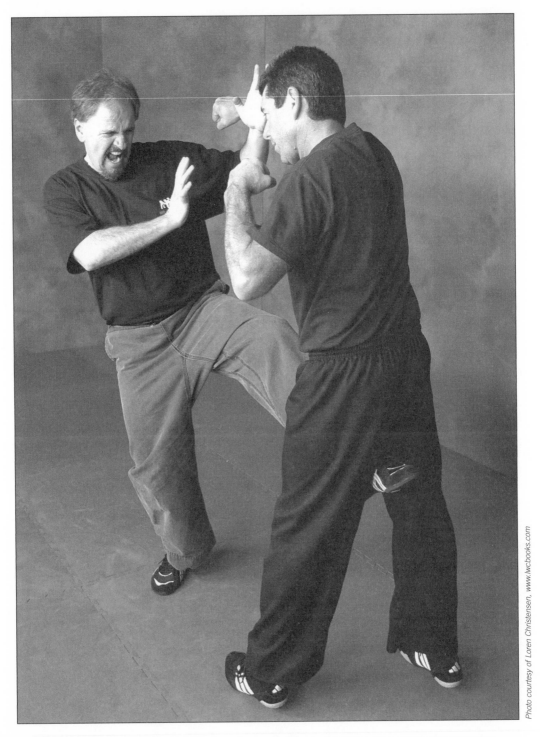

BLOCK/GROIN KICK. IN THIS APPLICATION THE OPPONENT'S LUNGE PUNCH IS BLOCKED WITH A SIMULTANEOUS COUNTERATTACK TO HIS GROIN. NOTE THAT THE KICK RISES FROM BELOW MAKING IT MUCH HARDER TO BLOCK THAN A STRAIGHT-IN TRAJECTORY.

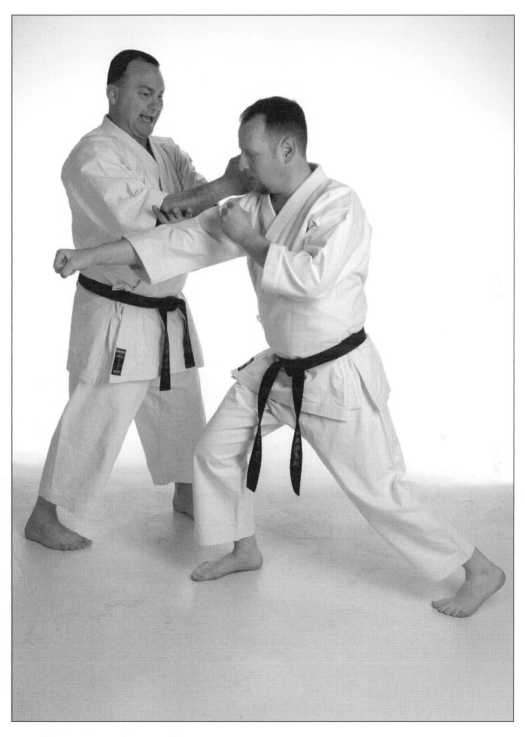

KURURUNFA OSAI UKE/SHITA TSUKI. THIS MOVEMENT FROM *KURURUNFA KATA* COMBINES A PRESS BLOCK WITH AN UPPERCUT.

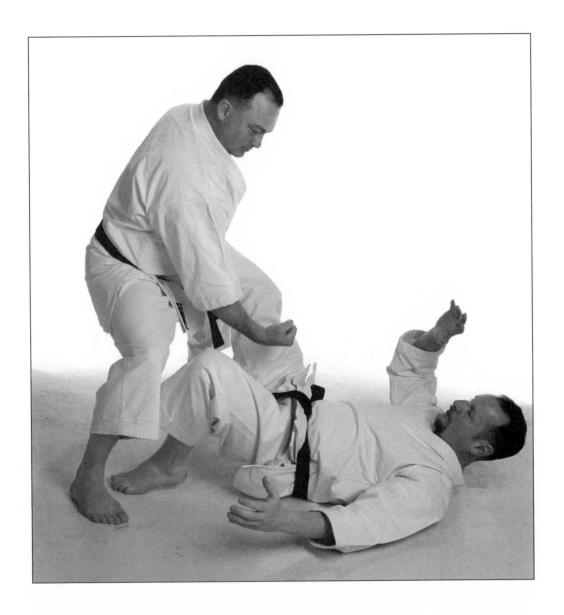

KIBISU GAESHI. THIS IS A REVERSE HEEL TAKEDOWN FOLLOWED IMMEDIATELY BY A BACKFIST TO THE GROIN.

CHAPTER 4

Rules

"Chojun Miyagi taught me this theory [kaisai no genri] just before his death and recommended that I not make it public. However as karate became popular around the world, I felt it would not benefit true karate if I were to hide it as a secret in my Shorei-kan school. I regret that the public has lost confidence in traditional Okinawan karate and may not understand the true value of karate kata."[45]

– Seikichi Toguchi

As we know by now, *bunkai* are fighting techniques found in *kata*. When executing the *kata*, however, such movements are typically stylized with the most formidable applications obscured. Although a formal set of applications, or *kata bunkai oyo*, have been developed for most *kata*, nearly limitless interpretations may apply.

While *kata* are always done exactly the same way, *kata bunkai* allow for more spontaneity and experimentation within a standard framework. In performing *bunkai oyo,* practitioners use techniques in prearranged manners with partners to understand better the emphasis and meaning of the various *kata* that they have learned. Almost all *kata* in *Goju Ryu*, as with many martial arts, have predefined *bunkai oyo* associated with them.

These standard sequences, however, are only the beginning. There are numerous correct interpretations for each movement of every *kata*, each demonstrating a functional real-life application. The work to uncover hidden techniques in *kata* is called *kaisai*. Since it offers guidelines for unlocking the secrets of each *kata*, *kaisai no genri* (the theory of *kaisai*) was once a great mystery revealed only to trusted disciples of the ancient masters in order to protect the secrets of their systems. As Toguchi *Sensei*'s quote from his book *Okinawan Goju Ryu II* indicates, this information has only recently become available to a wider audience.*

Using the rules of *kaisai no genri* practitioners can decipher the original intent of *kata* techniques by logically analyzing each specific technique to find their hidden meanings. After finding what one believes is the application of a *kata* technique, it must be examined to determine whether or not it would be effective in actual com-

---

* Interestingly, Taguchi *Sensei's* book was completed shortly before he passed away in 1998 and published posthumously in 2001, reinforcing the tradition of karate masters who only revealed their secrets shortly before their deaths. In this case, however, the *shuyo san gensoko* (three main or basic rules) of *kaisai no genri* were made widely available beyond his close circle of disciples.

bat. To do this, practitioners can practice the technique in a *kumite* situation with a partner; in essence reverse engineering the original *kata*. This is how many of the original *kiso kumite* were developed. This type of analysis goes a long way toward strengthening a practitioner's ability to understand and apply concepts found in the various *kata* that they practice to real life situations.

The *shuyo san gensoko* (three main or basic rules) of *kaisai no genri* are as follows:
1. Do not be deceived by the *enbusen* rule.
2. Advancing techniques imply attack, while retreating techniques imply defense.
3. There is only one enemy at a time.

The *hosoku joko* (supplementary or advanced rules) of *kaisai no genri* are as follows:
4. Every movement in *kata* has martial meaning/significance and can be used in a real fight.
5. A closed hand returning to chamber usually has something in it.
6. Utilize the shortest distance to your opponent.
7. If you control an opponent's head you control the opponent.
8. There is no "block."
9. Pay attention to the angles.
10. Touching your own body in *kata* indicates touching your opponent.
11. Contour the body—strike hard to soft and soft to hard.
12. There is no pause.

---

1) Do Not Be Deceived by the Enbusen Rule

"The rule of enbusen was created in order to make kata concise. This was the first rule the ancient masters created for the last stage of kata." [46]

– *Seikichi Toguchi*

Enbusen literally means "lines for performance" of fighting techniques. *Kata* are choreographed using artificial symmetry to ensure that the practitioner never takes more than three or four steps in any one direction, a process of conserving required practice space. These short movements obviously have nothing to do with real fighting situations. Techniques performed to the right do not necessarily imply an opponent on your right side. Similarly, attacks performed to the left do not necessarily mean that the practitioner is fighting against an enemy on his or her left side.

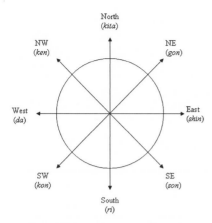

ENBUSEN (LINES OF PERFORMANCE) DIAGRAM.

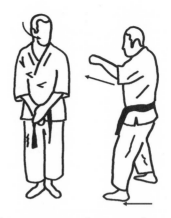

GEKISAI KATA: FROM YOI (WHICH MEANS "PREPARE")
STARTING POSITION, BEGIN THE KATA BY
LOOKING TO THE SIDE.

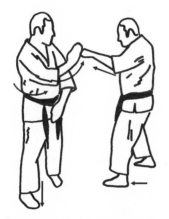

GEKISAI KATA: SHIFT OFF-LINE, MOVING YOUR
BODY AWAY FROM THE ATTACK.

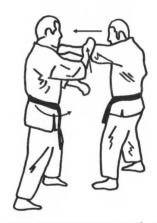

GEKISAI KATA: CHECK BLOCK THE OPPONENT'S STRIKE.

For example, at the beginning of *gekisai kata*, an elementary *Goju Ryu* form, practitioners turn left and head block. While one may occasionally be surprised by an attack, violence tends to escalate so we generally see it coming. Does it seem logical then, that the first movement of a basic *kata* would make an assumption such as responding to an ambush by turning toward the attacker? Perhaps, but more than likely not.

A closer examination of this movement indicates that the turn actually moves the practitioner off of the attacker's line of force. That is the real meaning of this turn. Get off line, shifting your body out of the way, then block (simultaneously of course). That way you are twice as likely not to get hit. If the shift fails, there is still a block. If the block fails, there is still a shift.

This redundancy is important for inexperienced new *karateka*. Viewed in that light, this turn obviously has nothing to do with what direction the attack is coming from and everything to do with moving to avoid the opponent's main force.* The *enbusen* for this, and every other movement in *kata*, must be analyzed before proper applications can be accurately interpreted. Do not be deceived by the *enbusen* rule.

2) Advancing Techniques Imply Attack, While Retreating Techniques Imply Defense.

"If kata's hyomengi [apparent movements of fighting techniques] are not for real fights, how then do we find clues of real fighting techniques in it? The second rule [of kaisai] gives us the answer." [47]

– Seikichi Toguchi

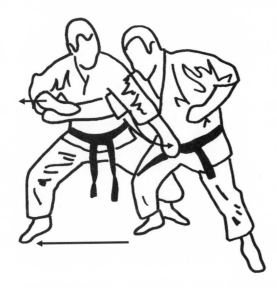

SEIYUNCHIN KATA: ARM GRAB, PULL/GROIN STRIKE. THIS IS AN OFFENSIVE INTERPRETATION OF WHAT INITIALLY APPEARS TO BE A DEFENSIVE BLOCKING TECHNIQUE. THE DEFENDER IS ON THE LEFT, ATTACKER ON THE RIGHT.

Kata technique executed while advancing should be considered an attack, even if it appears to be defensive. Similarly, those techniques executed while retreating should imply defensive or blocking techniques, even if they look like attacks.

The first half of the statement, "Advancing techniques imply attack," is fairly obvious, as pretty much everyone understands the definition of an attack. For example, as discussed in the introduction to this book, *seiyunchin kata* shows forward moving *gedan uke* (low blocks) performed in *shiko dachi* (*sumo* or straddle stance). It seems somewhat odd to be blocking while moving forward, especially in this low, immovable stance. According to the second rule of *kaisai*, these must be offensive rather than defensive techniques. Using this rule, *kata* applications become usable in real life situations.

Important nuance lies in the second half of the statement, *"retreating techniques imply defense."* This concept is not quite as simple as it sounds. In actual

---

* In fact, the block itself is actually an offensive technique, but we'll discuss that later on in Rule 8—*there is no block.*

combat, there is no retreat. A perceived retreat is really a technique executed to control distance.

You may move your body away from an opponent, but only to better your position or control the attacker's movement. The simple rule is to *always give pressure, give pressure always*. Through this commandment, your hands or feet will always be in contact with the enemy. Disengaging cedes momentum to your opponent, allowing him to control the fight. Since he who controls the momentum of the fight ultimately wins, that is just not something that *kata* would teach us to do.*

As we will discuss in more depth in Rule 8,† there really is no block in traditional martial arts. The word *uke* in Japanese translates most accurately to "receive" than it does to "block." Your defensive technique receives the attack and makes it your own. Once you own the attack, you can do with it what you will. A hard block (defensive technique) has the potential to drop an opponent just as easily as any offensive strike. Defensive techniques are supposed to be fight-stopping movements just as much as offensive techniques clearly are.

3) There is Only One Enemy at a Time.

"The origin of kata was a two-man tandem sparring form… It was the kumite of one vs. one. Therefore, when the ancient people rearranged it into a dance-like kata, they maintained its original concept of man-to-man combat." [48]

– *Seikichi Toguchi*

As practitioners face toward many directions moving along lines of *enbusen*, they might mistakenly believe that *kata* were created to emulate situations wherein one person fights against several opponents at the same time. The origin of *kata*, however, was in two-man tandem sparring. Consequently, the *bunkai* are also one-on-one. These dancelike direction shifts were created to keep the movement concise, not to imply multiple attackers.

Most forms take no more than three or four steps in any one direction prior to turning. Why did the movements need to be this concise? For a combination of reasons: First, a real fight simply does not take much room. While a confrontation might start at one end of a building and make its way to the other side of the building, the fact is that the physical fight can only take as much room as the range of a strike. By nature a fight is small. It swirls around the two (or more) combatants.

Second, to teach in private the practitioners had to be secluded. Physical space in Okinawa and Japan was (and still is) quite limited. Larger private spaces, as we have come to know them in the West, are a rather new occurrence. As a matter of

* For more information see Principle 10—*if you are not there you cannot get hit.*
† Rule 8—*there is no block.*

fact the Kodokan, the birthplace of modern judo, began with just six *tatami* mats (each mat is approximately 3' x 6') in a roughly 650-square-foot room.

Further, there is significant benefit in learning to move and turn while maintaining proper stance integrity and balance. To go a step further, even when engaged with a single opponent, *kata* turns may be demonstrating leg entanglement techniques such as sweeps and

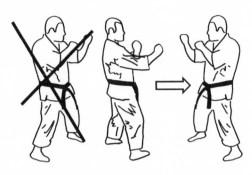

THERE IS ONLY ONE OPPONENT AT A TIME.

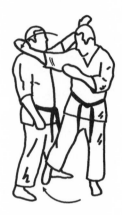

TURN IN STANCE. DEFENDER IS ON THE RIGHT.

throws.

In reality, from a street-fighting point of view, it is pretty much impossible to make a *kata* that is designed to fight against multiple attackers at once. One person cannot simultaneously execute many different techniques against multiple opponents except in well-choreographed movie stunts. The vast majority of *kata* techniques are designed to deal

with a single attacker who is directly in front of the practitioner. Although there are a few movements in certain *kata* where the imaginary enemy strikes from behind, there is always only one opponent at a time.

Dealing with multiple attackers is very challenging. Avoidance is obviously the best and most preferable alternative. If one is forced to fight, he or she can realistically only engage one opponent at a time. Once the first adversary has been defeated, a *budoka* can move on to defeat

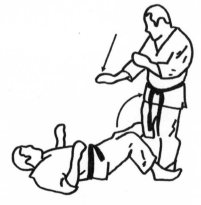

SWEEP THROW.

the next attacker. Defense against a large group is generally handled by strategically engaging one person at a time in a manner that confounds the other's ability to reach you.

Your response is a form of triage, striking for the greatest impact or taking on the most dangerous threat first. When Kane took an advanced defensive handgun course a few years back, the instructor emphasized taking cover, assessing the threat, and killing the most dangerous person (e.g., the guy with the shotgun*) first. If all are equally dangerous, take out the easiest target first (e.g., nearest aggressor, smallest person, the guy with no cover). The same concept holds true in a fistfight.

Several psychological factors can help you survive. In any large group of attackers, someone will be the primary instigator or leader of the pack. If you can instantaneously and dramatically disable that individual (or anyone else for that matter), blowing out a knee, shattering a nose, gouging out an eye, or otherwise leaving the leader huddled in a pool of his own blood, the psychological advantage will be enormous. We are not exaggerating here—the only way to survive assault from a large, determined group of thugs is to be more ruthless and violent than they are; a very good reason for avoiding such conflicts in the first place. Further, if you show no fear in the face of overwhelming odds your attackers may hesitate giving you the few seconds you need to disengage and escape.

In 1993 Kane had a young woman named Colleen working for him at the football stadium where he is a security supervisor. He recalls, "She was about 5'6" and perhaps 125 pounds—not intimidating by any stretch of the imagination. One day, as I was returning from escorting a couple of unruly football fans out of the stadium, I noticed a disturbance in east-end bleachers. From several hundred feet away, I saw Colleen racing up the stairs into the crowd. Against procedure and without regard for her personal safety, she had gone alone."

Fearing the worst, Kane says that he grabbed a couple of burly ushers and raced up after her. "By the time the three of us arrived, she was already heading back down the steps, grinning like the proverbial cat that had swallowed the canary. The unruly fans were no longer on the verge of fighting. In fact they just sat quietly in their seats, watching her walk away."

Kane asked, "How the heck did you manage to do that?" Colleen replied, "I told them to shut the @#*|@ up, sit their butts back down, and watch the damn game before I throw them out. When they started to argue, I told them that I'm a hockey player and I still have all my teeth. When I grinned at them they got the message and sat back down." While she was not actually a hockey player, but an assistant ice hockey coach, what she told them was more or less true.

Colleen also had four older brothers and was used to dealing with rough and tumble college and semi-pro players. Because the unruly fans did not frighten her in

---

* All things being equal (e.g., everyone has a gun, is equally skilled, and is approximately equal distance away), a shotgun-wielding assailant is the most dangerous (e.g., most likely both to hit you as well as most likely to kill you with his shot).

the slightest, she made *them* nervous. Faced with an authority figure who was not afraid of superior numbers, they complied with her request. This is an example of what the Japanese call *fudoshin* (or indomitable spirit). Miyamoto Musashi, arguably the greatest swordsman who ever lived, demonstrated the ultimate evolution of such spirit. In his writings he related that many opponents fell before his sword simply because they believed that they would, not necessarily because he was the better warrior.

By the time he finished his freshman year of college, Kane had climbed Mount Rainier, canoed the Bowron Lakes, hiked the Chilkoot Pass Trail, competed in numerous judo tournaments, rappelled out of a helicopter, and survived "hell week" to be initiated into a fraternity. Overcoming these mental and physical challenges had convinced him that he could accomplish nearly anything he truly applied himself to. All martial practitioners endure rigorous training, overcoming similar challenges. Take strength from your accomplishments, show no fear, and use your demeanor as an advantage when things get ugly. You may only be fighting one person at a time, but the way in which you dispatch them will psychologically affect other potential attackers in the crowd.

When engaged with the enemy, you must move constantly, controlling the momentum of the fight so that your attackers cannot dictate your movements.* Use balanced stances, deft footwork, and available cover (e.g., picnic tables, trees, or vehicles outside; tables, chairs, furniture inside) to minimize the number of people who can reach you at once.†

Defeat one adversary at a time. Employ applications from your *kata* to strike vital areas, spending the absolute minimum amount possible time dealing with each attacker. Do not ever let your enemies surround you, entangle you, or drive you to the ground. Loss of mobility quite often equates to loss of life in multi-opponent encounters.

---

4) Every Movement in Every Kata Has Martial Significance

> *"Once a form has been learned, it must be practiced repeatedly until it can be applied in an emergency, for knowledge of just the sequence of a form in karate is useless."* [49]
>
> – *Gichin Funakoshi*

Every movement of every *kata* has at least one application that can successfully be used in a real fight.‡ The ancient masters did not waste effort on pretty; they were concerned with functional. There were no *kata* tournaments or sparring competi-

---

* See Principle 10—*if you are not there you cannot get hit.*

† Perhaps the most famous example of this strategy was the battle of Thermopylae (480 b.c.) where King Leonidas and 300 Spartan hoplites held back the entire Persian army of roughly 250,000 men, defending a narrow pass for several days. The Persians eventually crushed this small force, defeated the Greek army, and sacked Athens, yet the valor of those heroic soldiers is recounted to this day. An epitaph at the battle site reads, "Friend, tell the Spartans that on this hill we lie obedient to them still."

‡ Also see Principle 2—*every technique should be able to end the fight immediately.*

tions where they could win fancy trophies to line their *dojo* windows. There were only life and death struggles to survive. Not only were they concerned about random violence from robbers, extortionists, murderers and other thugs, but also about *kakidameshi*, the tradition where *budoka* routinely tested each other's fighting skills in actual combat.

Remember, too, that they did not have the benefit of modern medicine. Even minor injuries could become life threatening. A broken jaw might cause a person to starve to death. A broken arm or foot might preclude his ability to earn a living. And since there was no welfare in feudal times and most folks lived in agrarian society, not having work could be life threatening as well.

Even a minor infection could be fatal. Antibiotics had not been invented yet. Consequently *kata* were developed to crush the life out of an attacker as efficiently and ruthlessly as possible.

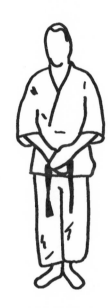

Even *yoi* (which means "prepare"), the very first preparatory movement in *kata*, has martial meaning. Gogen Yamaguchi* wrote, "When the leader calls *yoi*, you have to cross both hands in front of your body while you breathe in; and then, while you are breathing out, bring both fists to your sides as if you are tightening your belt, then tighten both armpits like you are pushing at the floor with your fists and put power in your whole body. The reason you cross both hands in front of your body is to cover the groin area from a sudden attack; at the same time, you show the opponent that you will not attack suddenly. As in the etiquette of the *samurai* in which they take off a *katana* (sword) from the waist and change it to the right hand showing that no cowardly act, such as

YOI (PREPARE), THE STARTING POSITION FOR MOST *KATA*.

slashing the opponent without notice, will occur. From that meaning, the inside of the hand that is crossed has to be your dominant arm."[†]

When examining *kata* for applications, practitioners cannot discount *any* movement. In the old days when most *kata* were developed, each contained a fully integrated fighting system. Nothing was superfluous. Every technique had to have real-world offensive or defensive applications, usually more than one. For example, another interpretation of the *yoi* movement at the beginning of a *kata* could be a neck crank takedown, while the similar movement at the end of a *kata* might represent a double clavicle strike (e.g., as defense against a tackle). As with any other *kata*

---

* Known as "The Cat" for his speed and athleticism, Yamaguchi *Sensei* (1909—1989) was an influential *Goju Ryu* karate master. Among his many accomplishments, he is credited with developing modern freestyle sparring in 1936. *Jiyu kumite* did not exist in karate before that time.

† Traditionally this is shown as left over right regardless of whether or not you are right-handed, since almost all *budo* applications are taught as though the practitioner was right hand dominant.

movement, applications for *yoi* are only bound by a practitioner's creativity and imagination.*

Creativity is required in other areas too. For example there are many *kata* in which techniques appear to be shown more than once, perhaps to the left side followed by the right or vice versa (e.g., *yoi* at the beginning and ending of each *kata*). Most times such applications are not truly mirror images; they are actually asymmetrical. In other words, they are not simply showing the same thing from two directions but are actually describing two similar-looking yet functionally different techniques.

For example, in *gekisai kata dai ni,*† there are two *mawashe uke* (wheel or circular blocks) shown in *neko ashi dachi* (cat stance), one at 45 degrees to the right of your starting position and one at 45 degrees to the left. While they look nearly the same, one demonstrates a closing technique while the other shows an opening technique. Even in this basic *kata* there is much more going on than the untrained eye can perceive.

The only exception to this rule is found in the *kihon* (basic) forms. On occasion a diagonal step called *yanjigo*‡ is required to re-center practitioners back to the *kiten* point from which their performance originated. This is technically not part of the *kata* hence it has no application. Similarly if *kata* performance ends facing any direction other than *shomen* (front) there will be a realigning shift or turn at the finish. Again, this movement is purely to ensure that practitioners finish their *kata* in an aesthetically pleasing manner, ending in a location from which they may repeat the sequence or start another *kata* without any additional superfluous movements.

5) A Hand Returning to Chamber Usually Has Something in It

"A block is often used to parry and set up a grab (immobilization or pulling-in) before a strike. The hand returning to chamber after a block simply slides down the arm to grab it and yank backwards, or locks an arm in place." [50]

— *Victor Smith*

In Principle 14,§ we learned that both hands are utilized in almost all *kata* applications. Frequently the hand returning to chamber at the practitioner's side has something captured in it, especially if it is shown closed when performing the *kata*. Applications that include trapping an opponent's hand or foot consist of grabs, locks, joint dislocations, takedowns, and throws.

When analyzing *kata*, it is important to pay attention to the off-hand, the one not executing an obvious technique. As it returns to chamber it will frequently grab,

* Within the bounds of practical reality and logical reasoning, of course.
† An introductory *Goju Ryu* form.
‡ Translating to the number forty five or "45 degrees" since this diagonal step moves the practitioner roughly 45 degrees from where they were.
§ Principle 14—*use both hands.*

pull, or trap an opponent's limb. Though often underrated and underutilized in the striking arts, grabs are an essential component of karate. They facilitate posting an opponent's weight over his or her leg so that a practitioner can effectively apply a joint kick, levering an arm for a lock or takedown, and whipping an arm to snap the head up and back, exposing the throat. Important techniques such as these are often lost in modern sparring due to use of protective equipment, which precludes full use of the fingers. Practitioners must uncover such applications through tandem drills or other practice methods.

On occasion a *kata* will show combinations that appear to be two defensive techniques at the same time, an unlikely occurrence in real-life, self-defense applications. If a practitioner trains to make multiple defensive movements without an offensive counterattack they would, by plan, assume a struggle against a vastly superior enemy—a rather doubtful assumption.

Take, for example, a simultaneous up and down block, a common enough movement in *kata*. Since Principle 2* states that every application must be able to immediately end a confrontation, there must be more going on than meets the eye. Further, Rule 8† states that there really is no such thing as a "block" in practical application anyway.

Seiyunchin kata shows a simultaneous *chudan uke* (chest block) and *gedan barai uke* (down block) performed with a 45-degree turn—a

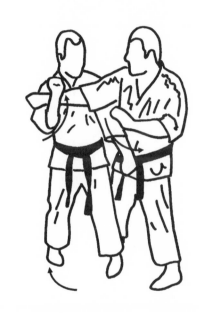

SEIYUNCHIN KATA APPLICATION: ARM BREAK/GROIN STRIKE.

good illustration of this odd dual-defensive movement. One practical interpretation would be blocking an aggressor's punch with a right-hand *uchi uke* (inside forearm block) , and then slip hooking with the left arm to trap the opponent's wrist or forearm while simultaneously striking his groin with the right arm (the one that performed the initial defensive movement). Using the turn, you hope to break or hyperextend your opponent's trapped arm using your chest or shoulder. In this case the limb is trapped rather than grabbed, an important consideration when analyzing other *kata* techniques. While it looks the same as a simultaneous upward and downward block in performance of the *kata*, this application is clearly a much more impressive technique.

* Principle 2—*every technique should be able to end the fight immediately.*
† Rule 8—*there is no block.*

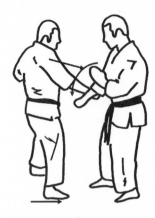

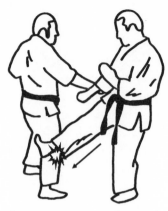

Seisan kata: arm grab. Defender is on the right.   *Seisan kata: kensetsu geri* (joint kick).

There are numerous other examples in *kata* where the hand returning to chamber captures an opponent's limb. An obvious application appears in *seisan kata,* where the practitioner's arm drops to his or her side just prior to a *kensetsu geri* (joint kick). Clearly this is a more traditional grab performed as the practitioner's hand returns to chamber. Its purpose is to post the opponent's weight on one leg prevent so that he cannot escape from the follow-on kick to his knee.

6) Utilize the Shortest Distance to Your Opponent

"In attacking techniques such as oi tsuki (lunge punch) or choko tsuki (straight punch), the movements must be straight and quick, so as to take the most direct path to the opponent." [51]

– *Morio Higaonna*

In geometry, the shortest distance between two points is a straight line. In business, the shortest distance between two points is integrity. In friendship, the shortest distance between two points is trust. In martial arts, the shortest distance between two points is where you strike.

To have the greatest opportunity for success, practitioners must strike or defend with their closest body part. Defensive techniques must cut off the attacker's blow before it gains too much speed and power, catching it as close to the opponent's body as possible. Offensive techniques must afford the adversary as little reaction time as possible. The shorter the distance, the faster you get there.

Karate punches, for example, shoot straight out from chamber (usually at the practitioner's side). With rare exceptions, such as *furi uchi* (swing strike), there is

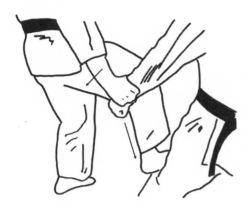

SEISAN KATA: CLOSE-UP OF ARM GRAB AND *KENSETSU GERI* (JOINT KICK).

no curve involved in a punch. Traveling at equal speed, the John Wayne-style haymaker commonly seen in barroom brawls takes a lot longer to land than a traditional karate punch because its curved path covers more distance to reach the opponent. Remember, however, that linear punches are more effective when they come in at an *off angle* as opposed to directly into the opponent's *enbusen.*

This concept is corollary to the *Goju Ryu* principle of not using two steps. The essential point is that extra movements take extra time. In a real fight, speed kills.* You must both be fast and efficient. Utilize your closest weapon (nearest limb to the attacker) and keep striking until he or she is no longer a threat. A simple tandem drill helps demonstrate how:

Work with a partner. One person will be the attacker (*tori*) and one the defender (*uke*), trading roles after each set. Initially work at half speed using a scale of 4:1 (four responses to one attack). Utilize your closest weapon (limb) for each attack and defense. Your partner must only defend against your last technique; then it becomes his or her turn to employ three unimpeded techniques followed by a fourth one which you get to block.

Here's how it works: After the initial attack (e.g., punch, kick, whatever you agree upon), *uke* gets four moves before *tori* gets to move again. The emphasis is on technique, so you do not have to go fast. Be sure to strike lightly so no one gets hurt while they are unable to defend themselves. Each technique (e.g., punch, kick) a person employs counts as one move. Movement such as a shift or step performed simultaneously with a technique is not counted as a separate "move." If your defense involves a technique (e.g., block) that counts as one of your four moves. An example of how this might go follows:

You attack with a chest punch. I block (1), shift and punch (2), elbow strike (3), and backfist (4). You absorb the first three attacks, and then block the backfist (1), perform a knee strike (2), thrust kick (3), then shift and lunge punch (4). I block the lunge punch and the cycle repeats. Any combination of techniques may be used. Each partner honors the other's techniques, responding as if they were actually struck forcefully. The goals of this drill include establishing flow, targeting your opponent with your closest weapon, and practicing the principle of continuous attack.

* See "Speed Kills!" in chapter 5 for more information.

After you perform this drill a few times and get it running smoothly, change the scale to two to one, then finally to 1:1. As long as each practitioner gets at least two movements per turn, it's pretty easy to trade techniques back and forth, blocking then counterstriking. As soon as the scale gets to one to one, you should notice a *big* difference. Conjunctions have been removed. You can no longer block and then strike because your turn ends with the block.

In this manner, once you get behind, it is almost impossible to do anything other than defend yourself—just like a real fight. Remember, he who controls the momentum ultimately wins the fight almost every time. The objective of this drill, of course, is ultimately to find ways to simultaneously defend and attack. It might go something like this:

You attack with a head punch (1). I drop to *shiko dachi* ducking below your strike and punch your ribs (1). You pivot, elbow striking my side, which simultaneously deflects my punch and counterattacks (1). I pivot out of the way and spin kick (1). You shift inside my range and straight punch (1), I straight punch back to your solar plexus inside your strike (1). Because I'm on the inside, my blow lands while yours glances off my shoulder. Since I connected with a vital area (the solar plexus), the round ends. We begin the drill again.

Any combination of techniques can be employed. Go slow enough that you are able to use proper stances, adhere to your style's strategy, and employ its tactics in a safe and controlled manner. In this fashion we learn the value of stance, position and angle in approaching an opponent. We learn that there is no time in a real fight for two steps when one will do. Ultimately, the only way you can win is by firing again and again with your closest weapon until you break through your opponent's defenses and disable him.

7) Control an Opponent's Head and You Control the Opponent

"Those skilled at making the enemy move do so by creating a situation to which he must conform." [52]

– Sun Tzu

If you can incapacitate an attacker's vision, breathing, or movement, you are in an excellent position to defeat your enemy. Any two out of three will pretty much guarantee success. Control a person's head, and you have direct access to his vision, breathing, and movement simultaneously. Consequently, if you can control an opponent's head you control the opponent.

Many techniques in *kata* take advantage of this fact. In fact, the head is often the primary target in a real fight. For both psychological and physiological reasons, most first strikes are directed there. When deciphering *kata*, practitioners will find a wide variety of techniques that target the eyes, ears, neck, and head.

Take, for example, the eyes. Nothing is scarier to most human beings than becoming blind. Our eyes are extremely sensitive even to speck of dust, a bit of smoke, or an errant eyelash. If you have ever stood down wind from a campfire or sliced a pungent onion you'll have a pretty good idea of how this feels.

The natural human blink reaction is nearly impossible to overcome. Try keeping your eyes open when you sneeze to get a feeling for what we mean. Further, most individuals instinctively flinch away from a strike to the face, a reaction that can open opponents to an unavoidable follow-up blow or even a neck twist takedown.

Using a check/control methodology* you parry or deflect an opponent's blow with your outstretched arm, then control him with what most people perceive as the block. A natural extension of such movements is an eye gouge or rake, particularly when the block is performed open handed such as *chudan hiki uke* (pulling/grasping open-hand chest block). The tips of your fingers need only travel upward a few extra inches[†] to contact your opponent's eyes.

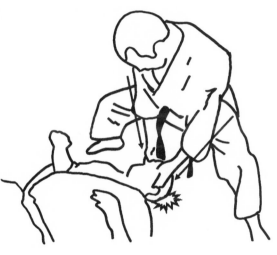

EYE GOUGE. THIS TECHNIQUE IS FACILITATED BY CONTROLLING THE DEFENDER'S HEAD—BOTH WITH THE GROUND AND BY CONTOURING WITH THE ATTACKER'S FINGERS. THIS IS CLEARLY NOT A TRIVIAL ATTACK AND SHOULD ONLY BE PERFORMED IN A TRUE LIFE OR DEATH ENCOUNTER!

If your attacker is standing, rakes[‡] will be much more successful than gouges since an unsupported head can be moved out of the way to avoid or lessen the blow. *Kata* accommodate this fact. Whether you brush the opponent's eyes with your fingertips or even scratch his eyebrows drawing blood, you can readily obscure his vision.

When an opponent is lying on the ground or you have control of the back of his head or neck, a gouge can be executed. This is generally done by contouring the side of the head with your fingers while your thumb is forcefully inserted into the inside edge of his eye socket displacing and popping out the eyeball. Excruciating pain

---

* See Rule 8—*there is no block.*

† See Rule 6—*utilize the shortest distance.*

‡ A rake sweeps across the eye to cause damage, while a gouge pushes into the socket displace the eyeball.

caused by this application will almost always render the victim unconscious.

Ear slaps are another easy extension of a traditional block. Cup your hand slightly and slap it against a heavy bag as fast and forcefully as you can (emphasis is on *fast*). The resulting blow sounds much like a gunshot. Now clap both hands together next to your ear. It does not have to be very loud to be uncomfortable. Imagine how much more painful the noise from a powerful slap would be. Further, displaced air from this technique can frequently rupture an opponent's eardrum. Pain and disorientation from this application is staggering.

Neck twist takedowns are another popular way to control the head. Although most practitioners develop very strong neck muscles through their training, when the head is tilted forward or backward the muscles that stabilize side to side become less effective (and vice versa). Opponents can often resist front to back or side to side, but not both at once. When the head turns beyond a certain point the body must follow. This is a popular application to defend against a tackle and shows up in many *kata*. If the twist is preceded by a disruptive eye or ear strike* it is even more likely to succeed. If the neck can be quickly stretched with a sharp pull before the twist, it becomes more effective still. Again, this is a potentially deadly technique that must be used prudently.

Grabs to the head are frequently misunderstood. Many practitioners believe that the target, especially in the *koryu* forms, was the *samurai*'s famous topknot. The simple fact that the vast majority of these *kata* originated in China, traveling through Okinawa before arriving in Japan, casts doubt on this theory. Further, many forms were not codified until after the Meiji Restoration. By 1876 the government had banned the wearing of the *katana* and *wakizashi* and the former *samurai* were forced to cut off their top knots in favor of Western-style haircuts, wear Western clothes, and take up jobs in business and other professions. Consequently, there were no longer any top knots to grab.

Beyond that, *kata* were designed to be fault tolerant. It is inconceivable that they would intentionally target an elusive strip of hair when a likely attacker could be bald, wearing headgear, or simply not be a member of the *samurai* class in the first place. The proper method of securing an opponent's head is most commonly a hook rather than a grab anyway.

To properly perform this technique, the fingers scoop up against the back of the head, neck, or center of the upper back rather than wrapping around it. This scooping maneuver is faster and easier to secure than a traditional grab that requires more dexterity and coordination to achieve.† There is certainly nothing wrong with grabbing the hair if it is available, it is simply not always the target of choice, nor must it be available to make such techniques work (fault-tolerant application).

A good example of this is found in *saifa kata,* which shows a sweep, stomp, *tetsui*

---

* See Principle 3—*strike to disrupt, disrupt to strike.*

† See Principle 5—*work with the adrenaline rush.*

uchi (hammerfist) followed immediately by a pull to the back of the head and simultaneous *shita tsuki* (palm-up center punch strike) to the throat. The sweep extends the attacker's leg so that your stomp might target the adversary's knee, ankle, or foot. Once an opponent's attention is drawn to his lower body, your *tetsui uchi* smacks him in the middle of the forehead.

While the opponent is still disrupted from this attack, your hand then snakes around to secure the back of his head,

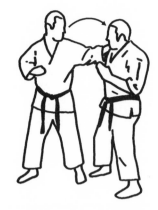

SAIFA KATA: SECURE BACK OF HEAD/STRIKE GALL BLADDER 20 SIMULTANEOUSLY.

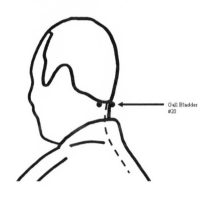

SAIFA: GALL BLADDER 20 CLOSE-UP.

then pulls forward and down to drive it into your *shita tsuki* punch. While this same grabbing technique could be performed using an opponent's hair or ear, the back of the head offers the most secure target. If your hook/grab impacts like a strike, it may achieve the additional benefit of lighting-up the adversary's gall bladder 20 nerve, a sensitive pressure point at the base of the skull on both sides.

Beyond the eyes, ears, and neck, the head is a target rich environment full of vital points that are relatively easy to break. These include *tendo* (the crown of the head), *tento* (fontanelle), *komekami* (temple), *miken* (summit of the nose), *seidon* (circumorbital region), *jinchu* (inter-maxillary suture), *gekon* (center of the jaw), *mikazuki* (mandible), *dokko* (mastoid process), and *hichu* (larynx). *Kata* frequently take advantage of these anatomically weak areas to disable an opponent.*

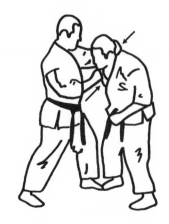

SAIFA KATA: FOLLOW-UP *SHITA TSUKI* (UPPERCUT) PUNCH.

* See "Vital Points," in chapter 5, for more information.

8) There is No Block

"Action is always faster than reaction. You should always aim to take control of a situation and never fight in a defensive fashion. Blocks simply do not work in real situations. However, in sport-based sparring, blocks work fairly well. This is because the combatants use complementary techniques at an exaggerated distance. Real fighting is much closer and more chaotic. In a real situation, blocks are rarely of any use and hence the kata rarely contain them. However they do contain many techniques that are misleadingly labeled as blocks." [53]

— Iain Abernethy

True blocks do not exist in most traditional martial arts. As we have discussed previously, the word *uke* means "receive." Your defensive technique receives the attack and makes it your own. Once you own the attack, you can do with it what you will. A fast, hard block has the potential to drop an opponent in his or her tracks, ending the fight before you even need to throw a blow.

When receiving attacks from an opponent, most martial systems use a check/control methodology. The hand that is closest to the adversary (e.g., just punched) performs the actual check, jam, or deflection, while the hand that is in chamber executes a technique designed to control your opponent's limb. To be most effective the check must be an aggressive powerful technique, much more like a strike than a block. It must cut off the attacker's technique before it gains too much speed and power, catching it as close to the opponent's body as possible.

In his book, *The Truth About Self Protection*, retired police officer and self-defense expert Massad Ayoob wrote, "In police work, I found that karate-trained street cops didn't get into nearly as many brawls as their chiefs feared they would. On the contrary, they were less likely to get into fights. If the Bad Guy couldn't tell he was overmatched just by the way the cop was standing, he'd know it quick enough when he threw his best shot and the cop simply deflected it harmlessly with a forearm." As this example illustrates, a good defensive movement hurts the attacker, weakening his morale and willingness to continue the fight.

Controlling pressure applied to the outside of an opponent's arm should be above the elbow to jam/disrupt while protecting against a follow-up elbow strike. Pressure to the inside of an opponent's arm should be below the elbow so that they cannot strike around your block.

The shield (or *scutum* in Latin) of the Roman foot solider was not a defensive part of their armament as one might assume from its name. It was used to attack the enemy in the same way a professional football* player uses his shoulder pads to push

---

* We are referring to American or Canadian league football, as opposed to European soccer which is played differently. Shoulder pads are not worn in that type of football.

an opposing player. The shield could be used to catch the attacker's weapon by allowing the tip of the blade or spear to be driven hard into it. This kept the business end of the weapon in a known place and rendered it useless until removed. As the opponent struggled to recover his weapon, he would be stabbed to death by the Roman infantryman.

Further, the *scutum* had a metal dome (center boss) projecting out of the center of the shield that protected the hand that held it. This metal boss could be used to punch-block, offensively intercepting a weapon with a violent strike. That same movement could also be used to smash an unarmored face or otherwise pound an enemy into submission.

Just as the Roman soldier used his shield as an offensive weapon, it is vital to look at a *budo* block in the same fashion. Even the most basic form of blocking is truly offensive in nature. Practitioners do not wait for an attack. They reach out and intercept it. In much the same way as the Roman soldier used his shield offensively; karate blocks are used to gain advantage over an opponent.

Try this drill with a partner to get a perspective on how this works: Take a large kicking shield and use it in the same manner a Roman soldier would. Have your partner

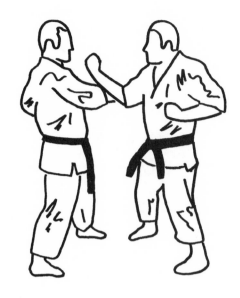

CONTROLLING PRESSURE TOO LOW ON THE ARM LEAVES YOU OPEN TO A COUNTER ATTACK. THE DEFENDER IS ON THE RIGHT.

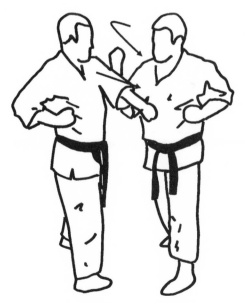

PROPER CONTROLLING PRESSURE REDIRECTS OPPONENT'S FORCE. THE DEFENDER IS ON THE RIGHT.

throw some punches and kicks and test your movement. Be sure that you are not moving away. Move into the attacks, jamming them. Once you get comfortable with the offensive movement, drop the shield and use your arms defensively. Block in the same manner you did with the shield, behaving as the Roman soldier would. You should discover that blocking is never passive. It is aggressive and violent.

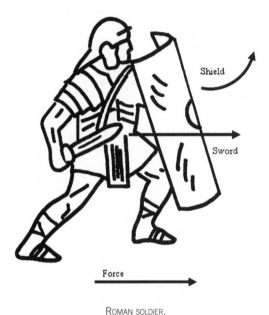

ROMAN SOLDIER.

In his famous *Book of Five Rings*, Miyamoto Musashi wrote, "Try to understand this. If you wait for the attack, defend against it, and only then go in the attack by parrying and striking, you are making extra work for yourself. Moreover, there is always the possibility of missing the 'block.' If you approach the enemy with the attitude of defeating him without delay and with utter resolve then you will certainly be a better position to finish him off."

Unlike what you have probably been led to believe, there are no blocks, at least not in the commonly understood sense. As Musashi so eloquently points out, if you wish to survive in actual combat you cannot wait for the attack to come to you. To reinforce this point, note a comment from Motoo Yamakura: "Focused, hard-hitting blocks can be attacking techniques."* The best defense really is a good offense (though we never provoke or start the fight in the first place, of course).

In Japanese, the term, *go no sen,* means to block and riposte (to receive the attack then strike back). *Sen no sen* means to intercept the attack once it is one its way. *Sen-sen no sen* means to cut off an attack before it even starts. *Sen-sen no sen* uses the tell† to sense that an attack will be forthcoming and then cut it short before the opponent has the chance to transform the mental desire to attack to the physical movement necessary to execute that desire. To the untrained observer, this looks a whole lot like a pre-emptive strike. Do not confuse the famous karate rule of "no first attack" with *sen-sen no sen*, however. Regardless of how it looks, *sen-sen no sen* is still a defensive movement.

Christopher Caile recounted on his web site, fightingarts.com, that "at first students learn to first block and then counter (two counts). Later a technique might

* From his book *Goju-Ryu Karate-Do Volume 1: Fundamentals for Traditional Practitioners.*
† Which we discussed in Principle 10—*if you are not there, you cannot get hit.*

first block and then continue on to become a counter (one and a half counts). Finally, more mastery can result in a single technique being a simultaneous block and counter (one count)." The ultimate goal, of course, is to execute techniques that both defend and attack at the same time.* Such applications do not have to be particularly complicated.

Try this quick exercise with a partner: Have *tori* hold out a head punch about an inch away from the your face. The first half of the drill shows the importance of distance in not getting hit. Since you wish to avoid a knuckle sandwich, you must push *tori*'s punch to one side or the other so that it will clear your face. If you push against *tori*'s fist, you must move it at least five or six inches to ensure a clean miss. If, on the other hand, you reach out farther and push against *tori*'s elbow, you need only move it one or two inches to ensure a clean miss.

The closer to your partner that you reach to intercept his blow, the easier it is to deflect—because his punch will be moving with less speed and power and also because he will have less mechanical leverage on his side. To run the drill, *tori* will punch at about half speed while you intercept his blows several times, progressively reaching closer to your opponent to see how this works. Switch roles and try it on the other side.

The second half of the drill takes advantage of this knowledge while removing the block entirely. This time as *tori* punches, so too should you. There are two tricks to making a simultaneous block/strike. The first, and most important, is to be inside of your opponent's blow. If your arm is outside of *tori*'s, you will get hit. If it is on the inside, you will be much safer. At worst the blow should glance off of your shoulder.

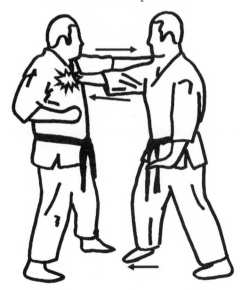

The second trick takes advantage of mechanical leverage shown in the first half of this drill. As soon you see *tori*'s arm begins to move, you must immediately throw your own blow.[†] The quicker you are, the closer your fist will be to *tori*'s body when your arms intercept and, therefore, the safer you will be. Once again, try this several times until it begins to become natural. Switch roles and try being the attacker.

A PUNCH TO THE INSIDE SIMULTANEOUSLY BLOCKS YOUR OPPONENT'S ATTACK. THE DEFENDER IS ON THE RIGHT.

---

* As we demonstrated in the 4:1, 2:1, 1:1 drill that was described in our explanation of Rule 6—*utilize the shortest distance to your opponent*.

† If cut off early enough, the counter becomes *sen-sen no sen*.

In actual martial combat, there really is no block. There is only attack. As you begin to analyze *kata* techniques through this lens, defensive movements can take on a whole new meaning.

---

9) Kata Demonstrate the Proper Angles

"The reason movements are performed at angles is to instruct the kata's practitioner that the technique in question requires the karateka to move at that angle in relation to their opponent." [54]

– Iain Abernethy

As stated earlier in Rule 1,* *kata* are choreographed using artificial symmetry to ensure that the practitioner never takes more than three or four steps in any one direction. While techniques performed to the right do not necessarily imply an opponent on your right side and vice versa, the angle demonstrated is very important. Advanced *budo* techniques generally avoid direct force to force. Practitioners move at an angle to their opponent's main strength, or *enbusen*, for attack or defense.

Turns in *kata* frequently suggest a particular angle of attack. Similarly, the distance from the practitioner's body at which the technique is displayed demonstrates the proper distance the practitioner should be from an opponent in order to perform the application effectively.

Shifting your body outside of an attacker's *enbusen* is safer than moving to the inside as you close distance to confront an aggressor. If you are outside, an opponent can only reach you with half his or her weapons—primarily one arm and one leg. The other limbs must cross the body to strike. While safer, this position limits your targeting opportunities. Conversely, being on the inside affords you free access to all vital areas; however, the opponent can directly attack yours as well.

The angle demonstrated in *kata* gives essential clues to your preferred approach for each technique in practical application. Unpredictable movements by an opponent may alter the tactic, of course, but practitioners will know what they should be trying to aim for. Further, the closer a technique is performed to the practitioner's body, the closer he or she will want to be to the opponent in actual combat (physical distance between opponents' bodies, not limbs). If the angle and distance are not carefully coordinated, practitioners will find that many techniques become untenable.

A good example of this is the *heiko hiji ate* (horizontal elbow strike), *osai uke* (press block), *uraken uchi* (backfist strike) sequence at the very beginning of *saifa kata*. To perform the *kata*, practitioners take a long step in *zenkutsu dachi*, shifting

---

* Rule 1—*do not be deceived by the enbusen rule.*

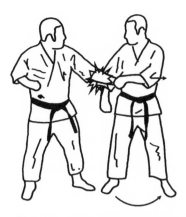

SAIFA KATA: ELBOW STRIKE, INCORRECT RANGE.

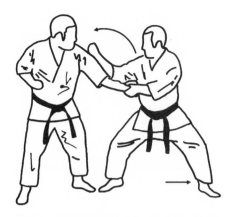

SAIFA KATA: BACKFIST, INCORRECT RANGE. NOTE THAT THE
ANGLE OF THE STRIKE MUST DEVIATE FROM WHAT IS SHOWN
IN THE *KATA* IN ORDER TO CONNECT WITH THE OPPO-
NENT—IT IS MUCH LESS VERTICAL. THE HEAD BECOMES A
VERY DIFFICULT TARGET AT THIS RANGE.

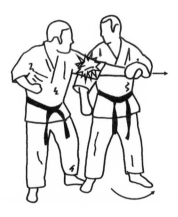

SAIFA KATA: ELBOW STRIKE, CORRECT RANGE.

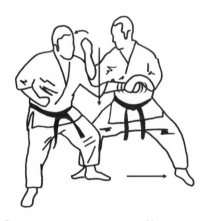

SAIFA KATA: BACKFIST, CORRECT RANGE. NOTE THAT NOT
ONLY DOES THE ANGLE OF THE STRIKE MATCH WHAT IS
SHOWN IN THE *KATA*, BUT ALSO THE TEMPLE BECOMES A
VIABLE, EASILY REACHED TARGET.

approximately 30 degrees from *shomen* (front), cover their chambered hand, and
then pivot forcefully 90 degrees to execute the elbow strike. This movement can be
interpreted as a shift in and slightly to the outside of an opponent to dodge his blow,
while checking his punch with your off-hand before delivering the elbow strike.

The follow-on *osai uke* and *uraken uchi* are performed very close to your body as
you do the *kata* indicating a very short distance to your opponent. In this fashion,
your leading elbow can strike down onto the opponent's upper arm snapping his

head into position for a killing backfist strike to the temple. If you have aggressive-ly stepped toward the attack ending up along side the opponent, all these move-ments make sense. Both the angles and the ranges are correct. Done at too far a range (away from the opponent) or at an improper angle (e.g., in front of the oppo-nent), this combination will not work.

In *seisan kata,* there is a 90-degree pivot preceding an arm wrap and throat grab. Once again the technique is performed very close to the practitioner's body in *kata.* In real life, it is virtually impossible to perform this movement from directly in front of an opponent without getting hit before you can pull it off. If, on the other hand, you have blocked an opponent's punch or otherwise shifted to the outside (any closing technique) and then attempt this maneuver the odds of success go way up. You sim-

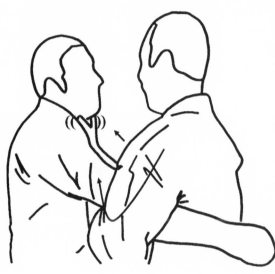

ply seek the attacker's second (far side) punch, intercepting it close to his body then ride the momentum of his punch back toward you with the arm wrap. As that arm pulls in the other shoots up to the oppo-nent's throat. The *kata's* pivot alerts practitioners to the off-angle approach while the close proximity of the technique to one's self in *kata* demonstrates that it must be a short-distance application.

Where your focus is directed in performance of the *kata* is also very important. Opponents are virtually always assumed to be directly in front of you, even when you approach at an angle to your attack-er's *enbusen.* Looking left or right in

SEISAN KATA: ARM WRAP/THROAT GRAB.

kata, therefore, denotes exceptions to that rule. For example, *saifa kata* shows a knee strike performed while looking to the side. This indicates that in practical applica-tion you must be standing *beside* rather than in front of your attacker.

10) Touching Your Own Body in Kata Indicates Touching Your Opponent

"If a man is offered a fact which goes against his instincts, he will scrutinize it closely, and unless the evidence is overwhelming, he will refuse to believe it. If, on the

other hand, he is offered something which affords a reason for acting in accordance to his instincts, he will accept it even on the slightest evidence." [55]

– Bertrand Russell

In sports, coaches signal plays to their teams by touching various parts of their bodies in predefined ways. In baseball, for example, typical signals might call for a sacrifice bunt, fake bunt, squeeze bunt, stolen base, straight steal, fake steal, delay steal, hit and run, or run and hit, among other possibilities. Such signals also indicate when an activity must occur (early or late in the count), or when it is the batter's responsibility to decide. The coach's signals must be simple enough to facilitate rapid communication with his or her players, but confusing enough to confound the opposing team.

The same thing happens in the martial arts. There are many examples of techniques in *kata* where practitioners touch their own bodies, placing their hands against their arms, cupping their elbows, crossing their forearms and so on. Like a baseball coach's signals, touching yourself in *kata* is an important indicator about what you should be doing to an opponent.

In practical application, *budoka* would never want to tie up two of their weapons (e.g., hands) in dealing with only one of an opponent's (e.g., punch). This cedes a huge strategic advantage to the attacker. Consequently, anything that looks like an augmented block is probably something else entirely. By creating such movements, the ancient masters were providing clues about hidden locks, holds, throws, arm bars, and other applications and how they might be applied on an opponent.

Some such instances are relatively obvious, while others are more obscure. For example, the augmented *chudan uke* (chest block) in *seiyunchin kata* can be applied as a grab to an opponent's hand or wrist with a simultaneous arm bar.

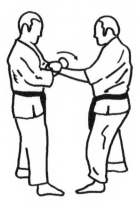

SEIYUNCHIN KATA: WRIST GRAB.

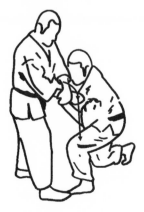

SEIYUNCHIN KATA: ARM BAR.

Another example is the *bensoku dachi* (cross-foot stance) turn performed in *saipai kata*. One interpretation of crossing the legs in that manner could be a foot entanglement or leg sweep against an opponent.

When deciphering *kata*, look for situations where your off-hand touches your own body to find hidden locks, holds, or throws. What appears at first blush to be an augmented block is almost certainly a lock, throw, or hold instead. Advanced practitioners often find that striking arts contain many grappling techniques and vice versa.*

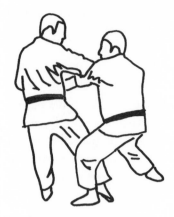

SAIPAI KATA: LEG ENTANGLEMENT.

11) Contour the Body—Strike Hard to Soft and Soft to Hard

"I'm not in favor of punching a person's jaw with a fist, since it's not much different than ramming your fist into a horseshoe. I've broken my hand doing it, and I know of others who have as well. Since I've never used my palm to strike someone in the jaw with the intention of knocking them out, I can't speak from experience as to the results. My guess is that it would do the job." [56]

– *Loren Christensen*

Contouring is an important and often overlooked component of deciphering *kata*. It helps identify the primary target for any given technique. In general, hard parts strike soft targets and vice versa. Anyone who has ever punched someone in the jaw with a closed fist knows how painful it is for both parties (hard fist vs. hard jaw). We have seen quite a few broken knuckles resulting from such folly. A palm heel strike to the jaw, on the other hand, can be quite effective (soft palm vs. hard jaw). It is vastly more painful for the recipient than for the person delivering the head punch when it is performed in this fashion.†

Kata are designed to make sure the strike applied fits the intended target. Consequently the type of strike demonstrated (e.g., fingers, palm, sword hand, one-knuckle, closed fist, heel, edge of the foot, or ball of the foot) along with its elevation in *kata* (high, middle, or low) identifies the appropriate vital target you should be aiming for.

---

* For more information about throwing and grappling applications in the striking arts (e.g., karate, tae kwon do) you might want to check out Iain Abernethy's *Throws for Strikers* (Summersdale Publishers, 2003) and/or his book *Karate's Grappling Methods: Understanding Kata and Bunkai* (Summersdale, 2001). These excellent books cover the throwing and grappling applications, respectively, in detail.

† Though Kane had a bruised palm for a week or so the last time he did hit someone in the jaw with a *shotei uchi* in a real fight, that sure beats a broken knuckle.

For example, the blade edge of the foot aligns best with a joint (e.g., knee), while the ball of the foot makes a nice upward arc into the groin or midsection. A single knuckle or finger strike fits the solar plexus better than the whole fist (even though you lead with the first two knuckles). A hammerfist aligns much better with the temple or the forehead than it does with the base of the jaw or stomach where an uppercut or palm-up straight punch might better apply.

As a general rule, techniques in *kata* are aimed at elevations equivalent to the practitioner's body. *Jodan* (head) punches are aimed at the level of one's own chin. *Chudan* (middle) punches are aimed level with the practitioner's solar plexus. *Gedan* (down) punches are aimed at *obi* (belt) knot level.

Kicks follow similar general logic for targeting *jodan*, *chudan* and *gedan*, though the type of kick is more enlightening than the general concept of *gedan* when aimed downward. For example, *kensetsu geri* always targets a joint (e.g., knee*). Kakato geri*, stomping heel kick, has, by physical necessity, targets limited to what you can stomp down onto such as a foot or ankle.* *Mae geri* swings upward, typically to the thigh or groin. *Mikazuki geri* (hook kick) often targets the kidneys from around the side.

Elevation by itself, however, can frequently be misleading. If an opponent is already on the ground, *gedan kakato geri* (downward heel kick) could quite easily target the head. Similarly, a *chudan oi tsuki* (chest-level lunge punch) performed in *zenkutsu dachi* (front forward stance) is often aimed *gedan*, since the lower stance frequently matches the practitioner's chest punch at waist or groin level with his or her opponent. Furthermore, while *budoka* must aim at the level of their own bodies in *kata* practice, they must adjust in actual combat to appropriately target opponents of greater or lesser height.[†]

With all this potential confusion, it is essential, therefore, to use body contour as the final arbiter of targeting. Specific techniques sometimes have special application rules. For example, *ippon ken tsuki* (single knuckle punches) performed with the index finger usually strike at a downward or horizontal angle. When executed with the middle knuckle, the *ippon ken* strikes upward into an opponent.

Consequently when applying the *ippon ken* double down strike in *saipai kata*, practitioners should realize that because they are using the knuckles of the middle fingers, their opponent must be lying on the ground. There is no other logical way to punch upward toward an opponent's head with a downward strike! That is why, as Morio Higaonna points out,[‡] the foot movement that immediately precedes this application is actually the most important component of the punching technique. It is what dumps the opponent onto the ground to allow this strike to take place at all.

Pay particular attention the type of strikes your *kata* demonstrates. Look for vital areas in the general vicinity (high, middle, or low). Once you find potential targets, look for the best match of hard to soft or soft to hard. Having found a possible

---

* Unless your opponent is already lying on the ground, of course.

† A good reason to pair up with others of different heights and weights during tandem *dojo* practice. Real life attackers are rarely identical in size to their victims.

‡ "For example, in the case of [*saipai*] striking *naka daka ippon ken*, the real meaning is in the foot stamp and not the punch."

match, try your new found application with a partner. The position of your hand or foot should easily fit into the area you are trying to strike, contouring the opponent's body. Since you are aiming for vital areas, we suggest that you conduct such experiments at slow speed for enhanced safety. It is bad form to break your training partner in during practice.

12) There is No Pause.

"Don't hesitate between techniques, waste time, or stop your movement. Try to do two or three things at once. Don't block then counter. Do both together. Don't kick in such a way as you have to recover your balance before you can punch. Combine them. Combine movement with a fast flurry of techniques that bridge all the ranges of distance to, or past, your opponent. Once practiced you should be able to execute 10 to 12 techniques in less than two seconds—about all the time you have in many situations."
57

– *Christopher Caile*

There is essential pacing and flow to the performance of *kata*. Pauses are incorporated for several important reasons including separating one section from another, emphasizing certain techniques or components of techniques, denoting expected actions by an opponent (e.g., falling down), or signifying the presence of hidden techniques between the more obvious movements. While these pauses must be demonstrated when practicing *kata*, it is utter folly to think that they exist in real-life applications.

Imagine a boxing match where a competitor, facing a former heavyweight champion like George Foreman or Mike Tyson, paused between each blow. He'd get his

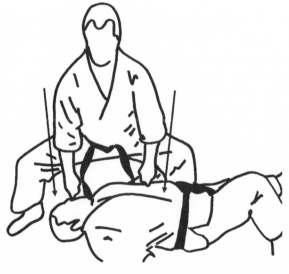

SAIPAI KATA: NAKA DAKA IPPON KEN (DOUBLE DOWNWARD ONE-KNUCKLE) STRIKE. PROPER CONTOURING INDICATES THAT THE OPPONENT MUST BE ON THE GROUND TO OPTIMIZE THIS TECHNIQUE. BECAUSE IT IS IMPRACTICAL AGAINST A STANDING ADVERSARY, THE FOOT SWEEP THAT PRECEDES IT IN THE *KATA* IS MORE CRITICAL THAN THE ACTUAL PUNCH. WHILE YOU DO NOT NECESSARILY NEED THE FOOT SWEEP IN A REAL FIGHT, THE OPPONENT MUST SOMEHOW ALREADY BE ON THE GROUND BEFORE YOU CAN USE THE *NAKA DAKA IPPON KEN* STRIKE.

lights punched out in no time. There may be a certain amount of jockeying for position or gauging each other's readiness at the beginning of a match, but once engaged in combat, boxers throw a constant flurry of jabs, uppercuts, and punches at their opponent until they are too exhausted to continue. There is no pause in the action until one combatant or the other takes a face plant onto the canvas, the bell rings at the end of each round, or someone forces a break by clinching or otherwise tying up an opponent.*

Similarly, full contact sparring matches in tae kwon do are equally fast and furious. Ultimate Fighting competitors do the same thing. Furthermore, in a real life-or-death confrontations, there are absolutely, positively no pauses in the action until one or both combatants disengages and escapes or is disabled, killed, or otherwise becomes unable to continue the fight.

When deciphering *kata*, practitioners should try to understand the reason for the pauses that are portrayed, but they should never be fooled into thinking that the pauses might exist in a real fight. For example, in *saifa kata* there is a *hiza geri* (knee kick) followed by a pause in *hakusura dachi* (crane stance) and then a *mae geri* (front kick). One obvious interpretation is that the practitioner strikes the attacker with a knee, waits for him or her to fall backward, and then launches the front kick as a follow-up strike.

This is a reasonable interpretation until you think about the physics involved. A properly thrown knee strike at close range is very powerful. It literally lifts the opponent off the ground, doubles him over, and hurls him backward immediately. If you pause as long as the *kata* demonstrates, your attacker would already be on the

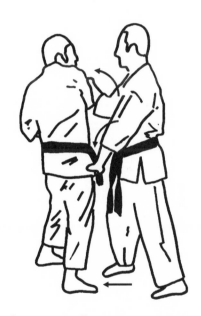

SAIFA KATA: BLOCK. THE DEFENDER IS ON THE RIGHT.

ground and you would send your follow-up kick over his or her head. A pause is completely unnecessary. It is only shown for emphasis. The knee attack is the prime objective for this particular application. The front kick that follows is bonus material, probably (hopefully) not even necessary.

* Something you should never attempt in a real fight since it works primarily due to the codified rules of boxing.

All karate kicks actually start with a knee lift necessary to achieve proper elevation followed instantly by the lower leg movement, so any leg technique could include a knee strike (or block) just before the kick. Whether it is utilized simply depends on how far away the *karateka* is from his or her opponent. In the *saifa kata* example, the knee strike is emphasized to demonstrate how close the practitioner is supposed to be to his or her attacker when executing the technique. Since there is no pause in practical application, practitioners throw the full kick anywhere in its effective range, regardless of how far from their opponents they actually are in real-life self defense situations. Pauses in *kata* are for emphasis, not to demonstrate a true pause in the action.

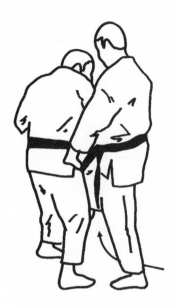

SAIFA KATA: HIZA GERI (KNEE STRIKE) STRIKE.

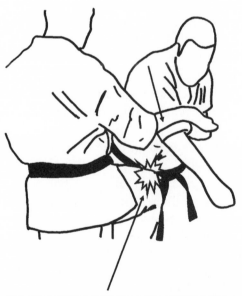

SAIFA KATA: REVERSE ANGLE/CLOSE-UP OF BLOCK/KNEE STRIKE.

Summary

"One of the things I like to do when analyzing kata is to say to myself, 'what if a kick is not a kick or a punch is not a punch or a block is not a block.' Then I like to construct applications that make use of the same movement, but give alternate explanations to the technique. Thus I attempt to develop the techniques in which kicking motions are utilized in ways other than the obvious manner." [58]

– Rick Clark

Although there are numerous "correct" interpretations for each movement of every *kata*, techniques are typically stylized with the actual applications obscured. The work to uncover hidden applications in *kata* is called *kaisai*. Since it offers guidelines for unlocking the secrets of each *kata*, *kaisai no genri* (the theory of *kaisai*) was once a great mystery revealed only to trusted disciples of the ancient masters in order to protect the secrets of their fighting systems.

Using the principles of *kaisai no genri* practitioners can decipher the original intent of *kata* techniques by logically analyzing each specific movement to find its hidden meaning. The first three conventions are called *shuyo san gensoko*, meaning main or basic rules. Rules 4 through 12 are called *hosoku joko*, which translates as supplementary or advanced rules. They are summarized as follows:

1. **Do not be deceived by the *enbusen* rule**
   Kata are choreographed using artificial symmetry to ensure that the practitioner never takes more than three or four steps in any one direction, a process of conserving required practice space. Techniques performed to the left do not necessarily imply an opponent on the left any more than techniques performed to the right imply an attacker in that direction.

2. **Advancing techniques imply attack, while retreating techniques imply defense.**
   Kata techniques performed while advancing imply attacks, even if they appear defensive in nature. As the second half of the rule implies, techniques performed while retreating are defensive in nature. In combat, however, there is no actual "retreat." The perception of giving ground is really a tactic executed to control distance while continuing to engage an opponent.

3. **There is only one enemy at a time.**
   In reality, from a street-fighting point of view, it is pretty much impossible to use the moves of a *kata* to fight against multiple attackers at once. The vast majority of *kata* techniques are designed to deal with a single attacker who is directly in front of you. Although there are a few movements in certain *kata* where the imaginary enemy strikes from behind, there is always only one

opponent at a time. Defense against a large group is generally handled by strategically engaging one person at a time in a manner that confounds the other's ability to reach you.

4. **Every movement in *kata* has martial meaning/significance and can be used in a real fight.**
Every single movement of every *kata* has at least one application that can be used to end a real fight quickly. The ancient masters did not waste effort on pretty; they were concerned solely with functional. There were no *kata* competitions or sports tournaments; only life and death struggles to survive. Without the benefit of modern medicine, even slight injuries in combat could become fatal so fights had to be ended quickly.

5. **A hand returning to chamber usually has something in it.**
Both hands are utilized in almost all *kata* applications. When analyzing *kata*, it is important to pay attention to the off-hand, the one not executing an obvious technique. Frequently the hand returning to chamber at the practitioner's side has something captured in it, especially if it is shown closed when performing the *kata*. This movement may imply grabs, locks, joint dislocations, takedowns, or even throws.

6. **Utilize the shortest distance to your opponent.**
In martial arts, the shortest distance between two points is where you strike. To have the greatest opportunity for success, practitioners must strike or defend with the closest body part. Defensive movements must cut off the attacker's technique before it gains too much speed and power, catching it as close to the opponent's body as possible. Offensive techniques must afford the opponent as little reaction time as possible.

7. **Control an opponent's head and you control the opponent.**
If you can incapacitate an opponent's vision, breathing, or movement, you are in an excellent position to defeat your enemy. Any two out of three will pretty much guarantee success. *Kata* frequently use control of a person's head to disrupt his or her vision, breathing, and movement simultaneously through a variety of eye, ear, neck, and head attacks.

8. **There is no block.**
Unlike what most beginners are taught, there really is no block in karate. The word *uke* in Japanese translates most accurately to "receive" than it does to "block." Your defensive technique receives the attack and makes it your own. Once you own the attack, you can do with it what you will. A fast, hard block has the potential to drop an opponent in his or her tracks, ending the fight before you even need to throw an offensive blow.

9. ***Kata* demonstrate the proper angles.**
Most *budo* techniques avoid direct force to force. While practitioners frequently intend to move at an angle to their opponent's *enbusen* for attack or defense, such turns in *kata* usually suggest an optimal angle of attack.

Similarly, the distance from the practitioner's body at which the *kata* technique is displayed demonstrates how far away he or she should be from an opponent when applying the application. An opponent is virtually always assumed to be directly in front of a practitioner, even when the practitioner approaches at an angle to the attacker's *enbusen*. Looking left or right in *kata*, therefore, denotes exceptions to that rule.

10. **Touching your own body in *kata* indicates touching your opponent.**

In practical application, practitioners would never want to tie up two of their weapons (e.g., hands) dealing with only one of an opponent's. This cedes a huge strategic advantage to the attacker. Consequently, anything that looks like an augmented block is probably something else entirely, typically a lock, hold, throw, or armbar.

11. **Contour the body—strike hard to soft and soft to hard.**

Contouring is an important and often overlooked component of deciphering *kata*. It helps identify the primary target for any given technique. In general, hard parts strike soft targets and vice versa. The type of strike demonstrated (e.g., fingers, palm, sword hand, one-knuckle, closed fist, heel, edge of the foot, or ball of the foot) along with its elevation in *kata* (high, middle, or low) helps identify what vital target you should aim for.

12. **There is no pause.**

There is essential pacing and flow to the performance of *kata*. Pauses are incorporated for several important reasons, including separating one section from another, emphasizing certain techniques, or signifying the presence of hidden techniques between the more obvious movements. While these pauses must be demonstrated when practicing *kata*, it is a mistake to think that they exist in real-life applications. An attacker will not hesitate between strikes and neither should you.

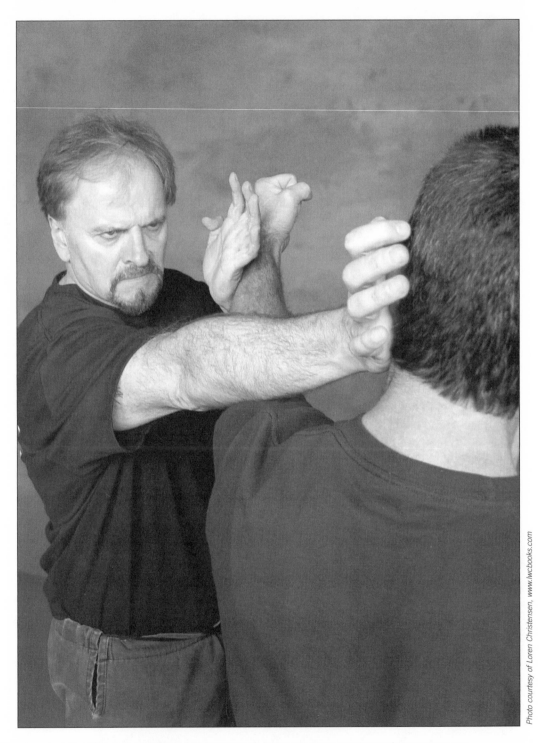

BLOCK/PALM HEEL TO STOMACH 6 (PRESSURE POINT). IN THIS APPLICATION THE OPPONENT'S ATTACK IS BLOCKED
WITH A SIMULTANEOUS STRIKE TO HIS JAW. LOREN CHRISTENSEN SHIFTS OFF-LINE AND CLOSES TO EXECUTE THIS
APPLICATION IN THE PROPER RANGE.

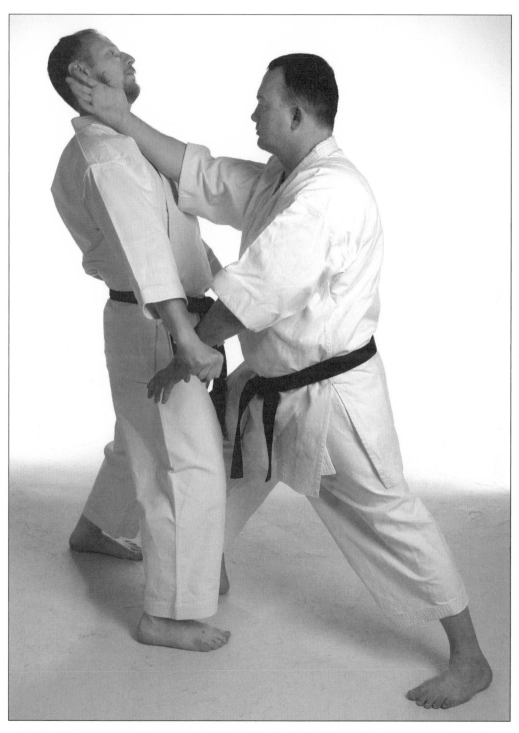

SHISOCHIN NECK STRIKE/BLOCK COMBINATION. THIS TECHNIQUE IS A SIGNATURE MOVEMENT OF
SHISOCHIN KATA. IT FEATURES A SIMULTANEOUS BLOCK AND RIDGE HAND STRIKE COMBINATION.

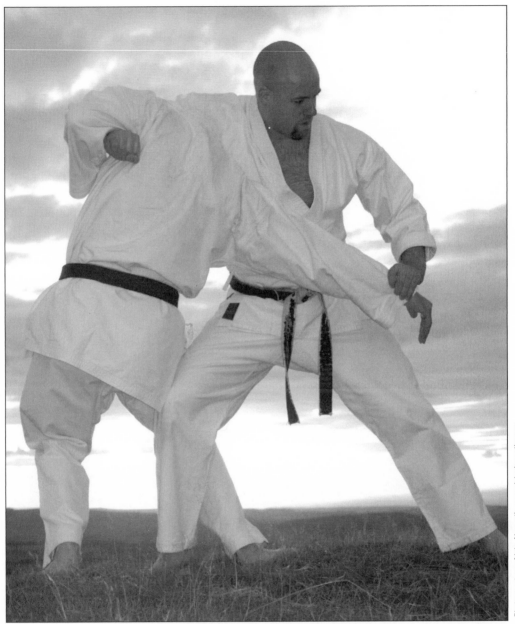

KUSHANKU NECK-CRANK AND TAKEDOWN. IAIN ABERNETHY APPLIES A NECK-CRANK AND TAKEDOWN FROM KUSHANKU (KANKU-DAI) KATA. THE RECIPIENT IS MURRAY DENWOOD. THE LOCATION IS THE LAKE DISTRICT IN CUMBRIA, NORTHERN ENGLAND.

CHAPTER 5

Physics, Physiology, and Other Considerations

"Do not let the body be dragged along by mind nor the mind be dragged along by the body." [59]

– Miyamoto Musashi

Now that concepts of strategy and tactics are understood, and the principles and rules for deciphering *kata* applications have been defined in the previous chapters, we provide a preview of the environment in which practitioners may need to use them. After all, *kata* forms the basis of a practical fighting art that you may have to use some day to defend yourself or protect a loved one from harm. This chapter covers a wide range of subjects, including the following:

1. Characteristics of violence, including the types of attackers you may ultimately find yourself confronting, the environment within which you may have to fight, as well as the escalation process that inevitably precedes violence in such encounters.

2. Physiological threat responses: a description of how the body reacts to these physical confrontations.

3. Brain activity in combat, including the four types of brain waves and how the concept of *zanshin*, or "continuing mind," can give you an edge in combat.

4. Non-diagnostic response: a training method that increases your changes of surviving violent encounters by predisposing your threat reactions.

5. Levels of response: a way to guarantee that techniques can be utilized in actual combat by ensuring that they conform to natural neurological reactions, sound tactics, and solid strategy.

6. "Catching bullets" and the importance of speed and timing in violent confrontations.

7. Stealing time: a method to help you overcome your opponent's speed by cheating to win.

8. Speed kills: a variety of tricks and tips for making yourself faster and ultimately more successful in combat or tournament competition.

9. Vital points: areas of the body where physiological damage is most likely to stop a determined opponent, your best targets in self-defense scenarios.

Because this information is rather broad, we think it will be useful to introduce this chapter with an overview of some of these concepts, relating them to the *kata* you practice, before we launch into explaining them in greater detail. In a real fight, the fastest person—whoever strikes and lands a solid blow first—is vastly more likely to win. Not only does this person keep an opponent off balance with rapid fire attacks, but as soon as an enemy is struck he becomes disrupted and increasingly vulnerable. While not all of us are gifted with naturally great speed, the good news is that anyone can train to enhance the ability that he or she already has.

Part of what makes certain martial artists fast are their abilities to react in a non-diagnostic manner. They do not think; they simply do. In the old days, traditional practitioners would spend many, many years learning a single *kata*. They would study it in great depth, learning all the subtle nuances and internalizing the movements until they became second nature. Conditioned muscle memory simply reacted to a threat instantly without conscious thought. Further, they were able to adapt to varied fighting environments because they understood every valid interpretation and subtle nuance of the *kata* techniques they studied.

Modern practitioners need to do the same thing. It is very important to understand how you might interpret applications from your *kata* should you be fighting on a hill, around furniture or other obstacles, in a stairwell, under water, in a crowd, or in any other unusual situation. While you need to be able to perform your techniques wearing a traditional loose-fitting *gi*, you must also know the restrictions of your street clothes as well. Training in the *dojo* is outstanding, but practicing outside the *dojo* on occasion can help realistically prepare practitioners for real combat.

Threat responses work like rungs on a ladder. The lowest rung, or base foundation, is built upon natural neurological responses, taking advantage of our hardwired fight or flight reaction. Tactics and strategy, the next higher rungs in ascending order, must work synergistically with the body's natural physiological reactions in order to be successful. The ancient masters took such things into consideration as they built their *kata*. In deciphering applications, we must understand them as well.

A famous quote from Sun Tzu reads, "To fight and conquer in all your battles is not supreme excellence; supreme excellence consists in breaking the enemy's resistance without fighting." The best self-defense is, of course, avoiding a fight altogether. Even if a person legitimately uses force in order to escape an imminent and unavoidable danger, he or she will still have to live with the physiological and psychological results of doing so, as well as the possibility of expensive and lengthy litigation that might follow.

In an e-mail interchange about this subject, *Goju Ryu* practitioner Nenad Djurjevic wrote, "My philosophy if it ever came to a fight is to avoid rather than check, check rather than hurt, hurt rather than maim, maim rather than kill, and kill rather than die. Anyone who goes straight for the final option as the default option is, in my opinion, a loose cannon in civilized society." We wholeheartedly agree. While martial practitioners may neither initiate aggression nor seek conflict, on occasion it comes looking for them nevertheless.

A good understanding of the characteristics of violence and insight into the criminal mind can help practitioners avoid dangerous confrontations. We'll begin examining these concepts in more detail, starting with the characteristics of violence. After all, the more you know about why fights occur, the better your odds of avoiding them.

Characteristics of Violence

"I remember seeing a young terrorist of about 17 describe the joy he felt when his knife or ax plunged into his victims' bodies. He liked slicing and chopping up his victims. He also relished performing these acts when his victims were tied down and after he had tortured them for days with bare electrical wires, gouged out their eyes, cut off their tongues, and castrated them. As I watched his smiling, innocent baby face, I realized what a severe disadvantage the normal, average person has in deadly combat with such creatures. Try to remember that when you make a decision on how to defend yourself from these dregs of humanity. Being sportsmanlike and humane to such murderers can get you and your family butchered." [60]

— Eugene Sockut

If someone is attacking you, you probably do not care much about who that person is or why he or she is doing it, at least not during the initial confrontation. You simply want to survive and be safe. It is useful however, to understand the types of violence and the types of criminals one might encounter, at least at an overview level. This information can give you an edge in surviving or avoiding a violent confrontation. Lots of good books have already been written on this subject so we'll be reasonably brief.

Types of Violence

In *A Professional's Guide to Ending Violence Quickly*, Marc MacYoung categorizes violence into four general groups. These types of aggression include fear, frenzy, tantrum, and criminal. Fear violence stems from feelings of personal threat, which lead to a countervailing response (justified or not). It is based on an individual's perception of a clear and immediate threat from which he or she will panic and attempt to fight to get free.

Frenzy violence stems from a lack of external limits or boundaries, hence the term "out of control." Individuals in this state look at any situation from an extreme point of view, disregarding anything that contradicts their perspective. They must have or do something and want it so badly that they will stop at nothing to achieve such an end. Typically they are reacting to internal perception rather than any specific external stimulus (e.g., intoxication through drugs or alcohol).

Tantrum violence comes from escalating fits of temper or uncontrolled fury, which is projected outward toward others. It is based on internalized anger that has reached a boiling point. Such individuals look for any excuse to explode and try to create a situation where they can do so. Demanding or bullying behaviors are common precursors to tantrum violence.

Criminal violence is used for coercion, to gain profit or power from (or over) others. Any time a person is placed in a situation where refusal to submit to another's demands would lead to personal injury they have encountered criminal violence.

While these various types of violence may overlap, responses can be tailored depending upon which type is encountered. The best response to fear-based violence is to present oneself in a non-threatening manner (e.g., unthreatening demeanor, empty hands held in front, reassuring tone of voice). Calming the fearful individual can frequently de-escalate and control the situation without the need to resort to physical confrontation.

Frenzy situations can be handled by providing stimuli that overrides the person's internal process and snaps them back into reality. An authoritative demeanor and commanding voice are often used. Limiting the person's options, forcefully if necessary, will demonstrate that compliance will limit or eliminate the negative consequences of the frenzied behavior. A good strategy is to control the frenzy.

Since tantrum-state violence is associated with negative attention, it is very difficult to handle. Either compliance or refusal with impossible demands will result in violence. It is important when dealing with such individuals to adopt an unemotional, professional demeanor—all while preparing to defend yourself should you be forced to do so. Do not be drawn into a confrontation by losing your cool or showing fear.

The best response to the threat of criminal violence is often to turn the tables. Attempt to remove the options of compliance versus victimization and replace them with, "leave me alone or I'll hurt you." Under personal and immediate threat, you need to be able to back up your assertion. Bullies will often back down from such threats.

Types of Criminals

Criminal violence has a variety of flavors that may vary depending upon the type of criminal you encounter. This list is presented simply to increase awareness, not to be definitive or all encompassing. The types of criminals you might encounter can include amateurs, professionals, psychopaths, drug addicts, sex predators, gang members, and terrorists. While they have some similarities, each is somewhat different and unique. It is important to keep things in proper context. Responding to a drunken fan at a football game as if he were a violent hardcore criminal could lead you to taking things a bit too far. Responding to a violent predator as if he was your intoxicated, somewhat ornery uncle, on the other hand, could get you killed.

Your most likely criminal encounter is with a rank amateur, someone who decides to rob a store that you are in, mug you, or otherwise make a few bucks with minimal effort. Such individuals are dangerous, unpredictable, and more often than not, armed. Their crimes tend to be spontaneous acts of opportunity. Simply being aware of your surroundings and staying out of bad neighborhoods is a good way to avoid such people.

While the aforementioned drunken football fan may fall into this category, odds are high that he is most likely someone with anger management problems rather than a hardened criminal who is really trying to kill you. In hundreds of violent encounters at the stadium, for example, Kane's life has been in danger only a handful of times. Countervailing force may not be necessary or even advisable in such situations, especially while the possibility of de-escalating the confrontation still exists.

Professional criminals, those who do actually make a living through their crime, frequently do not carry weapons, preferring fraud, deception, or other nonviolent means. These are the people behind telemarketing scams, stock fraud, real-estate swindles, bogus investment companies, and other cons such as e-mails telling you that a long lost relative has died in a foreign country and if you only send money to clear up the paperwork it will be repaid ten- or twenty-fold. They create fake web sites and e-mails phishing* for account numbers and other sensitive information online, steal identities, and do everything they can to get rich with other people's money . These individuals tend to plan their crimes carefully and methodically. Honest citizens with a reasonable degree of skepticism can frequently avoid such individuals. Even when they cannot, violence is rare when encountering such criminals.

Psychopaths could be random victimizers like the Green River Killer or the Son of Sam, or, more likely than not, abusers, stalkers, and bullies who are known to their victims. Dangerous and unfeeling, such individuals have a plan that makes perfect sense, if only to them. The single-mindedness and determination of such individuals makes them very dangerous indeed. Professional intervention is generally

---

* Pronounced "fishing." This term was coined in the mid-1990s by hackers who used this process steal America On-Line (AOL) accounts. Posing as an AOL staff member, the criminal would send an instant message to a potential victim asking for his or her password to "verify" the account or to "confirm" billing information. Once the victim gave over the password, the attacker could access the victim's account and use it for criminal purposes, such as spamming.

warranted when dealing with these people. Domestic violence, a lower level of psychopathic behavior, is the one of the last things police officers would like to respond too as such situations are so unpredictable and volatile. If you have a choice, it is preferable not to deal with such situations yourself. Get help.

While hard-core drug addicts may technically be medically ill and in desperate need of treatment for their maladies, they can be violent, dangerous, and unpredictable all the same. A naked man, high on crack cocaine, wrestled the gun away from a Bellevue, Washington police officer a couple of years ago and shot him dead in front of numerous witnesses. The jury, rejecting an insanity plea, found the defendant Ronald guilty of aggravated first-degree murder and put him away for life. Addicts looking for a few quick bucks to support their habits frequently vandalize vehicles and break into homes. Police crime statistics can help you avoid areas frequented by drug dealers and drug addicts. Neighborhood watch programs sponsored by local police agencies are a tremendous aid in cutting down this type of criminal activity.

Sex predators target specific individuals or types of individuals. Some are random encounters, though in many cases the victim may know or have met the attacker beforehand. While these types of individuals are violent, it is important to understand that this type of crime is generally more about control than it actually is about sex. Such people are difficult to rehabilitate and frequently re-offend. Consequently they often have to register with authorities as a condition of parole. Local police agencies usually have Web sites listing general geographic locations and the number of registered sex offenders by area. This is important information to have when buying a house, finding a school, or choosing what neighborhood to live in.

Gang members are often associated with drugs and violence. Sociologically people in large groups will frequently do things they would never dream of doing individually. Riots that broke out after the Rodney King trial are a good example. During a Mardi Gras celebration in the Pioneer Square area of Seattle, Washington, a few years back, roving gangs of thugs instigated several attacks on revelers. Random incidents that went on over the preceding couple of nights were well publicized on the local news, yet revelers continued to attend anyway. During one assault on the third evening, a young man named Christopher was beaten to death. His assailant claimed in court that he had simply been carried away by the party atmosphere and did not mean to seriously hurt anyone.

It is always good to avoid volatile situations, especially when you know in advance there have been problems. This includes bad neighborhoods, known gang hangouts (e.g., certain stores or nightclubs), and unpredictable crowds (e.g., raucous celebrations or violent political protests*). An additional consideration with true gang members (e.g., Crips, Bloods, Hell's Angels) as opposed to out of control crowds is

* For instance, Tiananmen Square in 1989.

that if you are forced to use countervailing force against one member, he or she will undoubtedly have unhappy friends who will want to pay you a visit later on.

Terrorists are a whole different animal. Somewhere around 400 B.C. the Chinese philosopher Wu Ch'i wrote, "One man willing to throw away his life is enough to terrorize a thousand." This sentiment is as true today as it was in ancient times. The world is becoming a more dangerous place, where anyone might become a victim of a random or a planned act of terror. Fortunately, instances of terrorist attacks, though headline grabbing, are still quite rare in most countries. While we certainly hope and pray it continues to be that way, it is important to be prepared.

Unlike other types of criminals, terrorists prefer to conduct their violence remotely. It is almost never a one-on-one attack. Improvised explosive devices such as remote roadside bombs, car or truck bombs are fairly common. Even when they do get personally involved (e.g., suicide/ homicide bomber), the goal is mass destruction rather than a single killing. Training in the martial arts is frequently insufficient, in and of itself, to deal with such threats.

Bomb Threats

According to the FBI Bomb Data Center, six pounds of explosives (cigar box) has a fragmentation range of 832 feet. Forty pounds of explosives (briefcase) has a fragmentation range of 1,129 feet. One hundred and sixty pounds of explosives (suitcase) has a fragmentation range of 1,792 feet. You can imagine how devastating a truck bomb twenty times that size could be.

Let's face it, only magicians can stop bullets with their teeth, and only via illusion. No matter how well trained a martial artist you are, you cannot fight a bullet or a bomb with your hands and feet and expect to win. The best defense is awareness, becoming conscious of and avoiding dangerous situations before it is too late.

Awareness can be used to protect not only yourself, but to save others around you as well. In his groundbreaking book, *The Gift of Fear*, Gavin DeBecker wrote, "Before the courageous FBI raid, before the arrest, long before the news conference, there is a regular American citizen who sees something that seems suspicious, listens to intuition, and has the character to risk being wrong or seeming foolish when making the call to authorities." This concept includes awareness of your environment as well as awareness of timing. When environment and timing converge, your level of alertness should be at its highest.

Awareness of environment includes listening to your intuition and being aware of what is going on around you. Identify and report suspicious unattended vehicles, luggage, or packages in high traffic areas. Monitor irregular activity, such as when someone leaves a large package in a trashcan across from a government building or other strategic location and report anything suspicious to the proper authorities.

Awareness of timing has to do with the time of day during which attacks are most likely to occur. Terrorists try to time attacks to inflict maximum casualties—typically during "rush" hour. For example, the April 19, 1995, Oklahoma City bombing and the September 11, 2001, attacks all took place during the workday when and where the highest number of potential victims congregated. Similarly, a crowded mall in daytime is much more likely to be hit than the same location late at night or just before closing. Awareness of timing in the United States can also include Department of Homeland Security threat level indicators (e.g., yellow, orange, red) that help predict likely attacks. The U.S. State Department also issues travel restrictions and warnings when they sense hazardous conditions in other countries.

Where environment and timing converge, it is prudent to take extra precautions by avoiding good places to hide explosives (e.g., unsecured trash cans, mailboxes) near likely targets to the extent practicable. You do not want to walk around in a state of constant paranoia, yet you should take prudent precautions and avoid clearly dangerous situations.

Kane works part-time as a security supervisor at a Pac-10 football stadium. A game was played there a couple of weeks after the 9/11 attacks. Right before that game, stadium officials got word that a local TV station was trying to plant a fake bomb in an unattended backpack to test the security. They were, of course, hoping to catch stadium employees unprepared and point out holes in their security.

While the event staff had always swept the stadium before each game, including a pass with bomb-sniffing dogs, extra diligence was taken due to a combination of the recent attacks and word of this so-called test. No such backpack was planted nor found at that time, but the incident was considered a good training opportunity.

This event led to drills in which suspicious packages were randomly left unattended to keep the event staff on their toes. Occasionally a timer would be set and left inside a package so that if it was not discovered expeditiously (that is, before the timer went off), it would simulate having already exploded. Similar drills can be duplicated in a *dojo* to help increase practitioners' levels of awareness.

Understanding Awareness

"Real fear," writes Gavin DeBecker in *The Gift of Fear*, "is a signal intended to be very brief, a mere servant of intuition. True fear is a survival signal that sounds in the presence of danger." It is very important to listen to these signals. As we discussed previously, even when you have a chance to win, avoiding danger is far better than fighting your way out of it.

True fear is a signal of the presence of danger. It is a good thing. If you listen to it, you can avoid a whole lot of unnecessary trouble. Unwarranted fear, on the other hand, is always based upon memory or imagination. It is a bad thing. Here are some brief suggestions about how to avoid unwarranted fear:

- When you feel fear or any intuitive signal, listen
- When you don't feel fear, do not manufacture it
- If you find yourself creating worry, explore and discover why

Avoidance

Although martial artists train to survive (or even triumph) in a fight, they should do everything they can to avoid violence in the first place. Gichin Funakoshi, the founder of *Shotokan* karate, once said, "When you leave home, think that you have numerous opponents waiting for you. It is your behavior that invites trouble from them." The only way to guarantee victory in a physical confrontation is to walk away before the first blow is thrown.

Criminals seek out easy victims. Your chances of being molested can be reduced simply by not looking like one. Lt. Col. (retired) Dave Grossman* reiterates this point, "Research conducted on convicts serving time for serous predatory acts of violence—assaults, murders, and killing law enforcement officers—found that the vast majority said that they specifically targeted victims by body language: slumped walk, passive behavior, and lack of awareness. They chose their victims like big cats do in Africa when they select one out of the herd that is least able to protect itself."

The way you carry yourself can help you avoid danger or, conversely, can call trouble to you like a magnet. Do you walk erect and alert like a warrior or hunched over and timid like an easy victim? Do your eyes move back and forth actively scanning the terrain for danger or are they unfocused as you drift along daydreaming? Are your hands poised for action and unencumbered, or buried in your pockets? Be aware of your surroundings and do your best to avoid unnecessary trouble.

Grossman continues, "However, when potential victims gave cues that indicated they would not go easily, the cons said that they would walk away. If the cons sensed the target was a counterpredator, that is, a sheepdog, they would leave him alone unless there was no other choice but to engage."

Grossman categorizes people into three major analogies: sheep, wolves, and sheepdogs. He argues that the vast majority of individuals are like sheep, happy productive citizens with neither a capacity for violence nor any interest in preparing for danger. Wolves, on the other hand, are the dregs of society who take advantage of that fact and prey upon the sheep. Sheepdogs are not only aware that predators exist but are willing and able to use violence when necessary to confront them. A critical difference between sheepdogs and wolves, however, is a moral and ethical code of conduct. Many are drawn to law enforcement or military careers. Some develop an interest in martial arts. Regardless, sheepdogs never commit violence for expedience

---

* A West Point psychology and military science professor and a retired Army Ranger, Grossman combined his experiences to form a new field of scientific endeavor which he has termed "killology." He is an expert in the psychological costs of war, the root causes of violent crime, and the process of healing the victims of violence, in war and peace.

or personal gain, only for self-defense, the protection of other citizens, or the preservation of order.

Swallowing your pride and walking away from a confrontation is a great tactic when you are able to use it. Always consider how your actions might look on the front page of your local newspaper or how they might be interpreted by a judge or jury before you act. Few things are really worth fighting for. Unless your life or the lives of your loved ones are in clear and immediate danger, your best course is to avoid violence altogether. Always remember that you are the good guy (or gal) and act like it.

Even if a person legitimately uses force in order to escape imminent and unavoidable danger, he or she still has to live with the physiological and psychological results of doing so, as wells the potential for litigation. Martial artists should never provoke confrontations. While there certainly are situations in which fighting is the only alternative, it is best to avoid physical altercations altogether whenever possible. Once a confrontation begins, however, we must do whatever it takes to end it quickly.

Escalation to Violence

According to Marc MacYoung, "Most amateur violence comes about because of this stupid game of *escalato*.* People have no clear-cut idea of what winning means, but by God they know they gotta do it. Think about how many times you have seen things escalate out of control. This simple pattern is behind nearly 90 percent of all conflicts you'll encounter. People get 'locked in' and begin raising the stakes. Each round is more intense. It's a basic human pattern no matter where you go. Escalato is the most dangerous game in the world… Anytime you step in to the arena of physical violence, you have to accept that it may not end until either you or your opponent, maybe both, are dead."

Glaring stares, verbal abuse, shoving, argument, or other clear signs of escalation precede the vast majority of violent encounters. As a trained martial artist, you simply cannot afford to play that game. Walk away. The more dangerous you are, the less you should feel a need to prove it.

While it is very common to experience an obvious escalation before a fight, ambushes do occur. In such situations, the escalation has already occurred, yet the victim is unaware of it because it has taken place within the mind of the attacker. These are probably the situations where you have no other alternative to fighting.

For example, in West Seattle (Washington) a few years ago, a homeless man approached a young couple who were sitting on a park bench watching the sunset. In a very friendly manner, he asked them what time it was. As the young man's attention was directed to his wristwatch, the transient reached up and slashed his

* Upward spiral of one-upmanship that almost invariably leads to violence.

throat with a knife he had hidden in his sleeve. He then proceeded to assault the female victim. Both died.

Sneak attackers may ask for the time, directions, a cigarette, or use any other dirty trick to get close enough to launch their assaults. It is exceedingly rare, however, for the victim to be caught totally unaware. Even when long-range weapons are involved (e.g., firearms), fights typically begin close up. Unarmed confrontations always take place at close range. If he or she can see an attacker, a trained martial artist should always have time to react. Regrettably, many practitioners are simply not mentally prepared to react to sudden violence, and thus may needlessly get hurt or killed.

In his column "The Karate Way," Dave Lowry* once wrote, "You don't want to live in a state of combat readiness 24 hours a day. It's not practical, and it isn't healthy. What you can do is train to eliminate your internal rules that say all aggressive acts must 'make sense.' Insisting that an attack make sense before you respond can get you seriously injured or killed." As always, he offers very sound advice.

Through years of diligent practice, *kata* training helps practitioners automatically respond to attacks without conscious thought. Given enough repetitions, the physical movements become hardwired into their subconscious. When the unexpected blow comes screaming toward your head, you can take advantage of your natural flinch reaction to instinctively intercept it and counterstrike. Only after you have safely dispatched the attacker need you wonder about their motivation.

Chivalry Is Dead!

No matter whom you are fighting or why you are doing it, chances are very good that it will not be a "fair" fight. Fair fights barely exist in sporting competitions and never on the street. Massad Ayoob in his book, *The Truth About Self Protection*, shares that "street fighting is not martial arts. It is between you and an enemy, who is trying to injure, maim, rape, or kill you. Whoever is attacking you has probably done it before and more than likely enjoys it. He has probably been hit hard before and has learned how to shrug off pain. You need to hurt him in a way that impairs his body's ability to function and takes him out of the fight."

Opponents on the street are not honorable. You cannot afford to be either. Too many martial artists who train with partners in the *dojo* or for tournament competition develop a rule-based mindset. You do not gouge out someone's eye because he or she is your training partner. You pull your punch so that you will not hurt anyone. You avoid joint kicks because they are against the rules. And so on...

Many years ago Kane attended an Oakland Raiders football game at the Kingdome in Seattle (Washington) with a martial arts instructor named Brad. Returning to his seat after purchasing refreshments, Brad accidentally spilled a small

---

* Dave Lowry regularly writes articles and columns for several popular martial arts magazines and Web sites. A highly skilled and knowledgeable martial artist, he is the author of *Autumn Lightning: The Education of an American Samurai*, Sword & Brush, Persimmon Wind, *Moving Toward Stillness, Traditions, and Clouds in the West* among other excellent books.

amount of beer on a female fan. Her boyfriend, a huge bodybuilder, took immediate offense, launching out of his seat with an explosive flurry of punches. Brad shifted gracefully out of the way of the first few blows, dropped his food and drinks on the floor (splashing the rest of the beer over several more people including the young lady), and then began to defend himself. He cut off the next punch with a powerful *uchi uke* (inside forearm block), immediately reposting with an *uraken uchi* (whipping back fist strike) so blazingly fast that Kane literally could not see it move until the blow landed.

The boyfriend let out a grunt of pain with the block, and then froze in surprise as the backfist gently touched his nose. Without missing a beat Brad looked him in the eye saying, "You really don't want to do this, do you?" The boyfriend grunted and sat back down. He spent the rest of the game glaring at the field, studiously avoiding both Brad and his beer covered girlfriend.*

Walking back to their vehicle after the game, Kane remarked how impressed he had been with Brad's impromptu karate exhibition. His friend looked at the ground chagrined, reddening slightly. He said, "I actually meant to clean his clock! I'm just so used to sparring with my kids (students) that I instinctively pulled the punch. The only reason I got away with it is that I had enough wits about me to pretend that's what I had intended all along. That and the fact that he was just sober enough to reconsider..."

This example was probably not a life or death encounter, but it serves as a valuable object lesson. The heavily built boyfriend launched an unprovoked ambush, well out of proportion to the perceived insult. There was no warning. He did not ask for an apology. He did not say anything at all. He just attacked—at full speed, with all the power his considerable muscles could generate—hoping to catch Brad unaware and knock him out.

When it comes to a real life combat, the rulebook has to go out the window. Clearly it is better to avoid violence in the first place but if you cannot, do not hold back. The bad guys certainly won't. You must do anything you have to in order to survive.

This story from Loren Christensen helps illustrate the necessity for quick and committed action in a fight. "A guy tried to tackle me one time when I was working as a police officer. His tackle didn't take me down, but he was able to wrap his arms around my legs in an embrace so tight that I was on the verge of crashing to the sidewalk. I'm not that skillful on the ground and as a police officer wearing a gun, I didn't want to go down and be at risk of losing my weapon. I had to act quickly. I flicked his closest eye with my fingertips. He instantly released his death grip on my legs and dropped to the sidewalk, clutching his face and yelping like a kicked dog. It worked like a charm."

---

* Who for some reason continued to watch the game without complaining though she did go to the restroom to dry off a little first.

While you certainly cannot physically strike your training partner's vital areas at full speed and power, you must learn to do so mentally. Eye gouges, joint kicks, groin strikes, ear slaps, throwing dirt, spitting, biting, and other "dirty tricks" are often a necessary part of defending yourself successfully. There are no rules in a real fight. What you train to do in practice is what you will most likely do under stress. Unless you get really lucky, pulling your blow in a life-or-death struggle will do you no good; it will simply encourage (or perhaps anger) your attacker. It takes serious physiological damage to stop a determined opponent.

Fighting Environment

If unprovoked attacks occur, you may not be able choose your fighting environment. In such cases you must remain flexible as Loren Christensen relates. "I can tell you that not one of them ever took place in a nice, wide-open space or on mats like those in your martial arts school. I've fought people on roof tops, on the edge of a dock over a river, in a slimy skid row bathroom, on stairways, inside of a car engulfed in flames, and many other places I had never thought of when I was learning my techniques."

It is very important to understand that real-life self-defense situations almost never occur in the *dojo*, though we are aware of a few isolated instances, including one where a martial arts instructor was assaulted in her studio. Practitioners must train with the understanding that should they be called on to apply their skills, it will most likely be in a totally different environment. Consequently it is important to practice your *kata* outside the *dojo* as well as in it.

Practitioners need to learn to interpret *kata* applications for fighting on a hill, around furniture or other obstacles, in a stairwell, under water, in a crowd, or in any other unusual situation. Not only do you need to be able to perform you techniques wearing a traditional uniform *gi*, but in street clothes as well. Tight fitting jeans or bulky jackets simply do not allow the freedom of movement one finds with a *gi*. Heavy boots or shoes affect kicking. Gloves affect one's ability to punch or grapple.

Kane once had to defend himself in a lift line during a driving snowstorm wearing heavy winter clothes, boots, and skis. He recalls, "In this situation, my legs were effectively useless. Thick, padded gloves hampered my ability to throw an effective punch. Lacking anything better to use, I simply stabbed the guy in the thigh with my ski pole. It was a very short, one-sided fight. Even better, since there were several witnesses who saw the guy attack me first I was not the one who got arrested afterward."

For more in-depth information about violence, the criminal mind, and staying away from trouble we highly recommend *The Truth about Self Protection* by Massad Ayoob and *The Gift of Fear* by Gavin DeBecker. Ayoob's book is a holistic guide to self-defense covering everything from walking down the street safely to effective defensive driving techniques. It also covers the physical, emotional, and legal ramifications of countervailing force. DeBecker's book, on the other hand, shows how to protect oneself from violence largely through one's own intuition. It also gives fabulous insight into the criminal mind and how to recognize and avoid dangerous situations. A couple of authors who have been forced to kill yet learned to remain human, Loren Christensen and Dave Grossman poignantly provide important insight into the psychological aspects of self-defense in their book *On Combat*, another tome well worth reading.

So far, we've discussed the characteristics of violence, briefly covering the mindset of those who may attack you. Now we'll shift gears a bit, and focus on how your body reacts during such encounters.

Physiological Threat Response

"One ought never to turn one's back on a threatened danger and try to run away from it. If you do that, you will double the danger. But if you meet it promptly and without flinching, you will reduce the danger by half." [61]

– *Sir Winston Churchill*

The amygdala is an almond-shaped region that sits in the brain's medial temporal lobe, a few inches in front of the ear (behind the eyeballs). It is also linked to perception of facial expressions, enhancing memory in emotional situations, fear response, and coordination of maternal behavior. The amygdala has also been associated with numerous psychiatric and neurological disorders ranging from epilepsy to anxiety disorders and social phobia to Alzheimer's disease.

For our purposes, we will focus on its role in threat response. In this role, the amygdala's job is to sound a siren call to action. When a threat is perceived the amygdala goes to work. This means the central nervous system is triggered to the threat with an "all-systems" alert, a chain reaction of physiological response designed to meet the threat.

Think of it this way—the body is saying, "If we don't get through this nothing else may matter, so everything goes to arming the body." All long-term projects and unessential functions are shut down.

The first step is for the hypothalamus, which regulates the vitals of the body, to trigger the pituitary gland. The pituitary gland, located near the bottom of the brain, produces thyrotropin to stimulate the thyroid gland and adrenocorticotropin (ACTH) that fires up the adrenal cortex, which shoots adrenaline throughout the body. This results in all non-essential body functions being shut down or reduced.

Arming the Body

When the adrenaline hits the body the pupils dilate. They open up to let in as much light as possible and thus aid in threat recognition. The eyes, the only exposed part of the brain, relay information directly to the thalamus. The thalamus acts as the mixing and incorporation superhighway of sensory information blending the sights, sounds, and other sensory intake into terms the brain can understand. The thyroid gland dumps thyroglobulin, an iodine-containing protein, into the body, raising the metabolic rate. The result is to make more energy available for the body to use as necessary to defend itself.

In the lungs, the bronchioles dilate. The walls of the air pipes in the lungs become larger to allow more air to pass into the lungs. Hair stands on end to give the body a little larger area of sensory reception. The liver breaks down glycogen, which is the main form in which carbohydrate is stored in liver tissue. This breakdown of glycogen provides additional instant energy that helps keep up with the higher metabolic rate the thyroid has delivered.

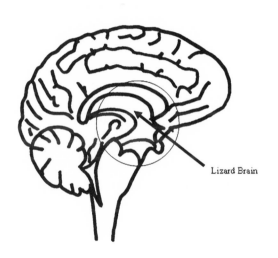

Lizard Brain

AMYGDALA.

The spleen, an organ located in the left of the abdomen near the stomach, which assists in the final destruction of red blood cells, filtration, and storage of blood, contracts, pumping out white blood cells to fight infection and platelets that assist in blood clotting. The skin vessels constrict causing sweat and cooling the body as it works above its normal operating limits. Meanwhile the adrenaline has hit the heart and blood pressure is up there as well. The body system is ready to perform, almost.

All Non-Essential Personnel

When the body goes on high alert, all bodily activities that don't have direct association with the "fight or flight" situation are reduced. The bladder that holds the urine and the colon that holds the feces prepare to void. The body does not need any extra weight and needs to reduce any infectious waste that could present a problem if it becomes injured. The stomach and the gastrointestinal tract constrict, redirecting blood to the muscles.

Now the body is, to use a military phrase, "locked and loaded." It is ready to respond to a threat. Since you are already adrenalized at this point, the more stressed you are through exertion, fear, or desperation in the face of danger, the harder it will be for you to perform appropriately in combat. Conversely, the more comprehensive and realistic your *dojo* training has been, the better you can expect to do. There are a lot of reasons why, some of which have been mentioned previously, but a paramount impact is the affect of adrenaline and elevated heart rate on your performance.

Due to the physiological effects we have discussed previously, your heart rate can jump from 60 or 70 beats per minute (BPM) to well over 200 BMP in less than half a second during a violent encounter. Here's how combat stress (accelerated heart rates) can affect you:

- For people whose resting heart rate is around 60 to 70 BPM, at around 115 BPM many people begin to lose fine motor skills such as finger dexterity, making it difficult to dial a phone, open a lock, or aim a weapon. While martial techniques requiring fine motor skills become less effective, those involving gross motor skills remain unaffected.

- Around 145 BPM, most people begin to lose their complex motor skills such as hand-eye coordination, precise tracking movements, or exact timing, making complicated techniques very challenging if not impossible to perform. Simple, straightforward applications, especially those involving pre-programmed muscle reflex actions, are quite feasible. Trained martial artists can operate very effectively in this range.

- Around 175 BPM most people begin to lose depth perception, experience tunnel vision, and sometimes even suffer temporary memory loss. It is very challenging to think logically at this point, yet conditioned gross motor responses are still effective.

- Around 185–220 BPM many people experience hyper-vigilance, loss of rational thought, and inability to consciously move or react. Without prior training, most people cannot function at this stress level. Even highly trained practitioners tend to experience degraded performance.

Brain Activity in Combat

"There are four brainwave states that range from the high amplitude, low frequency delta to the low amplitude, high frequency beta. These brainwave states range from deep dreamless sleep to high arousal. The same four brainwave states are common to the human species. Men, women and children of all ages experience the same characteristic brainwaves. They are consistent across cultures and country boundaries." [62]

– *Roger Traub, Ph.D.*

There are four levels of brain activity: beta, alpha, theta, and delta. Brain waves are scientifically recorded by measuring the fluctuating electrical impulses in the brain. Beta waves range from 14 to 30 cycles per second. Such pulses are indicative of a person who is fully awake, alert, excited, or tense. Alpha waves run from 8 to 13 cycles per second. They are characterized by deep relaxation, passive awareness, or a composed state of mind. Theta waves range from 4 to 7 cycles per second. They are indicative of a person who is drowsy, unconscious, or in a state of deep tranquility. Delta waves run from 0.5 to 3.5 cycles per second. They are characterized by sleep, unawareness, or deep unconsciousness.

The first two levels, beta and alpha, are the ones we are concerned with in martial arts. The brain discharges the beta wave when we are awake and intentionally focused; we are alert, ready for action, even irritated or afraid. This is because we are looking at the active mind. Beta is not as useful as alpha is to the martial artist. In a nutshell, beta is about thinking and thinking quite frequently gets you hit.

The alpha state is indicative of physical and mental relaxation, the relaxed, but alert mind. It is usually achieved during meditation. In the alpha state, we are aware of what is happening around us yet ultra-focused in our concentration. The professional athlete would call it being "in the zone," or being "in the flow." We have all heard of athletes that facing great impediments to their games such as the flu, an injury, or another tragedy, have excelled beyond what was expected. A large part of their success and performance directly results from an ability to shift into the alpha state of consciousness during competition.

One of the benefits to training in martial arts is the ability to switch between beta (waking brain waves) and alpha (or "the zone") brain waves. Multiple studies have shown that world-class athletes, no matter what the sport, have the ability to move their brain waves almost instantly from beta to alpha. This ability is also frequently demonstrated by martial artists as well. *Tamashiwara* (board-breaking) techniques are a good example. Concentration begins as the hand moves into chamber. By the time a practitioner's fist strikes a board or brick, his or her mind is fully in an alpha state. The target shatters effortlessly.

Zanshin means continuing mind. It is a state of enhanced awareness that should exist just before, during, and right after combat. A practitioner in this state should be hyper-aware of his or her surroundings and prepared for anything. He or she is working in an alpha state. A refined sense of *zanshin* can even help practitioners avoid conflict altogether.

Kane was once involved in a tournament where he was matched up against a competitor named David to whom he had lost to several times in the past. He recalls that on that particular day, however, his mental focus was absolute. While he may not have been as skilled or experienced as his opponent, he virtually knew what

David was going to do before it happened, easily defeating him. On that day his focus allowed him to defeat all challengers. Kane recalls, "Later on that afternoon David asked me for an unofficial rematch, complaining that he had not performed his best during the competition. I obliged, and then proceeded to win five straight matches in a row before he acknowledged defeat and bowed out. Such is the power of *zanshin*."

Non-diagnostic Response

"There is timing in the whole life of the warrior, in his thriving and declining, in his harmony and discord." [63]

– Miyamoto Musashi

Non-diagnostic response is unthinking awareness of and reaction to a threat. It literally means not having knowledge of what is going on.* We are not concerned with motives, thinking process, or anything else beyond the immediate. We are aware only that something threatening is happening to us.

For example, the amygdala does not care what kind of snake it sees slithering toward you in the grass, it is only concerned that you jump out of the way—get distance to protect yourself—and do it immediately. There is no assessment as to the age, size, or type of snake, it is just a snake. The advantages of non-diagnostic behavior are that you do not have to think.† One action solves many problems at the same time.

The brain screams, "Snake!" The immediate physical reaction is to clear distance and only then to assess. The same thing happens when a bee, wasp, or hornet buzzes by our ears. We jump first, and then figure out why. This is a natural evolutionary defense mechanism. Horses, deer and other animals do the same thing in response to a perceived threat—run, clear distance, then assess.

The exciting news is that it is possible to train this non-diagnostic stress response. If, for example, a soldier is under enemy fire and his or her gun jams, the immediate reaction is to clear the chamber. Compatriots screaming and bleeding around him, mortar rounds exploding, bullets whizzing, and shrapnel flying, are irrelevant. The soldier does just what he was trained to do.

The soldier does not analyze the problem. Training simply takes over. The gun is jammed; therefore he pulls back the slide, clears the chamber, aims and fires. This autonomic clearing action solves, perhaps, 19 of 20 common problems. If it does not work the first time, he does it again. Automatically. Finally, if it still does not work there are more procedures to follow. Most soldiers can fieldstrip their weapons by touch without even looking at them.

---

* And for our purposes not really recognizing anything outside of the blatantly obvious either.

† At certain elevated stress levels (e.g., above ~ 175 BPM, which is fairly common in combat), it is virtually impossible to think rationally anyway.

This is a life saving non-diagnostic response; the result of hundreds of hours of intense training and repetition. It is very similar to what martial artists go through when they practice *kata*. The concept of a non-diagnostic response translates readily to any martial art. After all, once you are engaged in combat, there is no time for thinking, only time for doing.

Wilder recalls an instructor at a seminar who was being peppered with questions from students such as, "should we move this way or that way," or "do we close here or open there?" He simply replied, "Just hit 'em!" This response cut right to the heart of the matter with a non-diagnostic response. This concept is at the very center of all martial arts. It can be applied to anything from fists to firearms.

Levels of Response

> *"Jiyu-kumite refers to the practice of using all the techniques you have learned until now against an opponent. You cannot be off your guard even a second. This is a very serious training method... You have to respect any opponent you have when you practice. In kumite, it is forbidden to attack your opponent with direct contact. As a principle, any technique you use will have to be stopped before it connects. However, when you are in defense, you have to practice as if you are actually being attacked. Any injuries in kumite are usually because of carelessness."* [64]

> – Gogen Yamaguchi

Levels of response in combat work like rungs on a ladder: starting with a natural neurological response, building upward to tactics, strategy, and finally culminating with control. The natural neurological response or twitch is the body's instinctive reaction to a threat. If a bee flies by your ear, you automatically shy away, ducking your head and throwing your arms up toward the noise. This flinch reaction happens whenever the lizard brain perceives a threat, the body moves out of the way and the hands rise to intercept danger.

Good defense tactics build upon the natural neurological reactions. So if the natural reaction is to duck and throw up your arms, the training would involve dropping into a controlled defensive posture with your arms up. While the gross physical movement is virtually identical, subtle details elevate the response from an unfocused flail to a defensive posture.

Strategy, as we have discussed, is the overarching architecture that coordinates tactics, helping us know how to choose the best tactic for any given situation. For example, it takes a much higher level of skill to move toward a threat (closing distance) rather than flinching away, even in a defensive posture. We move another step up the ladder of response by learning to work within a strategy.

Control is the highest form of response. By control we mean adapting strategy and choosing tactics as appropriate for a given situation. In sparring, for example, we must modify the strategy of controlling through physiological damage if we do not wish to injure our training partners. We consciously withhold the lethal aspects of our art physically while mentally knowing that it is there when we need it in a real life confrontation.

To assess any technique, the first and most critical test is to be absolutely sure that the control, strategy and tactics are built upon a natural neurological response. The natural response is based on the

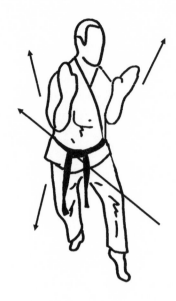

NATURAL FLINCH (STARTLE) REACTION—MOVING BACK WITH ARMS FLAILING UPWARD.

lowest level of the brain. The archipallium, often called the lizard or primitive brain, is the center of self-preservation and aggression. When the lizard brain is threatened it takes over. Any technique that counters this natural response cannot be executed swiftly or efficiently in the stress of actual combat.

Catching Bullets

"The effect known as the Bullet Catch has claimed the lives of at least 15 magicians who were killed in connection with this potentially lethal trick. In the effect, a bullet is fired directly at the performer, and he (or she) catches the bullet in the teeth, hopefully without any ill effects. There are a number of ways to perform this trick, and those that perform it as a stunt invite disaster. Sometimes things go wrong—equipment fails or worse. The most famous bullet-catching death was that of Chung Ling Soo (William Robinson), shot dead on stage in 1918." [65]

– Ben Robinson

Catching a "bullet," as we will use the term, refers to the idea of avoiding a blow without getting hit by moving your body out of the way, or by catching an opponent's fist with your hand. That's a very challenging thing to do. Your body is bigger than a

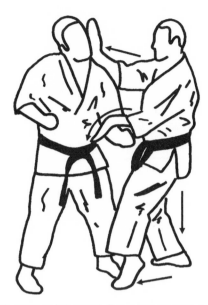

NEKO ASHI DACHI (CAT STANCE). THIS TRAINED REACTION HAS VIRTU-
ALLY THE SAME GROSS PHYSICAL MOVEMENTS AS THE NATURAL FLINCH
BUT CAN BE AN EFFECTIVE SELF-DEFENSE MOVEMENT SINCE THE BODY
IS PROPERLY ALIGNED TO RESPOND OFFENSIVELY OR DEFENSIVELY TO A
THREAT. BECAUSE THIS MOVEMENT FLOWS NATURALLY FROM THE NAT-
URAL FLINCH RESPONSE, IT BECOMES EASY TO PRACTICE, CONDITION,
AND ULTIMATELY UTILIZE IN COMBAT.

fist and Newton's first law of motion states that a body will remain at rest unless acted upon by some external force. There are two ways to get it moving—to let the impact of the blow move you, or to move all by yourself.

Clearly the latter is the best choice, yet a difficult one to pull off nevertheless. First you are moving a whole lot more mass than the fist coming toward you. Second, reaction is always slower than action. Third, you need to cover enough distance to avoid or cut off the blow.

Unless you are massively faster than your opponent, trying to dance away from a blow is virtually impossible. The only chance you have is to match hand to hand, because your and your opponent's hands have same mass and are the quickest parts of your body. You match speed-to-speed, mass-to-mass, and level-to-level.

It is impossible for a person to catch a punch that has been unloaded without a tell, something we commonly call a "sucker punch." A sucker punch gets its name because it catches the victim totally by surprise. Two critical elements are required for such a blow to be successful—close distance and pre-emptive strike. Close distance is touching range. Pre-emptive strike is jumping ahead in the aggression dance, an escalation process that typically contains name calling, pushing, and then ultimately striking, as opposed to simply hitting first.

That means you are going to stand in place until you need to move. Your body is bigger than a fist and needs more energy to move it, or even to get it started moving. Since you may not see a blow coming, and certainly will have little time to react, you must be extremely cautious about the range between you and a potential opponent.

Magicians routinely catch bullets in their mouths through the art of illusion. It's a dangerous trick where equipment failures have led to several deaths as the quote at the beginning of this section relates. They cannot do it for real, so they cheat.*

---

* Entertainers Penn and Teller make a big deal about this fact in their magic act, partly for comedic value and partly for fear that some goof-ball in the audience will try to shoot one of them for real. (At least one magician, Raoul Curran, died that way in 1880 and one or two oth-ers may have had similar fates.) Even though everyone knows it is just an illusion, their bullet catching act is suspenseful, entertaining, and carries an element of real danger. If you want to know how it is done, one partner pretends to load a gun with a marked bullet, palms the real cartridge, and then fires a blank round at the other through a pane of glass that is rigged to shatter with the shot, giving the appearance that a real bullet was discharged and traveled through. While the audience is distracted, the other slips a "marked" bullet into his mouth to complete the illusion. Many other illusionists have been injured by flying glass shards while performing this trick.

Similarly, there are tactics that martial arts practitioners can use to cheat, helping them catch the metaphorical bullets of their enemies' blows. One method is what we call "stealing time."

Stealing Time

"Sharp reflexes are absolutely mandatory for self-defense. Without them you are just a walking heavy bag for anyone wanting to do a little bag work. The good news is that sharp reflexes are not hard to develop and they are even easier to maintain. But you do have to make the effort." [66]

– Loren Christensen

Action is by definition faster that reaction. One of the reasons that martial artists are taught never to retreat straight backward is that such movements cede all advantage to the attacker. Moving backward can give action performed more time to be completed. It increases the amount of time the attacker has to execute what he or she already has set in motion. Giving the attacker the luxury of more time is unwise strategically as well as tactically.

If you move straight back, it would appear that you have given yourself more time to defend. While you have, the challenge is that such movements add time equally to both the attacker *and* the defender. Since action is still faster than reaction, the advantage remains with the attacker. You just delay the inevitable by a tiny fraction.

However if you can move in a way that steals time, you can gain an instant of advantage. If you can take time away from the attacker, you even the odds. This is most commonly done by moving into the attack and cutting it off. If you can intercept an attack before it builds up to full speed you not only buy yourself time, but you reduce the damage caused should you actually get hit.

Moving into an attack may seem counterintuitive. Let's use the analogy of a demolition derby* to explain: For the sake of argument, there are two cars in this hypothetical demolition derby. Car 1 is stationary, while Car 2 is behind it and moving forward. Car 2 takes a bead on Car 1 and accelerates to full speed before impact. The driver of the attacking car judged the time and distance and set out to crash his car into the stationary car per the rules of the derby. Car 1 takes the brunt of the damage.

Now let us change that formula a little. Car 1 sees Car 2 bearing down on it from behind and begins to pull away. Even at full speed, the impact is less, as Car 1 was moving away from Car 2 and its energy. Less energy was available to transfer from Car 2 into Car 1.

---

* For those who don't already know, a demolition derby is a motor sport. While rules vary from event to event, the typical demolition derby event consists of ten or more drivers competing by deliberately ramming their vehicles into one another to render them inoperable. The last driver whose vehicle is still operational is declared the winner.

Now a third version: Car 1 sees Car 2 starting to accelerate from out his rear window. Car 1 drops into reverse and accelerates crashing into Car 2 before Car 2 could get much speed. The result is that Car 2 was never able to get to top speed and make the most damage possible from the impact. Further, the initial amount of time Car 2 determined it would take to strike Car 1 was cut in half. Car 1 stole time from Car 2.

Just as Car 1 stole time from Car 2 by meeting its force head on, so too blocks can cut off an attacker's technique before it gains too much speed and power. Reach out and meet the attack, catching it as close to your adversary's body as possible. There are several drills that can get you better acquainted with this concept. Our favorite is called, "up against the wall." Here is how it works:

Choose a partner. *Uke*, the person defending (performing the techniques) stands about a half a foot away from one wall of the *dojo* (not too close to a corner). *Tori* (the attacker) begins throwing punches at *uke*, starting at about half speed. *Uke*'s job is to not get hit. The trick is that *uke* is not allowed to use his or her hands or arms for defense. *Uke* must dodge each blow. Since there is a wall at his or her back, *uke* is unable to back away. After a few repetitions the partners should switch roles.

Practitioners should quickly discover that moving out toward the attacker at an angle is the best defense. Not only does it keep them safe from being hit, but it also puts them in a strategic position to counterattack.*

Once both partners have tried this as a moving drill at half speed, the tempo can gradually be cranked up. The next step is to allow *uke* to use his or her arms. Combining body shifting with aggressive blocking, *uke* should be able to cut off and avoid any attack. Once again, the diagonal body shift closes distance while keeping *uke* safe.

Once both parties are able to successfully perform this maneuver at full speed without getting hit, they can slow things down again and begin working on counterattacks—blocks that work like strikes. Because we do not recommend protective gear, it is best not to do this at full speed until both practitioners are competently skilled.

Speed Kills!

> *"Response time combines the time it takes you to perceive a threat, choose a response, set that response in motion, and complete the motion… All the scientific studies, not to mention just pure logic, tell us that the fewer choices we have to make, the faster our reflexes will be offensively and defensively."* [67]

> – *Loren Christensen*

---

* If they were allowed to use their arms at this point in the drill.

Speed kills! And we mean that in a good way. In a fight, the fastest person is vastly more likely to win. Your speed keeps an opponent off balance with rapid-fire attacks, and also disrupts your enemy and makes him or her increasingly vulnerable. Training for speed is critical for survival in a violent encounter.

To become fast you cannot leave any part of your body behind. While it is critical to attack strongly, swiftly, and with intent to end the fight immediately, an incorrect attempt to do so may cause you to become slow, unduly exposing yourself to danger. The whole body must move in one coordinated (and fast) assault.

For example, many practitioners leave their fist in chamber when stepping in *zenkutsu dachi* (front forward stance), so what you see is step *and* punch rather than step/punch. This is a bad habit! It leaves you exposed because your attacking fist is held in chamber too long before being deployed at the completion of the step.

In martial arts, the fist is technically neutral; it is neither attacking nor defending. It is possible for an attack to be a defense if it is swift, cutting off the aggressor's attack before it reaches the target. But you cannot do that if you leave your limb behind you. The punch should lead slightly with your whole body following immediately behind.

In the ancient world, the Spartans, the Romans, and the army of Alexander the Great all used variations of a phalanx.* The phalanx (or "pikeman's square" as it later evolved) was a well-coordinated group of infantrymen who attacked or defended themselves from behind an interlocking wall of shields. Protruding from behind this wall of shields was a veritable forest of swords and spears, all of which pointed directly toward the enemy.

Once assembled the phalanx began moving toward the adversary's army, grinding through them in a disciplined killing march. The significant point for the modern martial artist is that all the weapons were forward toward the enemy with nothing held back. The weapon and the platform, in this instance the infantryman, all moved in unison. Clearly the phalanx in its various incarnations was extremely effective in battle. If not it would have been quickly discarded in favor of something else.

The phalanx was used by the most successful armies of the times. The significant point of the phalanx is to lead with the weapon and protect the platform from which it is launched, striking fast and repeatedly. This lesson should not be lost on the martial artist. To engage in a violent situation with the intention of stepping and striking is as foolish as a Spartan meeting the enemy with his sword still in his sheath, waiting to brandish it once he has arrived in contact with his enemy.

So how does one get faster? Connecting all the parts, moving as one with all weapons pointed at the enemy, is the first piece of the puzzle. There are no tricks or traps to lure your attacker into some secret technique. A skilled opponent will use the opportunity provided by your feint to overwhelm and defeat you. In a real fight,

---

* Derived from the Greek word *phalangos*, meaning "line of battle"

there is only attack, attack, and attack! Keeping all your weapons on target allows any to be used at the point of attack or defense.

To be fast, you must close distance and stay in range. You do not need to get there to defend or attack if you are already there. Because action is faster than reaction, if you need to get there you are already too late. Be there already, or at the least be close. Do not leave your weapon behind. You need to have it move at the same rate or even faster than the rest of your body.

Control your falling. Take charge of your body to avoid any uncontrolled actions. When you walk over a flat surface, for example, you are really just putting yourself in a state of balance from imbalance—standing on one foot, leaning your center of gravity slightly forward, and then gently falling onto your next foot. It is a slight motion, yet it is done so frequently that most people do not think or feel it as such. If you step over an unexpected curb or misjudge the height of a stair, however, it becomes instantly obvious that normal walking is an imbalanced movement.

Budo walking, on the other hand, involves gliding across a surface. The foot never really leaves the ground; hence there is little or no imbalance. If you are leaning during movement or throughout a technique, then you are falling, even for a split second, thus you are out of control. Do not lean! It is easy to lean into a technique in that it allows you to conserve muscle activity. Whenever you are out of control, however, you can be taken advantage of. There is little you can do about it except try to recover (e.g., the missed stair step). Once again, in reacting and trying to recover, you are damned by the fact that action is fast and reaction is slow.

It is clear then that a practitioner must move as one unit, but how do we do so really fast? The most essential ingredient is relaxation. Loose, relaxed muscles move much more quickly than hard, tensed ones. Try this drill: pick a stance, any stance, lock down all your muscles straining as hard as you can. Force your breath out and hold it. Now, try to take a step forward without staggering like Frankenstein's Monster. It cannot be done. Until you relax your muscles and breathe, you cannot move smoothly. The only time a *budoka* should be tense is at the moment of impact, when his or her blow strikes the enemy. All other movements should be relaxed and flowing. From this comes maximum speed.

Chojun Miyagi *Sensei*, the founder of *Goju Ryu* karate was said to be obsessed with *sanchin kata*, believing it to be the core of all martial teaching. In *sanchin kata*, practitioners perform the movements slowly in a precisely controlled way. It is, in essence, a moving meditation as much as it is a *kata*. All body parts are aligned and integrated in the best method for each technique. Breathing is forceful and exaggerated, timed exactly with each movement such that exhalation matches hard techniques (e.g., punch, block) and inhalations match soft techniques (e.g., movement, return to chamber). Punches and blocks are slow and precise, demonstrating the essential relaxed movement followed by a tensing of the entire body at the moment of impact. In this fashion practitioners can enhance their ability to move their whole body at once, learning maximum speed and power.

Not all of us have a high propensity of fast twitch muscles.* Even if we do, the older we gets, the slower we become. To be really fast, you have to reduce your response time. Response time is a summation of the amount of time it takes you to perceive a threat, choose a response, set that response in motion, and then complete that motion. This concept is frequently explained as the OODA (Observation, Orientation, Decision, and Action) loop, or Boyd's law.†

Here's how the Boyd's law works: each party to a confrontation begins by observing themselves, their physical surroundings, and their adversary. This takes a quantifiable amount of time, which delays immediate action, even if only by milliseconds. Next each combatant must orient himself by making a mental image of the tactical situation, building on past experiences to interpolate the current environment before deciding how best to respond. Because it is impossible to process information as quickly as we perceive it, there is also an orientation delay that precedes any action a person chooses to take. This decision ultimately takes into account the various factors present at the time of the orientation. Once deciding upon an appropriate response, there is another delay between thought and action.

A person who can consistently go through Boyd's cycle faster than his or her opponent gains a tremendous advantage. By the time the slower person reacts, the faster one may already be doing something different so the defensive action is less effective than anticipated. With each OODA cycle, the effectiveness of the slower party's action becomes more and more diminished. Boyd's theory dictates that the aggregate resolution of these cyclic episodes will eventually determine the outcome of a conflict. Consequently, the better trained a person is and the fewer choices he has to make, the faster his response time will be, both offensively and defensively. The key is to keep it simple.‡

In the old days, traditional practitioners would spend many, many years learning a single *kata*. They would study it in depth, learning all the subtle nuances and internalizing the movements until the techniques became second nature. Conditioned muscle memory would simply react to threat without delay, setting a response in motion without any conscious thought. This type of training dramatically shortens the OODA cycle. Today, many systems require practitioners to learn a dozen or more *kata* by *shodan* level, something typically attained in a mere four to six years (on average).

While there is nothing wrong with knowing a lot of *kata*, at some point practitioners should focus primarily on one or two for use in self-defense situations. Most

---

* Fast twitch muscles provide rapid movement for short periods of time, giving you strength and speed in a fight. They use glycogen rather than oxygen, requiring anaerobic enzymes to produce power. Glycogen is stored in the muscles and liver and is synthesized by the body using carbohydrates. Slow twitch muscles, on the other hand, have a slower contraction times. They use oxygen for power and have a predominance of aerobic enzymes. These types of muscles are large muscles found in the legs, thigh, trunk, back, hips and are used for holding posture, body alignment, and similar tasks. Genetic differences can determine the propensity of fast or slow twitch muscles for each individual person.

† Named for military strategist Colonel John R. Boyd who codified it as a way of quantifying reaction times in combat.

‡ Remember the Decision Stick in chapter 2?

will not be ready to do that until they have completed the core curricula of their system and really know the key features and functions of each and every *kata*. Regardless, with as few as two or three *kata*, you can get a good feeling for what works with your body type, physical condition, personality, and predilections.

Choose one *kata* and practice it aggressively, doing it repeatedly until you can go through it without thought. Like typing by touch or riding a bike, eventually it should happen naturally. Do the *kata* in various conditions (e.g., darkness, daylight, rain, direct sun) and terrain (e.g., indoors, outdoors, hills, sandy beaches, rocky riverbeds, stairwells). Try it blindfolded. Reverse the pattern, performing techniques originally shown to the left on the right and vice versa. Change the *enbusen*; if you normally begin facing north, practice performing the *kata* facing south or east or west.

Break it down into component parts and try them with a training partner. Think about it throughout the day. Study it thoroughly, and decipher all of its secret applications. The end result of all your hard work should be a simple, well-understood, and neurologically preset group of applications from your favorite *kata*. Such applications are your "get out of danger free" card, helping you survive most any violent encounter.*

Vital Points (Kyushu)

"For many, that missing ingredient is a true and thorough knowledge of the body's vital points: what they are, where they are, how to quickly find them under duress, how to use them, constructively or for destruction—and how to recognize them in kata, hyung, or forms they thought they knew so well." [68]

– Rick Clark

By now we have drummed into your head that every movement in *kata* has practical self-defense applications. If you accurately strike or grab an attacker's vital area you can elicit pain, temporary paralysis, dislocation or hyperextension of a joint, knockout, or possibly even death. Vital areas are different than pressure points. They are mechanically weak areas that are easy to break on anyone, regardless of size, build, or conditioning. As we have previously discussed, *kata* demonstrate the proper angle, direction, and preferred target of attack for each application.

Because the strategy of *Goju Ryu* (as with most martial arts) recognizes that only physiological damage is guaranteed to stop a determined opponent, it is essential to understand weak areas of the human body that can be targeted. Since there are only a limited number of vital areas on the human body, almost all martial styles target these same points in similar ways:

---

* Bill Burger wrote a fascinating book about this concept called *Five Years, One Kata: Putting Kata Back Into The Heart Of Karate* (Martial Arts Publishing, 2003). It is well worth a read.

Vital Area Descriptions

Kyushu waza (vital area attacks) is extremely dangerous stuff. Please do not abuse this knowledge. Such areas should only be forcefully struck in true life-or-death, self-defense situations from which you can only escape through violence. It is wise to avoid such confrontations altogether, of course, but if you are forced to fight kata, demonstrate how to end such confrontations quickly. The shorter the fight the more likely you are to survive.

Name	Description
Tendo	The *Bubishi* calls the *tendo/tento* region the "sacred gates," restricted areas that should not be struck due to the fatal affects of doing so. *Tendo* is located at the crown of the head, at the coronal suture. If struck hard enough, the frontal bone can dislocate causing severe damage to the motor regions of the brain, which will result in paralysis or death.
Tento	Located at the fontanelle, or space between the crown of the head and the forehead. A hard blow to this area will cause fatal damage to the brain and cranial nerves.
Komekami	The temple. Located at the sides of the head, about two finger-widths back from the eye on each side. This is the weakest structural area of the skull where it flattens because curves are architecturally much stronger than flat surfaces. A hard strike to the temple can cause massive hemorrhaging of the meningeal artery, coma, and eventually death.
Mimi	Ears. A concussive slap to the ears can cause pain, disorientation, and severe trauma to the eardrum.
Miken	The summit of the nose in the center of the forehead. A strong blow here will shock the frontal lobes causing unconsciousness, while a severe blow will cause death.
Seidon	Circumorbital region above and below the eyes. Strikes to this area can transmit shock to the frontal lobes of the brain resulting in unconsciousness.
Gansei	Eyeballs. Clearly a weak point; eye strikes can cause anything from watering to blindness depending upon the severity. When the opponent is standing the eyes are usually attacked with a raking motion. When he or she is on the ground such that the head can be immobilized, gauges or displacements may be used. This is frequently done by pressing the thumb or a finger into the side of the socket, which displaces and ejects the eyeball. Excruciating pain and psychological trauma from this type of application usually render the victim unconscious.
Jinchu	Intermaxillary suture just under the nose. The nerves are very close to the surface in this area such that even a light blow can cause pain, watery eyes, and disruption in most people. Strong blows

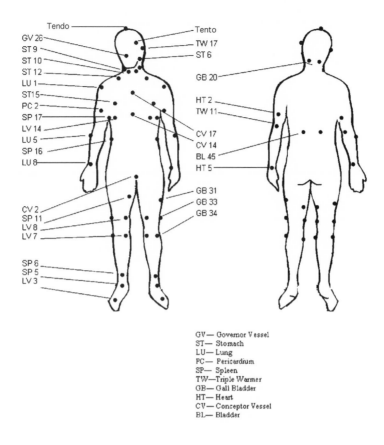

Tendo
GV 26
ST 9
ST 10
ST 12
LU 1
ST15
PC 2
SP 17
LV 14
LU 5
SP 16
LU 8

Tento
TW 17
ST 6
GB 20
HT 2
TW 11
CV 17
CV 14
BL 45
HT 5

CV 2
SP 11
LV 8
LV 7

GB 31
GB 33
GB 34

SP 6
SP 5
LV 3

GV— Governor Vessel
ST— Stomach
LU— Lung
PC— Pericardium
SP— Spleen
TW—Triple Warmer
GB— Gall Bladder
HT— Heart
CV— Conceptor Vessel
BL— Bladder

COMMON VITAL AREAS ATTACKED IN *GOJU RYU KATA.*

transmit shock through the upper jawbones into the braincase causing unconsciousness or death.

Gekon   Center of the lower jaw just beneath the lower lip. A blow here
transmits shock through the jaw into the inner ear, shaking the
brain. Injuries can include broken teeth, dislocation of the jaw,
whiplash, dizziness, or unconsciousness. Really severe blows such
as those from mass weapons (e.g., baseball bat, *bo*, *tonfa*, hammer)
or vehicle accidents could dislocate the skull from the top of the
spinal column resulting in instant death.

Mikazuki   Base of the jaw or mandible. Like *gekon*, blows to this location can
break or dislocate the jaw. If the angle is correct, a good stiff blow
will lead to unconsciousness. Shock to the facial nerve may addi-
tionally cause temporary or permanent paralysis in whichever side
of the face was struck.

* Throws which use the opponent's head for control/leverage.

Dokko	Located at the mastoid process, behind the ears at the side of the neck. Blows to this area affect the facial nerve, cause pain, and rapid disorientation. Neck "cranks"* are often performed in this area as well.
Keichu	Back (or nape) of the neck. Located at the third intervertebral space, this is the weakest point of the spinal column. A strong blow here will cause disorientation, unconsciousness, paralysis, or death depending on severity.
Matsukaze	Carotid Sinus. Located at the side of the neck in front of the sternocleidomastoid muscle, a blow to this area can disrupt the baroreceptors, which regulate blood pressure (flowing through the carotid artery) into the brain. This causes the heart rate to instantly, though temporarily, drop leading to disorientation or unconsciousness. This point is also used for strangulation techniques where applying pressure can cut off the blood flow leading to unconsciousness or death. It has also been used by emergency room technicians and paramedics to temporarily stave off dangerously high blood pressure until medication can be administered.
Hichu	Base of the throat at the Adam's apple, or projection of the thyroid cartilage of the larynx, or suprasternal notch. The windpipe is very vulnerable at this location. A blow here can crush the cartilage of the trachea leading to suffocation and death. A finger jab or push can elicit severe pain.
Danchu	Located at the summit of the breastbone, where the manubrium and sternum meet. A strong blow here can cause trauma to the heart, bronchus, lungs, thoracic nerves, and/or pulmonary arteries leading to unconsciousness or death.
Kyosen	Xiphoid process. Striking this point (particularly with a rising blow) can bruise the heart, liver, and/or stomach leading to unconsciousness or possibly even death.
Suigetsu	Solar plexus. Just below the xiphoid process, a blow to this area can shock the diaphragm rendering the recipient temporarily incapable of breathing. A powerful blow in this area can cause internal bleeding in the stomach and/or liver leading to severe pain, unconsciousness, and even death.
Kyoei	Located at the subaxillary region below the armpits, approximately the spot between the fifth and sixth ribs. A strong blow here, especially when performed with a single knuckle, can cause trauma to the lungs disrupting breathing. This area can also be raked with a knuckle causing considerable pain in many, but not all, people.
Ganchu	Spot below the nipples at the ends of the fifth and sixth ribs. Blows to this area can fracture the ribs and/or cause lung trauma, disrupting breathing.
Denko	Located at the hypochondriac region between the seventh and eighth ribs, approximately one hand width below the solar plexus. A blow to the right side can severely damage the liver causing inter-

nal bleeding. A blow to the left side can damage the stomach and/or spleen, once again causing internal bleeding. Either blow can have fatal consequences.

Ushiro Denko   Kidneys. A strong blow to this region can cause internal bleeding, shock, and death. This area is frequently targeted via kicking techniques.

Inazuma   Floating ribs. The eleventh and twelfth ribs are only attached at one end making them more vulnerable than other ribs to breakage. Similar to *denko*, a blow to the right side can damage the liver while a blow to the left can damage the stomach and/or spleen.

Myojo   At the *tanden*, approximately one inch below the navel (where your *obi* knot is tied). A strong downward blow to this area can damage the bladder and large intestine causing extreme pain and loss of bladder control. This is the primary aim point for a basic *gedan tsuki* (down punch).

Wanshun   Back of the arm, located at the top of the outside edge of the upper arm. A strike to this area can affect the radial nerve, causing pain and weakness. A forceful rub in this area affects the triple warmer (plexus of the radial, ulnar, and medial nerves), causing pain in many individuals and an involuntary rotation of the arm, which facilitates controlling techniques such as an arm bar.

Hijizume   Elbow joint. A strike to the area about an inch above the elbow will affect the ulnar nerve (this area is sometimes referred to as the funny bone), causing pain and weakness. The joint itself can be dislocated or hyperextended rendering the arm unusable for combat.

Kote   Wrist. The joint itself can be dislocated or hyperextended resulting in temporary or permanent loss of use of the hand. The wrist is much harder to damage using joint manipulation techniques than the elbow or shoulder, however.

Uchijakuzawa   Located at the inside of the wrist where the pulse can be felt. A blow here can affect the median nerve eliciting pain and weakness. Arteries are very close to the surface in this area making them vulnerable to damage, especially from edged weapons. The joint itself can be dislocated or hyperextended.

Sotojakuzawa   Outside (back) of the wrist. A blow to the back of the wrist can affect the median nerve eliciting pain and weakening the grip. The joint itself can be dislocated or hyperextended.

Shuko   Located on the back of the hand. The radial nerve is exposed between the thumb and index finger, and the radial and ulnar nerves meet between the knuckles of the middle and ring fingers. A sharp blow to these areas will cause additional pain and weakness, though a powerful strike to anywhere along the back of the hand can damage delicate bones. Digging the knuckles into the back of an opponent's hand can break his or her grip. The fingers themselves may be attacked as well.

Kinteki	Groin. An obviously delicate area of the male anatomy; severe blows to this region can elicit pain, shock, nausea, vomiting, unconsciousness, or even death. A firm grab to this area can also be incapacitating. Upward blows to the pelvic girdle of a female opponent can elicit similar results, though it takes a bit more force and accuracy.
Bitei	Base of the spine at the coccyx. Because the major nerves feeding the lower limbs originate in this sacral plexus region at the tailbone, a blow to this area can elicit severe pain. Further, the tailbone itself is fairly easy to break with an upward strike severely hampering an opponent's ability to move.
Yaku	Located at the inguinal region inside the upper thigh where it joins with the torso. A strike to this area can affect the femoral artery as well as the femoral nerve, weakening the whole leg. A severe blow can cause temporary paralysis.
Ushiro Inazuma	Gluteal fold, just below the buttocks. The sciatic nerve, the largest in the body, is located here. A solid blow will cause cramping, loss of control of the leg, and pain throughout the hips and abdomen.
Fukuto	Lateral part of the lower thigh, about halfway down on the outside of the vastus lateralis (the large muscle). A blow here can cause pain and temporary paralysis of the thigh. This target is commonly kicked with the practitioner's shin to break down an opponent and disrupt his or her balance and stance integrity.
Hizakansetsu	Knee joint. One of the weakest areas of the human body when struck from the proper angle, this joint can be hyperextended or dislocated to disrupt balance and effectively take an opponent out of a fight.
Kokotsu	Center point of the tibia (shin bone) and fibula (splint bone on the outside of the leg). A blow delivered about two-thirds of the way down the shin can hit the peroneal nerve, eliciting pain and weakening the leg.
Uchikurobushi	Ankle joint. This joint may be hyperextended, dislocated, or simply crushed by a solid blow, causing severe pain, disabling an opponent's balance, and reducing the ability to move and fight.
Kori	Instep. A blow to the upper surface of the instep can damage the plantar and peroneal nerves causing pain throughout the leg, hip, and abdomen, weakening the leg.
Kusagakure	Located at the outside edge of the top of the foot. Like the hand, small bones in the foot are easily crushed, disabling an opponent's balance and reducing the ability to move and fight.
Sobi	Base of the calf. Blows to the inside of the lower leg at the base of the calf can cause pain and temporary paralysis of the leg muscles.

Summary

"We sleep safe in our beds because rough men stand ready in the night to visit violence on those who would do us harm." [69]

– George Orwell

Traditional practitioners in Okinawa, Japan, and China spent many, many years learning a single *kata*. Many of the ancient masters only practiced two or three. They would study these in great depth, learning all the subtle nuances and internalizing the movements until they became second nature. Over thousands of hours of intense training and repetition, these practitioners could react in a non-diagnostic manner, letting conditioned muscle memory to respond to a threat instantly without conscious thought. After all, once you are engaged in combat, there is no time for thinking, only time for doing.

To attack or defend effectively, you cannot leave any part of your body behind. While it is critical to attack strongly, swiftly, and with intent to end the fight immediately, an incorrect attempt to do so may cause you to become slow, unduly exposing yourself to danger. The whole body must move in one coordinated assault.

To be really fast, you also have to reduce your response time. Response time is a summation of the amount of time it takes you to perceive a threat, choose a response, set that response in motion, and then complete that motion. This concept is frequently explained as the OODA (Observation, Orientation, Decision, and Action) loop, or Boyd's law. A combatant who cycles through the OODA loop faster than his opponent invariably wins the battle.

The ancient fighting arts were developed to deal with real violence. Modern practitioners too, must be able to use their martial skills to defend themselves in unavoidable real-life confrontations. Understanding the characteristics of violence and of the perpetrators thereof can help practitioners remain safe. Violence can stem from fear, frenzy, tantrum, or criminal aggression. Criminals include amateurs, professionals, psychopaths, drug addicts, sex predators, gang members, and terrorists.

The ancient masters practiced their *kata* in every conceivable environment and so too should we. It is important to understand how you might interpret applications from your *kata* should you be fighting on a hill, in a vehicle, around furniture or other obstacles, in a stairwell, under water, in a crowd, or in any other unusual situation. Not only do you need to be able to perform your techniques wearing a traditional loose-fitting *gi*, but in restrictive street clothes as well.

Response to a real threat works like rungs on a ladder. The foundation must be built upon a natural neurological response, taking advantage of our brain chemistry and autonomic reactions. You cannot train counter to these natural physiological responses and expect to be able to deploy your training in actual combat. Tactics and strategy build upon this foundation, synergistically working with the body's natural physiological reactions. Control, the highest form, brings these components together to create a martial art. By control we mean adapting strategy and choosing tactics as appropriate for a given situation.

The best self-defense is avoiding a fight altogether. Even when a person legitimately uses force in order to escape an imminent and unavoidable danger, he or she still has to live with the physiological and psychological results of doing so, as well as the potential for expensive and protracted litigation.

Once a conflict occurs, however, practitioners must do everything they can to end it quickly. They have to be at least as ruthless and violent as their attackers. Unlike sparring in the *dojo*, vital points are most certainly not off limits. They are the only targets that matter, required knowledge for survival in self-defense situations because nonvital targets will not stop a determined attacker.

Every movement in *kata* has practical self-defense applications. If you accurately strike or grab an attacker's vital area you can elicit pain, temporary paralysis, dislocation or hyperextension of a joint, knockout, or possibly even death. *Kyushu* (vital area attacks) is very dangerous stuff and should only be used in true life-or-death emergencies.

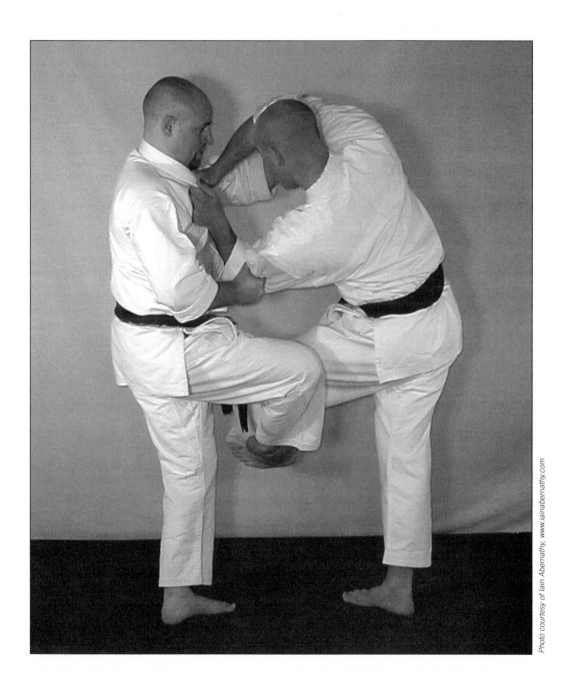

Photo courtesy of Iain Abernathy, www.iainabernathy.com

NAIHANCHI THROW. IAIN ABERNETHY APPLIES A SWEEP FROM *NAIHANCHI (TEKKI) KATA.* THIS TECHNIQUE IS AN APPLICATION OF THE "RETURNING WAVE KICK" AND "REINFORCED BLOCK" MOVEMENTS IN THAT *KATA.* THE RECIPIENT IS PAUL CARTMELL.

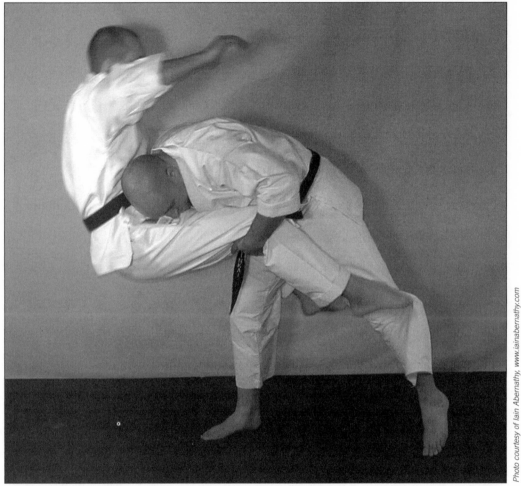

Photo courtesy of Iain Abernathy, www.iainabernathy.com

PASSAI TAKEDOWN. IAIN ABERNETHY APPLIES A DOUBLE-LEG-LIFT TAKEDOWN FROM *PASSAI (BASSAI-DAI) KATA*. THIS TECHNIQUE IS ATTRIBUTED TO *PASSAI* IN GICHIN FUNAKOSHI'S 1925 BOOK *RENTAN GOSHIN KARATE JUTSU*. THE RECIPIENT IS CRAIG STRICKLAND.

CHAPTER 6

Process

*"A process cannot be understood by stopping it. Understanding must move with
the flow of the process, must join it and flow with it."* [70]

– Frank Herbert

By now you should have a good understanding of strategy and tactics along with
the various principles and rules outlined herein that can help you identify the *okuden waza* in your *kata*. The simplest interpretation of most any *kata* sequence is, as
we know by now, almost always sub-optimal. If you adopt the guidelines we have
proposed and make them your own, you will have the power to get the most out of
your martial art. This chapter helps you understand more about how to do that.

Bringing It All Together

"It may seem difficult at first, but everything is difficult at first." [71]

– Miyamoto Musashi

To begin let's use one of the simplest movements in *kata*, a *jodan uke* (head
block). In *gekisai kata*, practitioners begin with a 90 degree turn to the left then execute the *jodan uke*. All but the newest of practitioners have practiced this movement
hundreds of times, yet few understand what it is truly telling them. For example, the
most commonly practiced *bunkai* is a simple block of a straight punch.* Here is
what this looks like. For this series of illustrations the attacker is on the right and
the defender is on the left:

Not a particularly strong application is it? Yes, it keeps you from getting hit, but
momentum is still in the opponent's court. You have done nothing to keep your
attacker from punching at you again. You have done nothing to end the fight, only
to survive. By now you understand that the ancient masters were a bit more proac-
tive than that. Let's analyze this technique using all of the materials outlined previously in this text to find out what is actually being demonstrated through this *kata*
movement.

---

* It is actually *henka waza* as it is done stepping back away from the punch rather than moving forward into it as implied by the initial
shift/turn in the *kata*.

181

Our first Principle* states that there is more than one proper application for any *kata* movement. Consequently whatever we decipher is only one interpretation. What we should strive for is to define the *best* interpretation for our own body types, personalities, and predilections. Our chosen tactic(s) must also be consistent with the strategy of the art. In *Goju Ryu*, that strategy is to close distance, imbalance, and use physiological damage to incapacitate an opponent. Since the simplest *bunkai* we offered initially does not seem to accomplish any of these things, it should to be discarded in favor of something better.

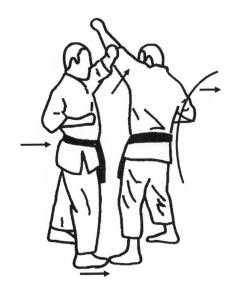

JODAN UKE (HEAD BLOCK). DEFENDER IS ON THE LEFT.

Principle 2[†] states that every technique should be able to end the fight immediately, hardly the case with the simple block. Combining this with Rule 8[‡] indicates that something more must be going on than the simple block that was initially taught. According to Rule 1,[§] advancing movements are offensive in nature. The initial 90-degree turn may be a bit misleading, but using Rule 1 to avoid being confused by the *enbusen*, it becomes clear that you actually do advance (slightly) prior to executing the head block technique. The pivot shows us the virtue of getting off-line, which is much safer than meeting an attack head on. As Rule 9[||] declares, our *kata* must demonstrate the proper angle.

Not only does the *Goju Ryu* strategy encourage attacking at an angle, but also because beginning practitioners need every advantage they can get, this *kihon kata* demonstrates a shift in its very first movement. Once the body is out of the way,[¶] the application can begin. To be clearer though, to the creator of the *kata* certainly did not expect the *budoka* to stand there like an idiot until the punch is on the way, then shift and counter. You are simply getting the hint that a straight on confrontation is unwise.

Taken together, these principles and rules beg you to find an offensive, fight ending interpretation for the technique. Rule 6** tells you to utilize the shortest dis-

---

* Principle 1—*there is more than one proper interpretation of any movement.*

† Principle 2—*every technique should be able to end the fight immediately.*

‡ Rule 8—*there is no block.*

§ Rule 1—*don't be deceived by the enbusen.*

|| Rule 9—*kata demonstrates the proper angle.*

¶ Principle 10—*if you are not there you cannot get hit.*

** Rule 6—*utilize the shortest distance to your opponent.*

tance to the opponent. So, prior to executing a head block with your left hand, the right hand actually performs a check or deflection of the opponent's punch (it's the closet limb). The block then, becomes a controlling movement. As Principle 14* declares, both hands are involved in the defensive technique. Further application of Principle 3† adds another layer to the technique showing the deflection prior to the block as more of an attack than a defense. In other words, using our check/control methodology while moving forward allows you to aggressively cut off the punch rather than passively waiting for it to arrive.

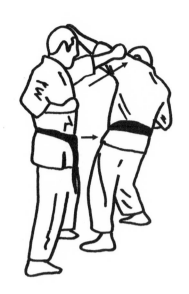

CONTROLLING WITH *JODAN UKE* (HEAD BLOCK).
DEFENDER IS ON THE LEFT

This is a much better interpretation; however, it is still way too defensive in nature. Only the arm has been attacked (by your check or deflection). An arm deflection is unlikely to stop a fight in and of itself, so let's delve a bit deeper using Principle 8‡ to examine this portion of the technique in depth.

There is no reason to assume that the strike to the opponent's arm with our hand is the only way to check or deflect the attacker's punch. We have an entire arm to use for defense. Since we have moved off-line to receive this attack, the goal is to shift to the outside and close the opponent. Obviously contact with the enemy in real life affords all sorts of opportunities to have plans disrupted or altered, but for the moment we will assume success. When closing an opponent, we strike at or above the elbow. That affords the greatest opportunity to cut off the attack and use mechanical leverage to overpower the opponent. It also protects against a follow-on elbow strike. When opening an opponent, we strike below the elbow to avoid a follow-on hammerfist or whipping attack.

So, if you are going to perform this deflection at full speed and power§ to stop a determined attacker,‖ you are probably aiming at or near the elbow. A good shot there will not only disrupt the attack, but if you are lucky it will also hyperextend the attacker's arm or otherwise damage the joint. Further, if this is done with your arm, your hand remains free to engage in more crafty fun.

* Principle 14—*use both hands.*
† Principle 3—*strike to disrupt; disrupt to strike.*
‡ Principle 8—*strive to understand how it works.*
§ Principle 6—*full speed and power.*
‖ Principle 7—*it must work on an unwilling partner.*

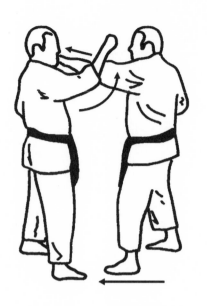

CHECK AS ELBOW STRIKE. AS THE PUNCH COMES IN THE DEFENDER (LEFT) STRIKES HIS OPPONENT'S LIMB WITH AN INSIDE CHECK/DEFLECTION TO THE ELBOW.

You know by now that between obvious movements in *kata* there are often hidden techniques. If the hand is free and you are close enough to the opponent, why not attempt to strike his temple using your closed hand as a hammerfist, or slap his ear if you prefer an open hand technique. This is a bit challenging, but it's just a continuation of the block so it really does not matter whether it works or not. The more disruptive your strike is to your opponent's elbow, the better the chance you have of getting that continuation attack to his head. Even if you cannot strike the head, your powerful blow to the elbow can be a fight-ending technique in and of itself. Now the simple check/deflection becomes an effective offensive action, and we have not even addressed the "block" or control half of this technique yet.

This is a fairly simple technique to execute. It works with the adrenaline rush* without being physically complex or mentally challenging. Just reach out and smack your attacker's arm. Since you naturally move faster from the outside to the inside, this check/deflection is a very natural reaction. Now, let's build even more techniques.

Since there is no pause as codified in Rule 12,† the controlling movement takes place immediately after the check/deflection (which is really a shot to the opponent's elbow joint). As that is happening, however, we must further consider Rule 5,‡ which says that the hand returning to chamber usually has something captured in it and Rule 7,§ which states that if you can control an opponent's head then you control the opponent.

In this application controlling the head technique is subtle. If instead of coming straight back down to chamber as the block moves up, use your right hand to drive the opponent's arm down with *muchimi*, it should snap the head back and up (assuming you do it properly). It is not really a grab, but it acts like one. You have already given the person a good strong shot to the arm and possibly an ear slap or hammerfist so he should be reasonably disrupted. Using *hikite* and proper body

* Principle 5—*work with the adrenaline rush not against it.*
† Rule 12—*there is no pause.*
‡ Rule 5—*a hand returning to chamber usually has something in it.*
§ Rule 7—*control an opponent's head and you control the opponent.*

mechanics to achieve this head whip will keep your attacker from avoiding the upward moving head block, which now becomes a forearm strike to his head. Pretty cool, huh?

So where should you be aiming? Applying Rule 11* you must be contouring the body, striking soft to hard or hard to soft. If you hit with the fleshy bottom of the arm, a soft part, your target is likely hard. The chin fits that bill nicely. But, if you consider the twisting motion of the *jodan uke* technique, the hard ulna bone really gets there first before the softer part of the arm arrives. Perhaps an ideal place to aim is at the larynx. It is a much more vital area than the chin, providing opportunities for a killing

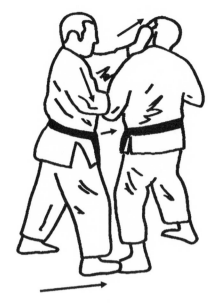

JODAN UKE (HEAD BLOCK) AS FOREARM SMASH. AS A FOLLOW-ON TO THE INITIAL CHECK/DEFLECTION, THE DEFENDER (LEFT) STRIKES HIS OPPONENT WITH A FOREARM SMASH. THIS MOVEMENT IS IDENTICAL TO A *JODAN UKE* HEAD BLOCK AS SEEN IN THE *KATA*; ONLY ITS APPLICATION IS MORE PROFOUND.

blow rather than a simple knockout. As you hit the throat with your arm it twists up higher into the neck.

You can see that this simple head block is a simultaneous arm strike and forearm smash into the throat. Who would have thought that *jodan uke* could be a devastating, fight ending attack?

But wait, there's more! We have not even addressed the lower half of the body yet. Principle 12† declares that stances are not just for *kata*, while Rule 4‡ states that every movement in *kata* has martial significance. Further, the *Goju Ryu* principle of working the whole body has not yet come into play.

The head block, we have been discussing is performed in *hidari sanchin dachi* (left foot forward, hourglass stance). In this stance, the foot of the forward leg turns inward while the knee points straight ahead. As you confront the attacker, you should be slightly off-line to the outside of your opponent with your left knee pointed directly at him. Assuming that he threw an *oi tsuki* (lunge punch), your left leg is in good position to assault his lower body. For example, you can hook his leg with your foot so that he cannot get away and attack the side of his knee with your own knee.

There are only two more components we have not already discussed. The first is Principle 13:§ breathing. Clearly, you must move swiftly and in a well-coordinated

* Rule 11—*contour the body.*
† Principle 12—*stances aren't just for kata.*
‡ Rule 4—*every movement in kata has martial significance.*
§ Principle 13—*don't forget to breathe.*

fashion to pull off this simultaneous upper and lower body attack. You must be fluid and relaxed to attain the necessary speed, tensing only at the moment of the strike. To facilitate this, you should breathe in while moving and exhale with the strike.

Rule 3* states that there is only one enemy at a time, which is absolutely true. Let's pretend, for a moment however, that your attacker has friends. Even though you can only deal with one person at a time, let's imagine the rest of the group's reaction to your technique. You step forward to meet the attacker's punch and the next instant he is lying on the ground, screaming in pain at worst, or unmoving and

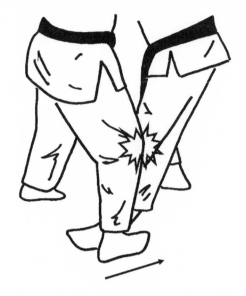

SANCHIN DACHI (HOURGLASS STANCE) AS HOOK/KNEE STRIKE. NOTICE HOW THE *SANCHIN* STANCE BOTH STRIKES AND OFF-BALANCES THE OPPONENT (RIGHT).

unconscious or perhaps even dead at best. And all you did was block! Now *that* is karate as it was meant to be.[†]

Once again, we only suggest utilizing this method when there is no choice but to fight. By now we hope that you viscerally know why: Martial arts teach, by definition, warrior skills. They are about expeditiously crippling or killing another human being. Once you have the power to do that, you also have the inherent responsibility to do your best to avoid doing so except as a last resort.

Dojo Practice

"Good ideas are not adopted automatically. They must be driven into practice with courageous patience." [72]

– Admiral Hyman Rickover

Dojo practice is inherently friendly. Martial artists train with partners rather than fight against opponents. Consequently minor bumps, bruises, or the occasional fat lip or bloody nose should be the only injuries expected. This is, of course, a completely unrealistic simulation of a real fight. After all, if no one ends up in the

---

* Rule 3—*there is only one enemy at a time.*

† And an important reminder of why we only use this stuff in the *dojo* and for legitimate self-defense purposes. Properly applied, the first technique of one of the first *kata* we learn can be deadly.

hospital, we are not performing street-worthy self-defense techniques realistically at full speed and power. That is exactly what we want to do in the *dojo*, of course, but it is important to be sure that everyone understands that what he or she is practicing is not actually street fighting.

Dojo practice affords practitioners a safe and sane way to learn new *kata*, decipher applications, and increase their skills through trial and error. It is an opportunity to understand strategy, tactics, principles, and rules to see what works and what does not work for you. One cannot expect that every session will overtly be about deciphering applications from *kata*. Some are simply about performing it, internalizing the movements, and timing. Others are about the *kihon*, or basic techniques that are strung together to form a particular *kata*. Sessions may focus on *ukemi* (breakfall techniques), *bunkai, kumite,* or any number of other subjects. Superior instructors provide a well-rounded curriculum.

While several different types of practice occur in the *dojo*, the best educational method for deciphering *kata* takes advantage of the fact that two heads are frequently better than one. In educator-speak it is called cooperative performance.

Cooperative Performance

"When a man says he approves of something in principle, it means he hasn't the slightest intention of putting it into practice." [73]

— Otto von Bismarck

In cooperative performance, practitioners work side by side on a task, engaging in practice along with a continuous discussion on how to do something or why it works (or does not work). To be most effective, both parties should already have a fair level of competency in the techniques being performed and discussed. We typically start students along this path at 5th *kyu* (green belt) level.

This teaching method can be a powerful tool to help practitioners understand how to apply martial tactics within the framework of their arts' strategy. It is useful to discuss what works, what does not work, and why that is the case in conjunction with application of the martial technique(s). This can help each practitioner develop a better understanding of which approaches are most effective for someone of his or her size, conditioning, skill level, and body type.

As practitioners build a repertoire of techniques to draw from, they will need to develop an understanding of how and when to combine or modify movements as they face varying tactical environments and prepare for real-life self-defense situations. While this could certainly be accomplished through trial and error during *kumite* or *randori*, cooperative performance adds significant velocity to the learning process. It is generally less painful that way too.

Tandem drills are excellent ways to practice deciphering *kata*. Once the paired practitioners have found what they believe is a valid interpretation for a particular technique, they can perform it with a partner who honors his or her technique, giving realistic pressure and appropriate feedback. They can discuss the strategic concepts, principles, and rules that apply for each given tactic, holistically evaluating its applicability and structure.

Practitioners can even find viable applications beyond traditional martial arts. For example, Black Belt Hall of Fame member George Chung works with NFL players, primarily members of the San Francisco 49ers, to enhance their performance on the football field through martial arts. Linemen learn hand-to-hand techniques, applying proper body mechanics to overcome brute speed and power. Running backs and safeties similarly improve their balance and coordination.

Defensive End Chike Okeafor, a student of *Sensei* Chung's, told *Seattle Times* reporter Greg Bishop that "all these forms are self defense. Is a man trying to put his hands on you? Yes or no? If it's yes, then you get his hands off you, you don't let him put them on you and you punish him for trying to. That's martial arts. That's football."

When they apply what they learn through cooperative performance, the next time practitioners perform a *kata* they will keep their newfound applications in mind so that they become natural extensions of the form. The *kata* itself does not change—only the practitioner's understanding of it. In this fashion both the practitioner and the art practiced may evolve and grow.

Formula

> *"Sometimes a block is not a block and a preparatory move is the meat of a technique. In diagnosing kata—trying to find what its self-defense applications are— every move should be examined in detail. Look beyond names, such as block or punch. The actual movements might be hiding in other applications."* [74]

> – *Don Sorrell*

Just because you *know* a *kata*, understand its various applications, and recognize its hidden techniques, this does not necessarily mean that you will want to rely on it in actual combat. Everyone is better at some things than at others. It is essential that during a life or death struggle practitioners personalize techniques, applying actions for which they have a natural affinity.

We suggest starting with a three-step approach. You already understand about strategy, principles, and rules that apply to the various tactics of your art, so we will build on that and take it a step further. Our formula is to (1) learn the pattern, (2) make any changes necessary, and then (3) incorporate them into your applications. Here is how it works.

Learn the pattern. Become familiar with the flow of the techniques. Understand the important ideas that the *kata* is trying to impart such as "load/release," "charge/bounce," "reduce," "spiral," or "always give pressure; give pressure always." These features build upon the principles and rules discussed earlier, highlighting the mechanical advantage that facilitates an application's ability to work. You can think of them as extensions of Principle 8* to understand why it works.

"Loading" forces an opponent into an undesirable position from which they feel compelled to push against. "Release" allows the opponent to move from a loaded position. The combination of "load/release" forces an opponent into an undesirable position that he will want to push against. As he responds, you release the pressure allowing him to move into a different yet still undesirable (hopefully *more* undesirable) position for him. It is one method of using an opponent's force against him to gain control, something commonly seen in most grappling arts.

A "charge" is when you move aggressively toward your opponent. "Bounce" is when you move with speed and your opponent's assistance from one position to another. While an opponent obviously does not want to assist you, you can nevertheless use his or her force to your advantage. With a "charge/bounce," you move aggressively toward your opponent then use his or her reaction to assist you in moving to another position, which gains you even greater advantage.

"Reduce" means to make smaller. It can apply to your body or your angle of attack. As discussed previously, the natural flinch reaction is to get small, protecting the vital core.

"Spiral" means to move in a circle while getting concentrically smaller and moving in the three dimensions of height, depth, and width. The vast majority of martial techniques are circular in nature. The spiral simply tightens and speeds up a circle, facilitating such applications as throws and arm breaks, or escapes from holds, locks, or throws.

"Always give pressure; give pressure always" is a foundational concept of *Goju Ryu* and many other martial arts. It means being relentless and aggressive in your offensive and defensive positions and using stances and body positioning to apply pressure to as many parts of the attacker as appropriate. It is a great disrupting tactic that can aid in both offensive and defensive techniques.

Every *kata* uses some or all of these concepts to apply its techniques. Understanding how and why they are used will elevate your ability to implement *kata* applications at a whole new level.

---

* Principle 8—*strive to understand why it works.*

Make changes as necessary. *Kata* and basic *bunkai* assume an opponent who has the same height, weight, strength and ability as the practitioner. When punching *jodan*, for example, practitioners are taught to aim at the level of their own chins. Mismatches in size or other factors may require tactical modifications as practitioners approach each individual opponent in real life confrontations.

We believe that it is essential to practice with as many different individuals as you have available. That way, encountering something unexpected or new will not slow your natural reaction. Your body will automatically compensate for such differences. Adults should practice with kids on occasion, and vice versa. Men should practice with women. Short, heavy practitioners should match up with tall lanky ones, and so on.

Line sparring drills are excellent ways to do this. Each practitioner has an opportunity to handle a known attack, spontaneously responding with techniques from his or her favorite *kata* in a safe and controlled manner. The drill is organized so that everyone makes a line across the *dojo*. The practitioner at the head of the line receives each technique, counterattacking any way he or she feels appropriate. The rest of the class files through one person at a time, each throwing one or more pre-assigned blows (e.g., head punch, front kick) for the *uke* to receive. Once *uke* has faced everyone else in the class, the next person in line takes on that role and the drill repeats once again until everyone has had a turn.

Line sparring not only affords practitioners an opportunity to tangle with *budoka* of other sizes, shapes, and abilities, but it also helps them learn timing and flow. Any defense is acceptable so long as the *uke* does not get hit. Similarly, any counterattack is okay so long as there is no pause. The goal is, of course, block/strike rather than block and strike. Although this drill is more controlled than *randori* sparring, senior practitioners still need to proactively assure the safety of their less-experienced juniors. Line sparring is conducted for a specific educational purpose and should not be allowed to devolve into a free for all.

Understand your tendencies and incorporate them. Your tendencies are built off of your natural reactions. Different practitioners gravitate toward different *kata*. Everyone eventually develops a personal favorite. Even within a *kata*, certain applications are generally more appealing than others. In a stress situation, you will naturally want to select something that works well for you. Therefore, you must make an extra effort to train with such techniques. However, that is not to say that you should completely avoid applications with which you are uncomfortable. Every technique in every *kata* should be practiced until you are minimally competent with it if for no other reason than understanding its strengths and limitations as potentially applied by your opponent against you.

The only other caution is that your natural reaction must serve as a foundation for good technique. This requires adherence to your style's strategy, along with the principles and rules for deciphering *kata*. Further, solid physiological integrity must be behind every technique. Even when you apply pressure point techniques or strike vital areas, you will want a clear physical advantage that can be applied in a stressful situation to expeditiously defeat an attacker.

Summary

"In the past it was common for a whole style to revolve around a single kata. The old masters would know, at most, two or three kata. However, they fully understood that within those kata was all the information they would ever need. Every single kata is a complete system of fighting in its own right!" [75]

– Iain Abernethy

The simplest interpretation of most any *kata* sequence is, as we know by now, almost always sub-optimal. When you adopt the principles, rules, and strategic guidelines outlined in this book and make them your own, you will have the power to get the most out of your martial art. Using a technique called cooperative performance, you can work with others in their *dojo* to experiment with their *kata*, identify what you believe are hidden applications, and ascertain whether or not they will work in a self-defense situation.

Although a practitioner may be able to perform a *kata* and understand its various applications and hidden techniques, he or she may still not want to rely on it in actual combat. Everyone is better at some things than at others. It is essential that practitioners understand how to personalize techniques, applying actions for which they have a natural affinity during a life-or-death struggle. *Kata* were developed as fighting arts. Practitioners must be able to apply them in actual combat. We suggest a three-step approach outlined in this chapter: (1) learn the pattern, (2) make any changes necessary, and then (3) incorporate them into your applications.

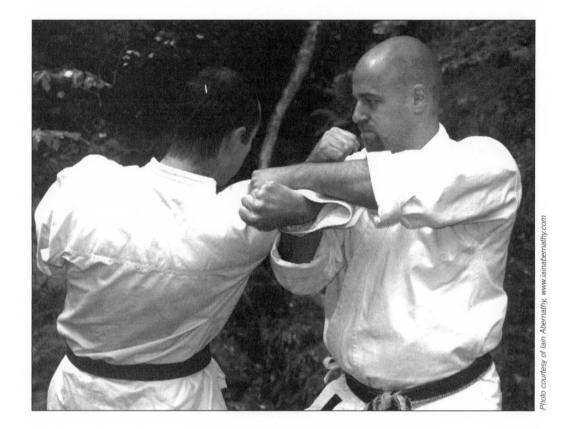

Pinan shodan armlock. Iain Abernethy applies a shoulder-lock from *Pinan shodan (Heian nidan) kata*. The recipient is Murray Denwood. The location is Holme wood, Loweswater, Northern England.

CHAPTER 7

Kata Examples

"Karate as a means of self-defense has the oldest history, going back hundreds of years. It is only in recent years that the techniques which have been handed down were scientifically studied and the principles evolved for making the most effective use of the various moves of the body. Training based on these principles and knowledge of the working of the muscles and joints and the vital relation between movement and balance enable the modern student of karate to be prepared, both physically and psychologically, to defend himself successfully against any would-be assailant." [76]

– Motoo Yamakura

This chapter uses *kata* from *Goju Ryu* karate to demonstrate how the previous material comes together. Using our examples, practitioners will have a leg up in deciphering the secrets of their own martial arts, analyzing their own *kata* in a similar fashion.

Using one technique from each of several *kata*, we demonstrate a commonly taught application then show a more optimal approach. We have tried to pick highly recognizable techniques that are frequently associated with each form demonstrated. Because more than one proper interpretation always exists, our examples are certainly not the only approach. They have, however, been proven effective. To help compare and contrast the various techniques we also include an application evaluation checklist, a blank version of which is available for your use in Appendix C.*

---

* Appendix C—*kata application evaluation checklist.*

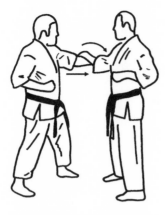

SAIFA KATA: URA UKE (WRIST) BLOCK.
DEFENDER IS ON THE RIGHT.

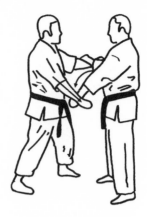

SAIFA KATA: SECOND BLOCK.

Saifa

"History is the version of past events that people have decided to agree upon." [77]

– *Napoleon Bonaparte*

The name *saifa* is commonly expressed in English as "smash and tear." Yet if you ask to have it translated, you will get a strained look as the original meaning is difficult to interpret. As it has moved from Chinese to Hogen (a regional Japanese dialect) to Japanese to English the actual meaning of the name has been lost. While the exact translation may have been lost to time it really does not matter. The commonly accepted name—"smash and tear"—suits this *kata* quite well.

Smash is defined by *The Merriam-Webster Dictionary* as, "A blow or attack, or the action or sound of smashing; especially: a wreck due to collision." As the name implies *saifa kata* does not propose waiting to receive an adversary's assault. It takes the attack to the opponent, closing to smash and tear into them.

Common Application:

This *kata* contains a somewhat unique up/down block combination followed by a *hiza geri* (knee strike) and *mae geri* (front kick). For the common application, we will focus on the blocking portion of that movement. As most frequently taught, this technique assumes that an attacker will stand static, punch once, leave that hand out, and then punch again before re-chambering the hand that initially attacked.

Once again this is too defensive to stop a fight. Even if followed by a knee strike, the next sequence in the *kata*, it is less than optimal as our checklist suggests.

Kata Application Evaluation Checklist—Saifa Common

To evaluate a potential kata application, check (✓) the boxes that apply:

Yes	No	Principles	Yes	No	Rules
✓		1) More than one proper interpretation exists			1) Do not be deceived by the enbusen rule
		2) Every technique should be able to immediately end the fight			2) Advancing techniques imply attack, while retreating techniques imply defense
		3) Strike to disrupt; disrupt to strike	✓		3) There is only one enemy at a time
		4) Nerve strikes are "extra credit"			4) Every movement in kata has martial meaning/significance
		5) Work with the adrenaline rush, not against it	✓		5) A hand returning to chamber usually has something in it
		6) Techniques must work at full speed and power			6) Utilize the shortest distance to your opponent
		7) Application must work on an "unwilling" partner			7) Control an opponent's head and you control the opponent
		8) Understand why it works		✓	8) There is no "block"
		9) Deception is not real			9) Kata demonstrate the proper angles
✓		10) If you are not there, you cannot get hit			10) Touching your own body in kata indicates touching your opponent
		11) Cross the T to escape			11) Contour the body—strike hard to soft and soft to hard
		12) Stances aren't just for kata		✓	12) There is no pause
		13) Don't forget to breathe	**Yes**	**No**	**Other Considerations**
		14) Use both hands		✓	A) Consistent with style's strategy
		15) A lock or hold is not a primary fighting technique			B) Built on natural physiological reaction

Valid applications should comply with principles, rules, and considerations above. Those that are not applicable should be left blank. If any "no" box is checked your potential application is sub-optimal.

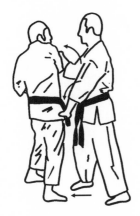

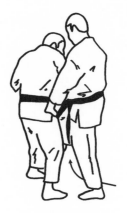

SAIFA KATA: CLOSING *URA UKE* (WRIST BLOCK) WITH
PRESSURE. DEFENDER IS ON THE RIGHT.

SAIFA KATA: KNEE STRIKE.

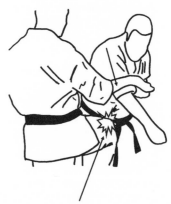

SAIFA KATA: CLOSE-UP/REVERSE ANGLE KNEE STRIKE.

Optimized Application:

Optimally, the practitioner moves directly into the attacker, choking down his or her opportunity for counterattack while striking simultaneously with the knee.

In keeping with the theme of *saifa*, this is a much more aggressive response. Even the block becomes a disruptive movement. As our checklist indicates, this is a far better interpretation.

Kata Application Evaluation Checklist—Saifa Optimal

To evaluate a potential kata application, check (✓) the boxes that apply:

Yes	No	Principles	Yes	No	Rules
✓		1) More than one proper interpretation exists	✓		1) Do not be deceived by the enbusen rule
✓		2) Every technique should be able to immediately end the fight	✓		2) Advancing techniques imply attack, while retreating techniques imply defense
✓		3) Strike to disrupt; disrupt to strike	✓		3) There is only one enemy at a time
✓		4) Nerve strikes are "extra credit"	✓		4) Every movement in kata has martial meaning/significance
✓		5) Work with the adrenaline rush, not against it	✓		5) A hand returning to chamber usually has something in it
✓		6) Techniques must work at full speed and power	✓		6) Utilize the shortest distance to your opponent
✓		7) Application must work on an "unwilling" partner			7) Control an opponent's head and you control the opponent
✓		8) Understand why it works	✓		8) There is no "block"
		9) Deception is not real	✓		9) Kata demonstrate the proper angles
✓		10) If you are not there, you cannot get hit			10) Touching your own body in kata indicates touching your opponent
		11) Cross the T to escape	✓		11) Contour the body—strike hard to soft and soft to hard
✓		12) Stances aren't just for kata	✓		12) There is no pause
✓		13) Don't forget to breathe	**Yes**	**No**	**Other Considerations**
✓		14) Use both hands	✓		A) Consistent with style's strategy
		15) A lock or hold is not a primary fighting technique			B) Built on natural physiological reaction

Valid applications should comply with principles, rules, and considerations above. Those that are not applicable should be left blank. If any "no" box is checked your potential application is sub-optimal.

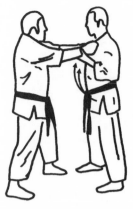

SEIYUNCHIN KATA: GRIP. DEFENDER IS ON THE RIGHT.

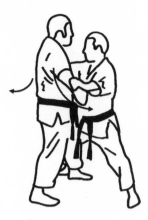

SEIYUNCHIN KATA: ESCAPE.

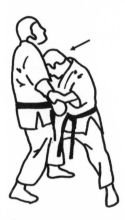

SEIYUNCHIN KATA: HEAD BUTT.

Seiyunchin

"Let the other guy have whatever he wants before the fight. Once the bell rings he's gonna be disappointed anyway." [78]

— George Foreman

Called the "storm within the calm," *seiyunchin* involves multiple means of un-rooting an attacker by pushing, pulling, or sweeping. It includes many different joint locks and arm hyperextensions as well. Even when *seiyunchin* appears to be retreating with a technique, it is still attacking in an uncompromising effort to keep the opponent off balance. This *kata* is unique in that it contains no kicks. It is believed to have originated in China.

Kata Application Evaluation Checklist—Seiyunchin Common

To evaluate a potential kata application, check (✓) the boxes that apply:

Yes	No	Principles	Yes	No	Rules
		1) More than one proper interpretation exists		✓	1) Do not be deceived by the enbusen rule
	✓	2) Every technique should be able to immediately end the fight		✓	2) Advancing techniques imply attack, while retreating techniques imply defense
	✓	3) Strike to disrupt; disrupt to strike	✓		3) There is only one enemy at a time
		4) Nerve strikes are "extra credit"			4) Every movement in kata has martial meaning/significance
		5) Work with the adrenaline rush, not against it			5) A hand returning to chamber usually has something in it
	✓	6) Techniques must work at full speed and power			6) Utilize the shortest distance to your opponent
	✓	7) Application must work on an "unwilling" partner			7) Control an opponent's head and you control the opponent
		8) Understand why it works			8) There is no "block"
		9) Deception is not real			9) Kata demonstrate the proper angles
		10) If you are not there, you cannot get hit			10) Touching your own body in kata indicates touching your opponent
		11) Cross the T to escape			11) Contour the body—strike hard to soft and soft to hard
		12) Stances aren't just for kata			12) There is no pause
		13) Don't forget to breathe	**Yes**	**No**	**Other Considerations**
✓		14) Use both hands		✓	A) Consistent with style's strategy
	✓	15) A lock or hold is not a primary fighting technique	✓		B) Built on natural physiological reaction

Valid applications should comply with principles, rules, and considerations above. Those that are not applicable should be left blank. If any "no" box is checked your potential application is sub-optimal.

Common Application:

Yama uke (mountain block) is introduced in this *kata*. The following is a common interpretation of that movement. It presumes that a practitioner using a reverse grip can break his or her attacker's grip, and then attack with a head butt to the opponent's sternum.

We suspect that it would be challenging to obtain sufficient leverage to expeditiously break a determined attacker's grip in this manner. Further, the rib cage, nature's shield for the chest, will most likely absorb this attack, rendering it ineffective. Our checklist shows that this interpretation could be improved.

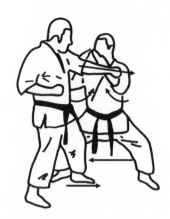

SEIYUNCHIN KATA: YAMA UKE (MOUNTAIN BLOCK).

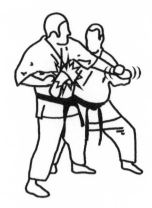

SEIYUNCHIN KATA: PULL/STRIKE.

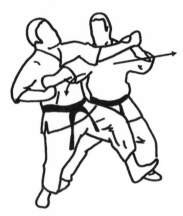

SEIYUNCHIN KATA: TANI OTOSHI (VALLEY DROP THROW).

Optimized Application:

Blocking *yama uke*, the practitioner covers his or her face while moving in behind the attacker in a swift unified movement. This technique is both defensive and, if done properly, uprooting as the practitioner crashes into his or her opponent's legs. The immediate follow-up is a simultaneous pull and strike to the ribs with the practitioner's elbow. This sequence ends with the practitioner throwing the attacker over his or her leg using *tani otoshi* (valley drop throw).

Our checklist indicates that this optimized version is more powerful.

Kata Application Evaluation Checklist—Seiyunchin Optimal

To evaluate a potential kata application, check (✓) the boxes that apply:

Yes	No	Principles	Yes	No	Rules
✓		1) More than one proper interpretation exists	✓		1) Do not be deceived by the enbusen rule
✓		2) Every technique should be able to immediately end the fight	✓		2) Advancing techniques imply attack, while retreating techniques imply defense
✓		3) Strike to disrupt; disrupt to strike	✓		3) There is only one enemy at a time
		4) Nerve strikes are "extra credit"	✓		4) Every movement in kata has martial meaning/significance
		5) Work with the adrenaline rush, not against it	✓		5) A hand returning to chamber usually has something in it
✓		6) Techniques must work at full speed and power			6) Utilize the shortest distance to your opponent
✓		7) Application must work on an "unwilling" partner			7) Control an opponent's head and you control the opponent
✓		8) Understand why it works	✓		8) There is no "block"
		9) Deception is not real	✓		9) Kata demonstrate the proper angles
		10) If you are not there, you cannot get hit			10) Touching your own body in kata indicates touching your opponent
		11) Cross the T to escape			11) Contour the body—strike hard to soft and soft to hard
✓		12) Stances aren't just for kata	✓		12) There is no pause
		13) Don't forget to breathe	**Yes**	**No**	**Other Considerations**
✓		14) Use both hands	✓		A) Consistent with style's strategy
✓		15) A lock or hold is not a primary fighting technique	✓		B) Built on natural physiological reaction

Valid applications should comply with principles, rules, and considerations above. Those that are not applicable should be left blank. If any "no" box is checked your potential application is sub-optimal.

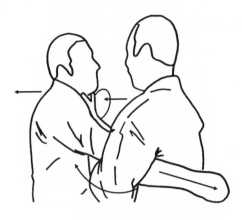

SEISAN KATA: THROAT GRAB WITH BACKWARD PRESSURE.

Seisan

"A ferocious counter-attack, especially when coupled with surprise, is the best way to throw your enemy off balance and win. Attack, attack, and then attack again. Never give up." [79]

— *Eugene Sockut*

Seisan translates to thirteen hands. Unlike much of Western thought, this number is considered lucky in China and much of the Orient. There are several versions of *seisan* and the relationships between those versions can vary from tangential to significant. Regardless, all versions of this *kata* use close distancing and short techniques to break down an opponent swiftly and brutally. The practitioner moves from attack to attack relentlessly. His or her opponent's joints are a primary target.

Common Application:

A throat grab is one of the most distinctive techniques in *seisan*. The difference between the common application and the optimized version of this procedure is quite subtle. As the standard approach is taught, this technique is used as a defense against a straight punch. The defender intercepts and wraps his or her attacker's arm in a pin while thrusting to and grabbing the attacker's throat, pushing him or her backward.

Upon reviewing our checklist, we can see that this is a pretty good interpretation.

Kata Application Evaluation Checklist—Seisan Common

To evaluate a potential kata application, check (✓) the boxes that apply:

Yes	No	Principles	Yes	No	Rules
✓		1) More than one proper interpretation exists			1) Do not be deceived by the enbusen rule
✓		2) Every technique should be able to immediately end the fight	✓		2) Advancing techniques imply attack, while retreating techniques imply defense
		3) Strike to disrupt; disrupt to strike	✓		3) There is only one enemy at a time
		4) Nerve strikes are "extra credit"	✓		4) Every movement in kata has martial meaning/significance
		5) Work with the adrenaline rush, not against it	✓		5) A hand returning to chamber usually has something in it
		6) Techniques must work at full speed and power	✓		6) Utilize the shortest distance to your opponent
		7) Application must work on an "unwilling" partner	✓		7) Control an opponent's head and you control the opponent
		8) Understand why it works	✓		8) There is no "block"
		9) Deception is not real	✓		9) Kata demonstrate the proper angles
		10) If you are not there, you cannot get hit			10) Touching your own body in kata indicates touching your opponent
		11) Cross the T to escape	✓		11) Contour the body—strike hard to soft and soft to hard
		12) Stances aren't just for kata	✓		12) There is no pause
		13) Don't forget to breathe	**Yes**	**No**	**Other Considerations**
		14) Use both hands	✓		A) Consistent with style's strategy
		15) A lock or hold is not a primary fighting technique	✓		B) Built on natural physiological reaction

Valid applications should comply with principles, rules, and considerations above. Those that are not applicable should be left blank. If any "no" box is checked your potential application is sub-optimal.

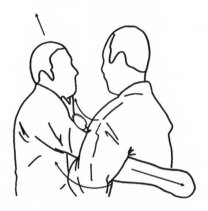

SEISAN KATA: THROAT GRAB WITH UPWARD PRESSURE.

Optimized Application:

Once again, the attacker delivers a straight punch. The practitioner intercepts and wraps his or her opponent's arm in a pin while thrusting to and grabbing the attacker's throat. The difference is that pressure is generated in an upward motion tracking the center line, lifting the attacker up on his or her toes. This subtle change in pressure makes the technique much more effective and significantly harder to counter.

Upward pressure is much more disruptive and effective than the standard approach of pushing an opponent backward. Our checklist indicates that it is superior.

Kata Application Evaluation Checklist—Seisan Optimal

To evaluate a potential kata application, check (✓) the boxes that apply:

Yes	No	Principles	Yes	No	Rules
✓		1) More than one proper interpretation exists			1) Do not be deceived by the enbusen rule
✓		2) Every technique should be able to immediately end the fight	✓		2) Advancing techniques imply attack, while retreating techniques imply defense
		3) Strike to disrupt; disrupt to strike	✓		3) There is only one enemy at a time
		4) Nerve strikes are "extra credit"	✓		4) Every movement in kata has martial meaning/significance
		5) Work with the adrenaline rush, not against it	✓		5) A hand returning to chamber usually has something in it
✓		6) Techniques must work at full speed and power	✓		6) Utilize the shortest distance to your opponent
✓		7) Application must work on an "unwilling" partner	✓		7) Control an opponent's head and you control the opponent
✓		8) Understand why it works	✓		8) There is no "block"
		9) Deception is not real	✓		9) Kata demonstrate the proper angles
		10) If you are not there, you cannot get hit			10) Touching your own body in kata indicates touching your opponent
		11) Cross the T to escape	✓		11) Contour the body—strike hard to soft and soft to hard
		12) Stances aren't just for kata	✓		12) There is no pause
		13) Don't forget to breathe	**Yes**	**No**	**Other Considerations**
✓		14) Use both hands	✓		A) Consistent with style's strategy
✓		15) A lock or hold is not a primary fighting technique	✓		B) Built on natural physiological reaction

Valid applications should comply with principles, rules, and considerations above. Those that are not applicable should be left blank. If any "no" box is checked your potential application is sub-optimal.

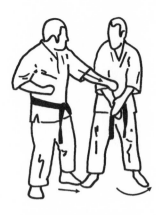

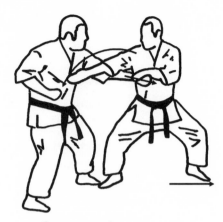

SAIPAI KATA: STEP BACK/BLOCK.
DEFENDER IS ON THE RIGHT.

SAIPAI KATA: GRAB/SPEAR HAND STRIKE.

Saipai

"There's nothing that cleanses your soul like getting the hell kicked out of you." [80]

– Woody Hayes

Saipai translates as the number eighteen or "eighteen hands." In context of the *kata* this number has been linked to the eighteen alms bowls outside of temples, eighteen sacred sites of Buddhism, and a multiple of the sacred number nine as well as other similar suggestions. *Saipai* comes from China, a fact which is stylistically reflected in its techniques (e.g., spinning moves, discriminating body positions similar to *Ba Qua Zhang*). Rotating the body into and away from an attacker, *saipai* uses many circular movements to achieve positional advantage while simultaneously damaging an opponent. This is a very non-linear *kata*.

Common Application:

The very beginning of this *kata* contains a very recognizable technique, the signature move of *saipai*. This application is commonly taught as defense against a straight punch. As the attacker steps in and strikes, the practitioner drops back, turning and blocking the punch with his or her arm. This is followed by a body drop and simultaneous spear-hand thrust to the solar plexus.

Although this is probably not the best interpretation, this application can be effective. We believe that significant finger conditioning is required to strike *nukite* without injuring your own hand though.

Kata Application Evaluation Checklist—Saipai Common

To evaluate a potential kata application, check (✓) the boxes that apply:

Yes	No	Principles	Yes	No	Rules
✓		1) More than one proper interpretation exists			1) Do not be deceived by the enbusen rule
	✓	2) Every technique should be able to immediately end the fight			2) Advancing techniques imply attack, while retreating techniques imply defense
✓		3) Strike to disrupt; disrupt to strike	✓		3) There is only one enemy at a time
✓		4) Nerve strikes are "extra credit"	✓		4) Every movement in kata has martial meaning/significance
✓		5) Work with the adrenaline rush, not against it	✓		5) A hand returning to chamber usually has something in it
✓		6) Techniques must work at full speed and power	✓		6) Utilize the shortest distance to your opponent
	✓	7) Application must work on an "unwilling" partner			7) Control an opponent's head and you control the opponent
	✓	8) Understand why it works			8) There is no "block"
		9) Deception is not real	✓		9) Kata demonstrate the proper angles
✓		10) If you are not there, you cannot get hit			10) Touching your own body in kata indicates touching your opponent
		11) Cross the T to escape	✓		11) Contour the body—strike hard to soft and soft to hard
✓		12) Stances aren't just for kata		✓	12) There is no pause
		13) Don't forget to breathe	**Yes**	**No**	**Other Considerations**
✓		14) Use both hands		✓	A) Consistent with style's strategy
		15) A lock or hold is not a primary fighting technique	✓		B) Built on natural physiological reaction

Valid applications should comply with principles, rules, and considerations above. Those that are not applicable should be left blank. If any "no" box is checked your potential application is sub-optimal.

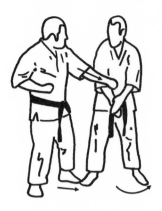

SAIPAI KATA: ADJUST RANGE/BLOCK.
DEFENDER IS ON THE RIGHT.

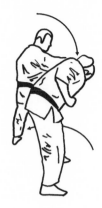

SAIPAI KATA: PIVOT/STRIKE.

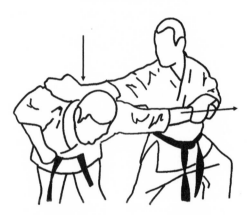

SAIPAI KATA: REVERSE ANGLE/CLOSE-UP OF STRIKE.

Optimized Application:

The optimized application can work against both a punch and a knife thrust equally well. Receiving the attack, the practitioner drops back and blocks with the outside of his or her arms while simultaneously pivoting out of the way (especially important against a knife). Grabbing the attacking limb, the practitioner continues his or her motion to deliver a *shuto* (sword hand strike) to the back of the attacker's neck, striking Gall Bladder 20.

Performing this technique at the correct range and angle makes a significant difference as indicated by our checklist.

Kata Application Evaluation Checklist—Saipai Optimal

To evaluate a potential kata application, check (✓) the boxes that apply:

Yes	No	Principles	Yes	No	Rules
✓		1) More than one proper interpretation exists			1) Do not be deceived by the enbusen rule
✓		2) Every technique should be able to immediately end the fight	✓		2) Advancing techniques imply attack, while retreating techniques imply defense
✓		3) Strike to disrupt; disrupt to strike	✓		3) There is only one enemy at a time
✓		4) Nerve strikes are "extra credit"	✓		4) Every movement in kata has martial meaning/significance
✓		5) Work with the adrenaline rush, not against it	✓		5) A hand returning to chamber usually has something in it
✓		6) Techniques must work at full speed and power	✓		6) Utilize the shortest distance to your opponent
✓		7) Application must work on an "unwilling" partner	✓		7) Control an opponent's head and you control the opponent
✓		8) Understand why it works			8) There is no "block"
		9) Deception is not real	✓		9) Kata demonstrate the proper angles
✓		10) If you are not there, you cannot get hit			10) Touching your own body in kata indicates touching your opponent
		11) Cross the T to escape	✓		11) Contour the body—strike hard to soft and soft to hard
✓		12) Stances aren't just for kata	✓		12) There is no pause
		13) Don't forget to breathe	**Yes**	**No**	**Other Considerations**
✓		14) Use both hands	✓		A) Consistent with style's strategy
✓		15) A lock or hold is not a primary fighting technique	✓		B) Built on natural physiological reaction

Valid applications should comply with principles, rules, and considerations above. Those that are not applicable should be left blank. If any "no" box is checked your potential application is sub-optimal.

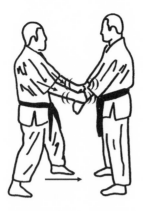

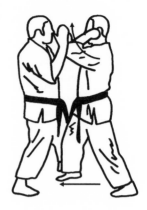

SHISOCHIN KATA: DOUBLE GRAB.
DEFENDER IS ON THE RIGHT.

SHISOCHIN KATA: ESCAPE.

Shisochin

"Learning is not compulsory... neither is survival." [81]

– *W. Edwards Deming*

Shisochin can be translated as "Battle in Four Directions," "Four Fighting Monks," or "Four Direction Fighting." It was brought back from China by Kanryo Higashionna *Sensei*. This *kata* is unique to *Goju Ryu* and is not used in other *Naha Te* styles.

This form uses the idea of cutting off lines of retaliation by confidently moving into the attacker with aggressive and powerful movements. Like western boxing, *shisochin* employs the concept of beating an opponent to the punch by using position and speed. One of the unusual features of this *kata* is a double-elbow strike.

Common Application:

The most commonly taught approach assumes a double grab to the practitioner's wrists by an opponent. The practitioner then breaks this grip by moving in, lifting his or her arms and delivering force against the attacker's thumbs.

If someone grabs both your arms, it is probably easier and faster to simply kick the attacker, among other alternatives. Our checklist indicates that this sequence is a sub-optimal interpretation.

Kata Application Evaluation Checklist—Shisochin Common

To evaluate a potential kata application, check (✓) the boxes that apply:

Yes	No	Principles	Yes	No	Rules
✓		1) More than one proper interpretation exists			1) Do not be deceived by the enbusen rule
	✓	2) Every technique should be able to immediately end the fight		✓	2) Advancing techniques imply attack, while retreating techniques imply defense
	✓	3) Strike to disrupt; disrupt to strike	✓		3) There is only one enemy at a time
	✓	4) Nerve strikes are "extra credit"			4) Every movement in kata has martial meaning/significance
		5) Work with the adrenaline rush, not against it			5) A hand returning to chamber usually has something in it
	✓	6) Techniques must work at full speed and power			6) Utilize the shortest distance to your opponent
	✓	7) Application must work on an "unwilling" partner			7) Control an opponent's head and you control the opponent
		8) Understand why it works			8) There is no "block"
		9) Deception is not real			9) Kata demonstrate the proper angles
		10) If you are not there, you cannot get hit			10) Touching your own body in kata indicates touching your opponent
		11) Cross the T to escape			11) Contour the body—strike hard to soft and soft to hard
		12) Stances aren't just for kata		✓	12) There is no pause
		13) Don't forget to breathe	**Yes**	**No**	**Other Considerations**
✓		14) Use both hands		✓	A) Consistent with style's strategy
		15) A lock or hold is not a primary fighting technique	✓		B) Built on natural physiological reaction

Valid applications should comply with principles, rules, and considerations above. Those that are not applicable should be left blank. If any "no" box is checked your potential application is sub-optimal.

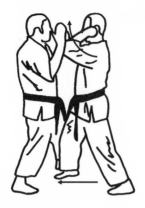 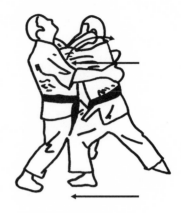

SHISOCHIN KATA: ESCAPE. DEFENDER IS ON THE RIGHT.   *SHISOCHIN KATA:* ELBOW STRIKE.

Optimized Application:

Our optimized version begins with an assumption that you will stop the opponent's grab before it succeeds. After all, if an attacker gets a hold of you, you are in a lot of trouble. The practitioner, therefore, lifts his or her hands up the center-line forcing the attacker's hands upward and away from his or her chest. The practitioner then drives his or her elbows directly into the attacker's chest without hesitation.

This interpretation is superior not only because it precludes the grab, but also because it is performed in the proper range.

Kururunfa

"All the art of living lies in a fine mingling of letting go and holding on." [82]

– Henry Havelock Ellis

Kururunfa is another *kata* of Chinese origin. It features *tai sabaki waza* (moving/shifting techniques) and very quick movement. It contains a wide variety of open-hand techniques, especially hand and hip coordination techniques.

The name *kururunfa* can translate to "holding your ground" and other variations along the same theme. It is explosive in its movements and requires deftness in shifting the body to execute the trapping, striking, dislocating, and breaking techniques included in the *kata*. One of the signature movements of this form is affectionately known as the "crocodile death roll throw."

Kata Application Evaluation Checklist—Shisochin Optimal

To evaluate a potential kata application, check (✓) the boxes that apply:

Yes	No	Principles	Yes	No	Rules
✓		1) More than one proper interpretation exists			1) Do not be deceived by the enbusen rule
✓		2) Every technique should be able to immediately end the fight	✓		2) Advancing techniques imply attack, while retreating techniques imply defense
✓		3) Strike to disrupt; disrupt to strike	✓		3) There is only one enemy at a time
✓		4) Nerve strikes are "extra credit"	✓		4) Every movement in kata has martial meaning/significance
✓		5) Work with the adrenaline rush, not against it			5) A hand returning to chamber usually has something in it
✓		6) Techniques must work at full speed and power	✓		6) Utilize the shortest distance to your opponent
✓		7) Application must work on an "unwilling" partner			7) Control an opponent's head and you control the opponent
✓		8) Understand why it works	✓		8) There is no "block"
		9) Deception is not real	✓		9) Kata demonstrate the proper angles
		10) If you are not there, you cannot get hit			10) Touching your own body in kata indicates touching your opponent
		11) Cross the T to escape			11) Contour the body—strike hard to soft and soft to hard
✓		12) Stances aren't just for kata	✓		12) There is no pause
		13) Don't forget to breathe	**Yes**	**No**	**Other Considerations**
		14) Use both hands	✓		A) Consistent with style's strategy
		15) A lock or hold is not a primary fighting technique	✓		B) Built on natural physiological reaction

Valid applications should comply with principles, rules, and considerations above. Those that are not applicable should be left blank. If any "no" box is checked your potential application is sub-optimal.

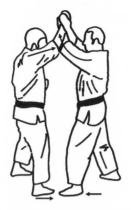

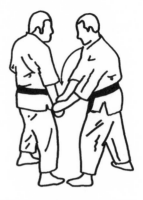

KURURUNFA KATA: JUJI UKE (CROSS-BLOCK).
DEFENDER IS ON THE RIGHT.

KURURUNFA KATA: ARM CAPTURE/PRESS.

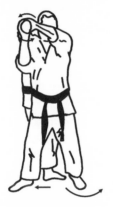

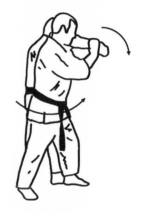

KURURUNFA KATA: TWIST/PIVOT.

KURURUNFA KATA: COMMENCE THROW.

Common Application:

The practitioner uses a *juji uke* (cross-block) to stop an overhead strike, pulling the arm down and spinning underneath his or her attacker's arm pit. As the attacker's arm is locked, he or she is thrown forward and down.

This application looks reasonable at first blush. It can both break an opponent's arm and hurl them to the ground with sufficient force to cause additional damage. Unfortunately it can be very

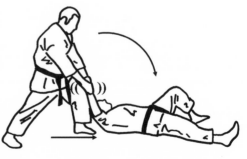

KURURUNFA KATA: COMPLETE THROW.

Kata Application Evaluation Checklist—Kururunfa Common

To evaluate a potential kata application, check (✓) the boxes that apply:

Yes	No	Principles	Yes	No	Rules
✓		1) More than one proper interpretation exists			1) Do not be deceived by the enbusen rule
	✓	2) Every technique should be able to immediately end the fight			2) Advancing techniques imply attack, while retreating techniques imply defense
	✓	3) Strike to disrupt; disrupt to strike	✓		3) There is only one enemy at a time
		4) Nerve strikes are "extra credit"			4) Every movement in kata has martial meaning/significance
	✓	5) Work with the adrenaline rush, not against it			5) A hand returning to chamber usually has something in it
	✓	6) Techniques must work at full speed and power			6) Utilize the shortest distance to your opponent
	✓	7) Application must work on an "unwilling" partner			7) Control an opponent's head and you control the opponent
	✓	8) Understand why it works		✓	8) There is no "block"
		9) Deception is not real			9) Kata demonstrate the proper angles
		10) If you are not there, you cannot get hit			10) Touching your own body in kata indicates touching your opponent
		11) Cross the T to escape			11) Contour the body—strike hard to soft and soft to hard
		12) Stances aren't just for kata			12) There is no pause
		13) Don't forget to breathe	**Yes**	**No**	**Other Considerations**
		14) Use both hands		✓	A) Consistent with style's strategy
		15) A lock or hold is not a primary fighting technique		✓	B) Built on natural physiological reaction

Valid applications should comply with principles, rules, and considerations above. Those that are not applicable should be left blank. If any "no" box is checked your potential application is sub-optimal.

challenging to perform this way in a self-defense situation where turning your back on an opponent gives him or her a moment of opportunity to counterstrike.

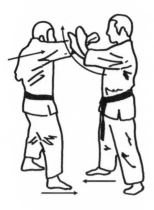

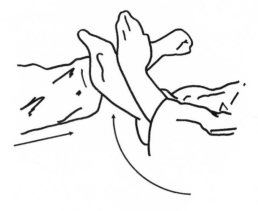

KURURUNFA: INITIATE *OSAI UKE* (PRESS BLOCK).
DEFENDER IS ON THE RIGHT.

KURURUNFA: INITIATE *OSAI UKE* (PRESS BLOCK)
CLOSE-UP OF HAND POSITION.

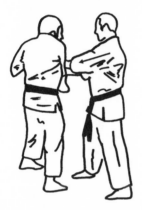

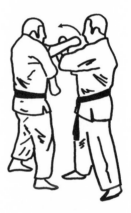

KURURUNFA: COMPLETE *OSAI UKE* (PRESS BLOCK).

KURURUNFA: HOLD GROUND/BLOCK FOLLOW-UP PUNCH.

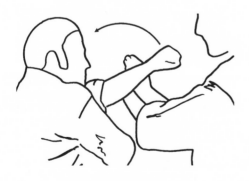

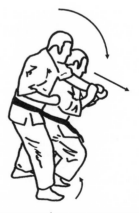

KURURUNFA: BLOCK SECOND PUNCH
CLOSE-UP OF HAND POSITION.

IPPON SEIO NAGE (ONE ARM SHOULDER THROW).

Kata Application Evaluation Checklist—Kururunfa Optimal

To evaluate a potential kata application, check (✓) the boxes that apply:

Yes	No	Principles	Yes	No	Rules
✓		1) More than one proper interpretation exists	✓		1) Do not be deceived by the enbusen rule
✓		2) Every technique should be able to immediately end the fight	✓		2) Advancing techniques imply attack, while retreating techniques imply defense
✓		3) Strike to disrupt; disrupt to strike	✓		3) There is only one enemy at a time
		4) Nerve strikes are "extra credit"	✓		4) Every movement in kata has martial meaning/significance
✓		5) Work with the adrenaline rush, not against it	✓		5) A hand returning to chamber usually has something in it
✓		6) Techniques must work at full speed and power			6) Utilize the shortest distance to your opponent
✓		7) Application must work on an "unwilling" partner			7) Control an opponent's head and you control the opponent
✓		8) Understand why it works	✓		8) There is no "block"
		9) Deception is not real			9) Kata demonstrate the proper angles
		10) If you are not there, you cannot get hit			10) Touching your own body in kata indicates touching your opponent
		11) Cross the T to escape			11) Contour the body—strike hard to soft and soft to hard
		12) Stances aren't just for kata	✓		12) There is no pause
		13) Don't forget to breathe	**Yes**	**No**	**Other Considerations**
		14) Use both hands	✓		A) Consistent with style's strategy
		15) A lock or hold is not a primary fighting technique			B) Built on natural physiological reaction

Valid applications should comply with principles, rules, and considerations above. Those that are not applicable should be left blank. If any "no" box is checked your potential application is sub-optimal.

Optimized Application:

Our optimized approach uses a double handed *osai uke* (press block) to the outside rather than a *juji uke*, pressing across the attacker's center line. As the attacker responds with a second punch, the same block is used again to the other side. While the second attack is not always on the way, we believe that it is reasonable to assume that it will be. The practitioner then drops into an *ippon seio nage* (one arm shoulder throw), hyperextending the attacker's arm while throwing him or her forcefully to the ground.

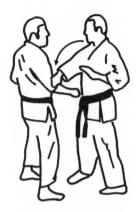 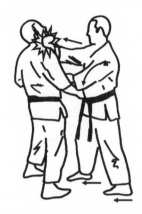

SANSEIRU KATA: PRESS BLOCK.
DEFENDER IS ON THE RIGHT.

SANSEIRU KATA: WRIST STRIKE TO THROAT.

This optimized approach takes advantage of the fact that a second punch from your opponent should always be expected and is probably on its way toward you. We believe that it is both safer to execute and more likely to be effective than the standard interpretation.

Sanseiru

"Making the simple complicated is commonplace; making the complicated simple, awesomely simple, that's creativity." [83]

– *Charles Mingus*

Sanseiru translates to the number thirty six or "thirty six hands." It is calculated by multiplying six time six. The number six represents the universe with the four points of the compass plus above and below, making six total directions. In Chinese culture there are also six senses: taste, touch, smell, sight, hearing, and mind. The *kata* pattern covers the four points of the compass using repetition of primary techniques. It is direct and ferocious. *Sanseiru* draws its strength through the powerful application of the rock-solid fundamentals of karate rather than in volumes of technique.

Common Application:
Our first example from *sanseiru* is a fairly basic yet highly effective down block with a bounce and counterstrike. It is drawn from a signature movement of the *kata*. The practitioner blocks downward with an open palm then follows the attacker's arm back up to execute a *koken tsuki* (wrist strike) to the throat.

Kata Application Evaluation Checklist—Sanseiru Common

To evaluate a potential kata application, check (✓) the boxes that apply:

Yes	No	Principles	Yes	No	Rules
✓		1) More than one proper interpretation exists			1) Do not be deceived by the enbusen rule
✓		2) Every technique should be able to immediately end the fight			2) Advancing techniques imply attack, while retreating techniques imply defense
✓		3) Strike to disrupt; disrupt to strike	✓		3) There is only one enemy at a time
✓		4) Nerve strikes are "extra credit"	✓		4) Every movement in kata has martial meaning/significance
✓		5) Work with the adrenaline rush, not against it			5) A hand returning to chamber usually has something in it
✓		6) Techniques must work at full speed and power	✓		6) Utilize the shortest distance to your opponent
✓		7) Application must work on an "unwilling" partner			7) Control an opponent's head and you control the opponent
		8) Understand why it works	✓		8) There is no "block"
		9) Deception is not real			9) Kata demonstrate the proper angles
		10) If you are not there, you cannot get hit			10) Touching your own body in kata indicates touching your opponent
		11) Cross the T to escape			11) Contour the body—strike hard to soft and soft to hard
✓		12) Stances aren't just for kata	✓		12) There is no pause
		13) Don't forget to breathe	**Yes**	**No**	**Other Considerations**
		14) Use both hands	✓		A) Consistent with style's strategy
✓		15) A lock or hold is not a primary fighting technique	✓		B) Built on natural physiological reaction

Valid applications should comply with principles, rules, and considerations above. Those that are not applicable should be left blank. If any "no" box is checked your potential application is sub-optimal.

This is a pretty good, direct application. It is quick and easy to execute, perhaps even capable of ending the fight.

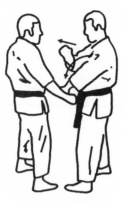

SANSEIRU KATA: DOWN BLOCK.
DEFENDER IS ON THE RIGHT.

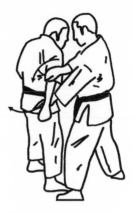

SANSEIRU KATA: ARM CAPTURE.

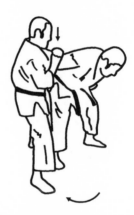

SANSEIRU KATA: SHOULDER DISLOCATION.

Optimized Application:

In our optimized solution, the practitioner blocks downward then reaches across the attacker's elbow, pulling to bend the attacker over. The immediate follow-up technique spins back both arms using the practitioner's body weight to separate the opponent's shoulder, a movement that is very difficult to counter. When executed with speed and power, this is movement causes crippling damage to an attacker.

Using our checklist, we can see that this application covers more ground than the standard interpretation. It is also more likely to immediately end a fight.

Kata Application Evaluation Checklist—Sanseiru Optimal

To evaluate a potential kata application, check (✓) the boxes that apply:

Yes	No	Principles	Yes	No	Rules
✓		1) More than one proper interpretation exists	✓		1) Do not be deceived by the enbusen rule
✓		2) Every technique should be able to immediately end the fight			2) Advancing techniques imply attack, while retreating techniques imply defense
✓		3) Strike to disrupt; disrupt to strike	✓		3) There is only one enemy at a time
✓		4) Nerve strikes are "extra credit"	✓		4) Every movement in kata has martial meaning/significance
✓		5) Work with the adrenaline rush, not against it			5) A hand returning to chamber usually has something in it
✓		6) Techniques must work at full speed and power	✓		6) Utilize the shortest distance to your opponent
✓		7) Application must work on an "unwilling" partner			7) Control an opponent's head and you control the opponent
		8) Understand why it works	✓		8) There is no "block"
		9) Deception is not real	✓		9) Kata demonstrate the proper angles
✓		10) If you are not there, you cannot get hit			10) Touching your own body in kata indicates touching your opponent
✓		11) Cross the T to escape	✓		11) Contour the body—strike hard to soft and soft to hard
✓		12) Stances aren't just for kata	✓		12) There is no pause
		13) Don't forget to breathe	**Yes**	**No**	**Other Considerations**
✓		14) Use both hands	✓		A) Consistent with style's strategy
		15) A lock or hold is not a primary fighting technique	✓		B) Built on natural physiological reaction

Valid applications should comply with principles, rules, and considerations above. Those that are not applicable should be left blank. If any "no" box is checked your potential application is sub-optimal.

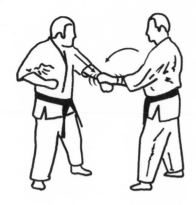

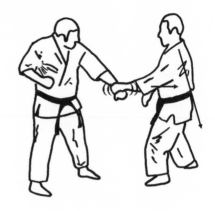

SUPARINPEI KATA: GRAB. DEFENDER IS ON THE RIGHT.

SUPARINPEI KATA: PULL.

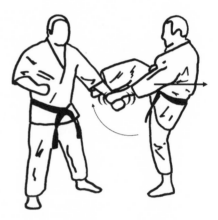

SUPARINPEI KATA: ELBOW KICK.

Suparinpei

"Forget goals. Value the process." [84]

– Jim Bouton

Suparinpei is another *kata* of Chinese origin. The name can be translated as "108 Hands" or "108 Techniques." The number 108 is significant in Buddhism as it is believed man has 108 evil passions. This number is also a multiple of other numbers found in *kata*, a point that delves into Chinese mysticism and numerology (all of which should be kept in the context of cultural significance). In almost all schools, *suparinpei* is the last *kata* that practitioners learn. The most likely reasons for this include the length of the form and complexity of techniques represented therein.

Kata Application Evaluation Checklist—Suparinpei Common

To evaluate a potential kata application, check (✓) the boxes that apply:

Yes	No	Principles	Yes	No	Rules
✓		1) More than one proper interpretation exists			1) Do not be deceived by the enbusen rule
	✓	2) Every technique should be able to immediately end the fight			2) Advancing techniques imply attack, while retreating techniques imply defense
	✓	3) Strike to disrupt; disrupt to strike	✓		3) There is only one enemy at a time
		4) Nerve strikes are "extra credit"	✓		4) Every movement in kata has martial meaning/significance
		5) Work with the adrenaline rush, not against it	✓		5) A hand returning to chamber usually has something in it
	✓	6) Techniques must work at full speed and power	✓		6) Utilize the shortest distance to your opponent
		7) Application must work on an "unwilling" partner			7) Control an opponent's head and you control the opponent
		8) Understand why it works			8) There is no "block"
		9) Deception is not real	✓		9) Kata demonstrate the proper angles
		10) If you are not there, you cannot get hit	✓		10) Touching your own body in kata indicates touching your opponent
		11) Cross the T to escape			11) Contour the body—strike hard to soft and soft to hard
		12) Stances aren't just for kata	✓		12) There is no pause
		13) Don't forget to breathe	**Yes**	**No**	**Other Considerations**
		14) Use both hands	✓		A) Consistent with style's strategy
✓		15) A lock or hold is not a primary fighting technique			B) Built on natural physiological reaction

Valid applications should comply with principles, rules, and considerations above. Those that are not applicable should be left blank. If any "no" box is checked your potential application is sub-optimal.

Common Application:

Suparinpei contains the movements of just about every other *kata* in *Goju Ryu*. One unique movement not found elsewhere in the system is a crescent kick. The most commonly taught application is a defense against a punch. After capturing the attacker's arm and pulling them off balance, the practitioner strikes the opponent's elbow with a kick.

As the checklist reveals, this is probably not the best interpretation of this technique. Among other things, it is executed at too great a range to be fully effective.

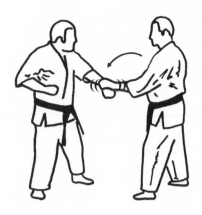

SUPARINPEI KATA: GRAB. DEFENDER IS ON THE RIGHT.

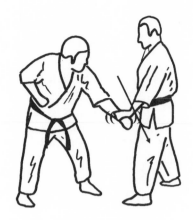

SUPARINPEI KATA: PULL.

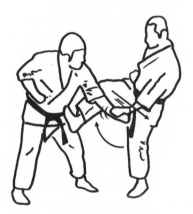

SUPARINPEI KATA: STRIKE.

Optimized Application:

Our enhanced interpretation uses the practitioner's shin to shatter the attacker's elbow. Not only is this a more powerful attack, but it frees the foot to strike the opponent's body simultaneously as well.

Using the checklist, this application fits our criteria much better.

Kata Application Evaluation Checklist—Suparinpei Optimal

To evaluate a potential kata application, check (✓) the boxes that apply:

Yes	No	Principles	Yes	No	Rules
✓		1) More than one proper interpretation exists			1) Do not be deceived by the enbusen rule
✓		2) Every technique should be able to immediately end the fight			2) Advancing techniques imply attack, while retreating techniques imply defense
✓		3) Strike to disrupt; disrupt to strike	✓		3) There is only one enemy at a time
		4) Nerve strikes are "extra credit"	✓		4) Every movement in kata has martial meaning/significance
		5) Work with the adrenaline rush, not against it	✓		5) A hand returning to chamber usually has something in it
✓		6) Techniques must work at full speed and power	✓		6) Utilize the shortest distance to your opponent
		7) Application must work on an "unwilling" partner			7) Control an opponent's head and you control the opponent
		8) Understand why it works	✓		8) There is no "block"
		9) Deception is not real	✓		9) Kata demonstrate the proper angles
		10) If you are not there, you cannot get hit	✓		10) Touching your own body in kata indicates touching your opponent
		11) Cross the T to escape			11) Contour the body—strike hard to soft and soft to hard
		12) Stances aren't just for kata	✓		12) There is no pause
		13) Don't forget to breathe	**Yes**	**No**	**Other Considerations**
		14) Use both hands	✓		A) Consistent with style's strategy
✓		15) A lock or hold is not a primary fighting technique			B) Built on natural physiological reaction

Valid applications should comply with principles, rules, and considerations above. Those that are not applicable should be left blank. If any "no" box is checked your potential application is sub-optimal.

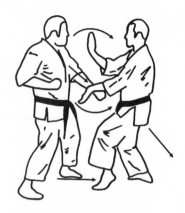

Gekisai Kata: Mawashe Uke (WHEEL BLOCK) COMMON.

Gekisai (Dai Ni)

"Education is simply the soul of a society as it passes from one generation to another." [85]

— *Gilbert K. Chesterton*

Gekisai means "attack and destroy." It was created by Chojun Miyagi and Nagamine Shoshin around 1940 to introduce karate to middle school students in Okinawa. This *kata* was specifically created to bring the standardization necessary for teaching martial arts in an education system. The design of *gekisai* is three fold: to create standardization, impart the basics of karate, and provide students a set of tools they can use for self-defense. In the second *gekisai kata* (*gekisai kata dai ni*), both the *neko ashi dachi* stance and the *mawashe uke* (wheel block) technique are first introduced.

Common Application:

As attacker steps in with a strike the practitioner shifts back into *neko ashi dachi* and performs a *mawashe uke* block.

This technique is far too defensive for a self-defense situation as our checklist indicates.

Kata Application Evaluation Checklist—Gekisai Common

To evaluate a potential kata application, check (✓) the boxes that apply:

Yes	No	Principles	Yes	No	Rules
✓		1) More than one proper interpretation exists		✓	1) Do not be deceived by the enbusen rule
	✓	2) Every technique should be able to immediately end the fight			2) Advancing techniques imply attack, while retreating techniques imply defense
	✓	3) Strike to disrupt; disrupt to strike	✓		3) There is only one enemy at a time
		4) Nerve strikes are "extra credit"	✓		4) Every movement in kata has martial meaning/significance
		5) Work with the adrenaline rush, not against it			5) A hand returning to chamber usually has something in it
	✓	6) Techniques must work at full speed and power		✓	6) Utilize the shortest distance to your opponent
	✓	7) Application must work on an "unwilling" partner			7) Control an opponent's head and you control the opponent
		8) Understand why it works		✓	8) There is no "block"
		9) Deception is not real			9) Kata demonstrate the proper angles
		10) If you are not there, you cannot get hit			10) Touching your own body in kata indicates touching your opponent
		11) Cross the T to escape			11) Contour the body—strike hard to soft and soft to hard
		12) Stances aren't just for kata		✓	12) There is no pause
		13) Don't forget to breathe	**Yes**	**No**	**Other Considerations**
		14) Use both hands		✓	A) Consistent with style's strategy
		15) A lock or hold is not a primary fighting technique			B) Built on natural physiological reaction

Valid applications should comply with principles, rules, and considerations above. Those that are not applicable should be left blank. If any "no" box is checked your potential application is sub-optimal.

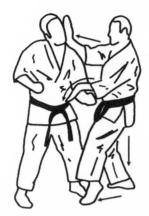

Gekisai kata: mawashe uke (WHEEL BLOCK) OPTIMAL.

Optimized Application:

Mawashe uke is actually a much more complex technique then it first appears. It is both offensive and defensive at the same time. As the attacker steps in with a strike, the practitioner drops in place into *neko ashi dachi* pinning and closing at the same time. When performing the *mawashe uke,* the practitioner executes a simultaneous *shotei uchi* (palm heel strike) to the face.

This interpretation is much more offensive in nature, thus more likely to succeed on the street.

Summary

> *"All men by nature desire knowledge... For the things we have to learn before we can do them, we learn by doing them."* [86]

> *– Aristotle*

Just because an application is commonly taught does not necessarily mean that it is always the best interpretation of a given technique. Practitioners are welcome to use the application evaluation checklist we have created, (a blank copy is available in Appendix C) to bring together all the principles and rules we have previously discussed and apply them to their own *kata.*

Back in the introduction of this book, we stated that *kata* is not dance practice nor is it aerobic training. It is the fundamental basis of a fighting art. Like a textbook, it contains all the applications you need to defend yourself in mortal combat. To get the most out of your martial art, you simply need to know how to "read" your *kata* like a book. By now you should be able to do just that.

Kata Application Evaluation Checklist—Gekisai Optimal

To evaluate a potential kata application, check (✓) the boxes that apply:

Yes	No	Principles	Yes	No	Rules
✓		1) More than one proper interpretation exists	✓		1) Do not be deceived by the enbusen rule
✓		2) Every technique should be able to immediately end the fight			2) Advancing techniques imply attack, while retreating techniques imply defense
✓		3) Strike to disrupt; disrupt to strike	✓		3) There is only one enemy at a time
✓		4) Nerve strikes are "extra credit"	✓		4) Every movement in kata has martial meaning/significance
		5) Work with the adrenaline rush, not against it			5) A hand returning to chamber usually has something in it
✓		6) Techniques must work at full speed and power	✓		6) Utilize the shortest distance to your opponent
✓		7) Application must work on an "unwilling" partner			7) Control an opponent's head and you control the opponent
✓		8) Understand why it works	✓		8) There is no "block"
		9) Deception is not real			9) Kata demonstrate the proper angles
		10) If you are not there, you cannot get hit			10) Touching your own body in kata indicates touching your opponent
		11) Cross the T to escape	✓		11) Contour the body—strike hard to soft and soft to hard
		12) Stances aren't just for kata	✓		12) There is no pause
		13) Don't forget to breathe	**Yes**	**No**	**Other Considerations**
✓		14) Use both hands	✓		A) Consistent with style's strategy
		15) A lock or hold is not a primary fighting technique	✓		B) Built on natural physiological reaction

Valid applications should comply with principles, rules, and considerations above. Those that are not applicable should be left blank. If any "no" box is checked your potential application is sub-optimal.

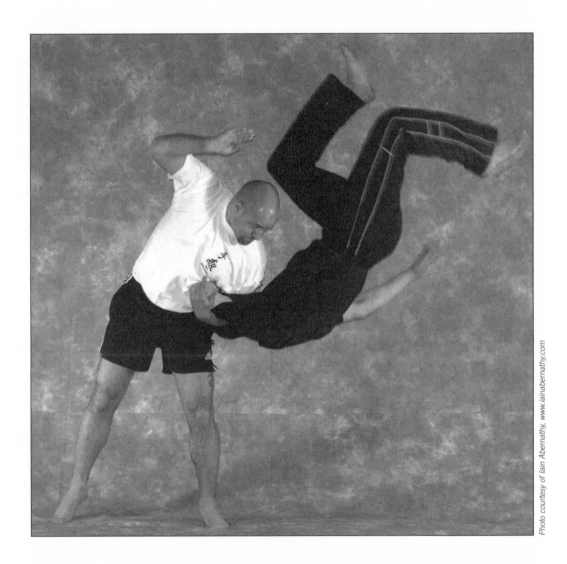

WANSHU THROW. IAIN ABERNETHY APPLIES THE SHOULDER WHEEL THROW
FROM *WANSHU (ENPI) KATA*. THE RECIPIENT IS MURRAY DENWOOD.

Conclusion

"The fact is that technique is no more or less important than physical fitness or mental conditioning. Many martial artists dislike this idea as it infers that those with poor technique can defeat those with good technique (if they lack the required mental and physical condition). A laborer on a building site (physically conditioned) who regularly gets involved in bar fights (mentally used to combat) could easily defeat the martial artist who concentrates on technique to the exclusion of the other forms of strength. If we are to be able to effectively defend ourselves then we need to ensure that our training also develops physical condition and mental strength in addition to technique. The key is to ensure that our training is intense enough to encourage growth in all three areas e.g., we drill our techniques with intensity and to the point of exhaustion (stimulates physical strength) and no matter how much we want to quit or ease off, we then drill them some more (stimulates mental strength)." [87]

— Iain Abernethy

In his book *Karate-Do Kyohan*, Gichin Funakoshi wrote, "Once a form has been learned, it must be practiced repeatedly until it can be applied in an emergency, for knowledge of just the sequence of a form in karate is useless." The same can be said for any martial art, of course.

When understood properly and performed correctly, *kata* form the heart of today's martial arts just as they did in ancient times. While this book provides the foundational principles and rules necessary for you to make the most out of your forms, we certainly don't believe that it contains all the answers. Mastering *kata* is a lifelong experience; one that is both intense and personal. Much must be discovered on your own. We encourage you to use this new information to continue your exploration.

When training together in a traditional *dojo*, both teacher and student bow to each other and say, *"Dozo one gaishimasu,"* which means, "Please teach me," as both expect to learn from each encounter. Similarly, at the end of training, both teacher and student say, *"Arigato gozaimashita,"* which means, "Thank you for teaching me," as both have learned. Now that we have shared our knowledge with you, we would appreciate your returning the favor. All comments are welcome. Your feedback may even be incorporated into the next addition of this book. We can be contacted through our publisher either by regular mail or through their Web site at www.ymaa-pub.com. Alternatively you may contact us directly via e-mail. Our e-mail addresses are listed at the end of this book next to our author bios. If you choose to go this route, please put *The Way of Kata* in the subject line so that your message will not be eaten by our spam filters.

Arigato gozaimashita.

Summary

"The recording of information through physical movement is an ancient practice. Even today, many cultures use 'dances' and sequences of physical movements to tell stories and to pass on their cultural heritage to the next generation. There can be little doubt that groups would also wish to pass on the fighting and hunting techniques they had refined and found to be most successful. When an individual learned the fighting and hunting skills of the group, they would be asked to copy the movements of those who were more experienced. The elders would demonstrate the various movements, and the younger members of the group would try to emulate these movements. These skills would eventually be further refined and then passed onto subsequent generations. It is in this way that the first kata were created." [88]

– Iain Abernethy

As martial forms evolved into sophisticated fighting systems, almost all Asian styles began to utilize *kata* in one form or another. A Japanese word meaning "formal exercise," *kata* consist of logical sequences of movements containing practical offensive and defensive techniques that are done in a particular order. The ancient masters embedded the secrets of their unique fighting systems in their *kata,* which became fault tolerant methods of imparting effective martial knowledge across the generations.

While there are almost unlimited combat applications in each *kata* movement, additional applications may be hidden *between* the movements of a *kata*. Every *kata* contains a significant number of secret techniques or *okuden waza* that are not obvious to the causal observer. Most of the truly dangerous, advanced routines are deliberately concealed. There are a couple of important historical reasons why these mechanisms are not readily apparent.

First off, when the Japanese conquered Okinawa, the birthplace of karate, in 1609 they banned the teaching of both armed and unarmed martial arts. Consequently the Okinawans had to conduct their training in great secrecy. Forms were passed between master and disciple through oral tradition with little or nothing written down. Much of the training was conducted indoors, at night, or otherwise shielded from prying eyes.

A second important reason for this secrecy can be found in the ancient custom of *kakidameshi*, a tradition where *budoka* in Okinawa routinely tested each other's fighting prowess with actual combat. Like the feudal *samurai* before or the old West gunfighters who would follow, the more famous the practitioner, the more often he would be challenged to combat by those seeking fame. Techniques not only had to be combat-worthy, but they also had to be held pretty close to the vest. It simply would not do for a competitor to know one's secrets before a fight.

Consequently there was often a two-track system of instruction, one that could be found in Japanese, Korean, and Chinese martial arts as well. The outer circle of students learned basic fundamentals, unknowingly receiving modified *kata* where critical details or principles were omitted. It was a significant honor to achieve even that level of training, as masters turned away all but the most dedicated of followers. Further, the heads of these martial ways universally expected instant obedience from their students, clarifying little and tolerating no questions. These practitioners had no idea that anything was missing.

The inner circle that had gained a master's trust and respect, on the other hand, could be taught *okuden waza*. Even within this inner circle, the rules and principles for deciphering all of a system's *kata* were frequently taught only to one student, the master's sole successor, rather than to the group as a whole. Often this instruction was withheld until the master became old or ill, shortly before his death. On occasion the master waited too long to pass along this vital knowledge and it was lost altogether.

In modern times *kata* was spread from Okinawa to the rest of the world, primarily by American GIs and Allied troops who learned karate during the occupation of that country at the end of World War II. Although locally high unemployment drove the many *budo* masters to teach the Westerners as a means to earn a living, most soldiers were not initiated into their inner circles. Further, even when instructors wished to share their secrets, language barriers often inhibited communication.

Later on, as karate was opened-up to society at large, it was frequently taught to schoolchildren. Many dangerous techniques were hidden from these practitioners simply because they were not mature enough to handle them responsibly. Consequently much of what made it to the outside world was intermediate level karate, devoid of principles and rules necessary to understand and utilize hidden techniques.

In Japanese martial arts understanding can be classified in two ways, *omote* and *ura waza*. *Omote* signifies the outer or surface training, while *ura waza* can be translated to denote the inner or subtle way. It is these critical details that make the more obvious succeed. Practitioners who never learn essential subtleties lack the tools required to make the most out of their martial art.

A deep understanding of strategy and tactics is a necessary prerequisite for being able to properly decipher *kata*. Like a house without a solid foundation, tactics without strategy will ultimately fail. To be effective, all martial applications must be grounded in a system's strategy. Picking and choosing individual techniques from a variety of different styles is almost always sub-optimal as there is no strategic concept binding them together.

We offer 15 specific principles that help practitioners identify effective techniques. They are the framework within which practitioners can identify valid interpretations of *bunkai*, *henka waza*, and even *okuden waza* from the *kata* they practice. These principles are summarized as follows:

1. **There is more than one proper interpretation of any movement**
   In actual combat practitioners transcend the artificial limitations of *kata*, finding near limitless interpretations for any given technique. Each practitioner should strive to find the interpretation which is most effective and practicable for him or her to use in a fight.

2. **Every technique should be able to end the fight immediately**
   Kata were developed before the advent of modern medicine which cures injuries that would have been fatal a century ago. Consequently the ancient masters designed every offensive technique and most defensive ones to immediately end a fight, dramatically reducing their changes of being crippled or killed.

3. **Strike to disrupt; disrupt to strike**
   An attacker is rarely going to stand there like a *makiwara* and let someone tee off on them. Practitioners need to disrupt an opponent's designs, get them off balance, and then move in for the kill.

4. **Nerve strikes are "extra credit"**
   Rather than relying solely on nerve techniques to stop a determined attacker, practitioners should consider them "extra credit", to be combined with other types of strikes. While generally effective, nerve attacks alone do not always work on everyone.

5. **Work with the adrenaline rush, not against it**
   Adrenaline limits practitioner's fine motor skills and higher thought processes so applications must be straightforward and simple to execute while causing incapacitating physiological damage sufficient to stop a resolute aggressor who is also hyped up on adrenaline.

6. **Techniques must work at full speed and power**
   While *kata* practice is about perfection, real fights are sloppy affairs. Practitioners must know what is necessary for success and not let the pursuit of perfection keep them from surviving a violent encounter.

7. It must work on an "unwilling" partner

Although practitioners cannot rely on unpredictable movements or specific techniques by an aggressor, *kata* applications do anticipate predictable anatomical responses. Real life opponents rarely fight fair and never cooperate with our techniques.

8. Strive to understand why it works

Ura waza are the subtle details that make the more obvious *omote* or surface training succeed. Understanding why an application works can help practitioners ensure that they will use it in the proper situations.

9. Deception is not real

Practitioners cannot count on deception during a fight. It must be used before a confrontation escalates to violence, preferably to avoid conflict altogether.

10. If you are not there, you cannot get hit

The only way to guarantee success in a fight is not to engage in combat in the first place. When forced to fight practitioners should be constantly moving, striking, and moving on such that by the time an opponent reacts to their strike the *budoka* should already have moved to the next technique.

11. Cross the T' to escape

"Crossing the T" is a historical nautical analogy describing a broadside cannon attack against the unprotected bow or stern of a sailing ship. This same concept is used to facilitate escapes from holds and throws in modern martial arts.

12. Stances aren't just for *kata*

Much *okuden waza* in *budo* uses stances and movement to unbalance and weaken an opponent. Combining simultaneous leg and hand techniques in one swift attack can be devastating.

13. Don't forget to breathe

For athletes in all types of sports, correct breathing is a vital component of energy management. *Budoka* are taught to breathe in through their noses and exhale through their mouths using their diaphragms to move the maximum amount of air possible through the lungs.

14. Use both hands

Both hands are used simultaneously in almost all techniques. When examining *kata* for *okuden waza* pay particular attention to the off hand, the one that is not executing an obvious technique.

15. A lock or hold is not a primary fighting technique

A lock or a hold is never a primary fighting technique in the striking arts. The goal is actually to drop the opponent with the initial strike, applying the lock or hold only when further control is required.

Traditional study of martial systems presumes the ability to perform techniques in actual combat. Sport and conditioning applications are more or less fringe benefits associated with such study. Individuals who learn an art's strategy and diligently practice its *kata* can develop real world fighting applications they may use to defend themselves. The theory of deciphering applications from *kata* is called *kaisai*. Since it offers guidelines for unlocking the true meaning of each *kata* movement, *kaisai no genri* was once a great mystery revealed only to trusted disciples of the ancient masters in order to protect the secrets of their systems.

Using the rules *of kaisai no genri*, practitioners can decipher the original intent of *kata* movements by logically analyzing each specific movement to find its *okuden waza*. The three main (or basic) rules are called *shuyo san gensoko* while the nine supplementary (or advanced) rules are called *hosoku joko*. Together these 12 rules are summarized as follows:

1. **Do not be deceived by the *enbusen* rule**
   Kata are choreographed using artificial symmetry to ensure that the practitioner never takes more than three or four steps in any one direction, a process of conserving required practice space. For this reason, movements to one side or the other do not necessarily imply an attacker on that side.

2. **Advancing techniques imply attack, while retreating techniques imply defense**
   Kata techniques performed while advancing imply attacks, even if they appear defensive in nature. As the second half of the rule implies, techniques performed while retreating are defensive in nature. In actual combat, however, there is no "retreat" per se. The perception of giving ground is really a tactic executed to control distance while continuing to actively engage an opponent.

3. **There is only one enemy at a time**
   In reality, from a street-fighting point of view, it is pretty much impossible to make a *kata* that is designed to fight against multiple attackers at once. Defense against a large group is generally handled by strategically engaging one person at a time in a manner that confounds the other's ability to reach the practitioner.

4. **Every movement in *kata* has martial meaning/significance and can be used in a real fight**
   Without the benefit of modern medicine, the ancient masters realized that even slight injuries in combat could become fatal. To ensure their survival, every *kata* technique was designed to end a confrontation as expeditiously as possible.

5. **A hand returning to chamber usually has something in it**
   When analyzing *kata*, it is important to pay attention to the off-hand, the one not executing an obvious technique. Frequently the hand returning to

chamber at the practitioner's side has something captured in it, especially if it is shown closed when performing the *kata*. This movement may imply grabs, locks, joint dislocations, takedowns, or even throws.

6. **Utilize the shortest distance to your opponent**
   To have the greatest opportunity for success, practitioners must strike or defend with their closest body part. Defensive movements must cut off the attacker's technique before it gains too much speed and power, catching it as close to their body as possible. Offensive techniques must afford the opponent as little reaction time as possible.

7. **Control an opponent's head and you control the opponent**
   Kata frequently use control of a person's head to disrupt their vision, breathing, and movement simultaneously through a variety eye, ear, neck, and head attacks. Simultaneous incapacitation of vision, breathing, and movement invariably assures victory in a violent confrontation.

8. **There is no "block"**
   Defensive techniques actively receive and take control of an attack. A fast, hard block has the potential to drop an opponent in his or her tracks, ending the fight before the practitioner even needs to throw an "offensive" blow.

9. ***Kata* demonstrates the proper angles**
   Turns in *kata* usually suggest an optimal angle of attack. Similarly, the distance from the practitioner's body at which the kata technique is displayed demonstrates how far away they should be from an opponent when applying the application.

10. **Touching your own body in *kata* indicates touching your opponent**
    By demonstrating a touch to one's own body, *kata* provides clues about locks, holds, throws, arm bars, and other applications and how they might be applied to an opponent. Augmented blocks are ineffectual in actual combat.

11. **Contour the body—strike hard to soft and soft to hard**
    When deciphering *kata*, contouring helps identify the primary or best target of any given technique. In general, hard parts strike soft targets and vice versa. The type of strike, along with its elevation in *kata*, is the essential clue you need.

12. **There is no pause**
    Pauses are incorporated into *kata* for several important reasons, including separating one section from another, emphasizing certain applications, or signifying the presence of hidden techniques between the more obvious movements. In combat application, however, there is no hesitation between techniques.

Using the principles and rules outlined previously in conjunction with a technique called cooperative performance, *budoka* can work with others in their *dojo* to experiment with their *kata*, identify what they believe are hidden applications, and ascertain whether or not they will work in an actual self-defense situation.

The best self-defense is avoiding a fight altogether. Once a conflict occurs, however, practitioners must do everything they can to end it quickly. They have to be at least as ruthless and violent as their attackers. If you accurately strike or grab an attacker's vital area you can elicit pain, temporary paralysis, dislocation or hyperextension of a joint, knockout, or possibly even death. Knowledge of such techniques can save your life in a fight.

It is also important to understand how you might interpret applications from your *kata* should you be fighting on a hill, around furniture or other obstacles, in a stairwell, under water, in a crowd, or in any other unusual situation. Not only do you need to be able to perform your techniques wearing a traditional loose-fitting *gi*, but in more restrictive street clothes as well. Training in the *dojo* is outstanding, but practicing outside the *dojo* on occasion can help realistically prepare practitioners for real combat.

Although you may be able to perform a *kata* and understand its various applications and hidden techniques, you may still not want to rely on it in actual combat. There are, after all, techniques you know, techniques you do, techniques you train, and techniques you'd stake your life on. It is essential to understand how to personalize techniques, applying things for which you have a natural affinity during a life or death struggle. We suggest a three-step approach: (1) learn the pattern, (2) make any changes necessary, and then (3) incorporate them into your applications.

When performed correctly and understood properly, *kata* form the heart of today's martial arts just as they did in ancient times. Alas, all too many practitioners overlook the importance of *kata* as a vital component of modern martial arts simply because they do not understand what their forms are trying to tell them. Everyone gains corollary benefits of improved physical conditioning, mental focus, and control through *kata* practice, yet only a select few truly unleash the full potential of their forms. By reading this book you are well on your way to becoming a member of that select group!

Bubishi Poem—Eight Precepts of Kempo

This is a Chinese *Kempo* poem found in the *Bubishi* (book of poems). *Goju Ryu* was named from the third line of this poem, which is sometimes translated as "Eight Poems of The Fist."

1. *Jinshin wa tenchi ni onaji*
    (The mind is one with Heaven and Earth)

2. *Ketsumyaku wa nichigetsu ni nitari*
    (The circulatory rhythm of the body is similar to the cycle of the Sun and the Moon)

3. *Ho wa goju ryu wo tondo su*
    (The way of inhaling and exhaling is hardness and softness)

4. *Mi wa toki ni shitagai hen ni ozu*
    (Act in accordance with time and change)

5. *Te wa ku ni ai sunawa chi hairu*
    (Techniques will occur in the absence of conscious thought)

6. *Shintai wa ha karite riho su*
    (The feet must advance and retreat, separate and meet)

7. *Me wa shiho wo miru wo yosu*
    (The eyes do not miss even the slightest change)

8. *Mimi wa yoku happo wo kiku*
    (The ears listen well in all directions)

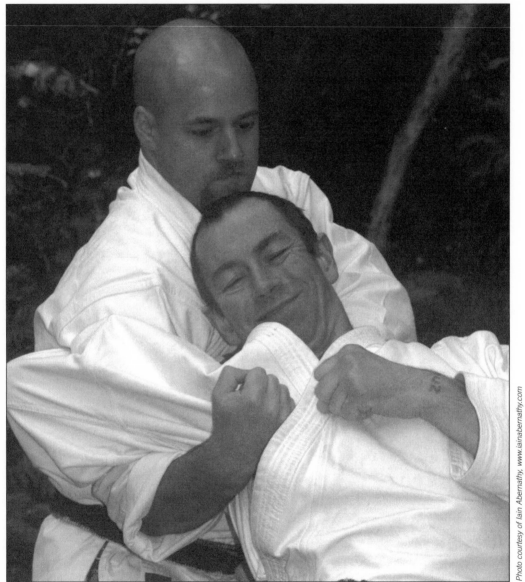

PASSAI ARMLOCK. IAIN ABERNETHY APPLIES A SHOULDER-LOCK FROM *PASSAI (BASSAI-DAI) KATA*. THIS MOVEMENT IS MOST COMMONLY LABELED AS A "HAMMER FIST STRIKE". THE RECIPIENT IS MURRAY DENWOOD. THE LOCATION IS HOLME WOOD, LOWESWATER, NORTHERN ENGLAND.

APPENDIX B

Kata of Goju Ryu

Goju Ryu has twelve core *kata* in its standard curriculum. These include *gekisai* (*dai ichi* and *dai ni*), *saifa, seiyunchin, seisan, saipai, shisochin, sanseiru, kururunfa, sanchin, tensho,* and *suparinpei*. In most systems practitioners learn all of these *kata* by *sandan* rank. Nine of the twelve are typically required for *shodan*, though the exact requirements can vary by school. The *Goju Ryu* kata are as follows:

Gekisai means "attack and smash, destruction." Created by Chojun Miyagi *Sensei* in 1940, *gekisai* are beginner's *kata*, the first to be learned in some styles. These *kata* introduce the fundamentals of *Goju Ryu* (e.g., stances, attacks, and blocks). Practitioners learn *dai ichi* first and then *dai ni*. The primary difference between the two is the introduction of open-hand techniques and additional stances in *dai ni*.

Saifa means "smash and tear" and is of Chinese origin, brought back to Okinawa by Kanryo Higaonna *Sensei*. It incorporates quick whipping movements and backfist strikes. *Seiyunchin*, another *kata* of Chinese origin, means to "pull off balance and fight." *Shiko dachi* (straddle or sumo stance) is emphasized and all of the movements are hand techniques (with no kicks), a distinctive feature.

Goju Ryu relies upon many grabbing and controlling techniques designed to unbalance an attacker and facilitate strikes to vulnerable parts of the body. Translated as "thirteen hands," *Seisan kata* emphasizes this principle with its eight defensive and five offensive techniques. This form stresses close-range fighting with short punches and low kicks to break through an opponent's defenses.

Another *kata* of Chinese origin, *saipai* translates as "eighteen hands," based on the formula of three times six. It contains many hidden techniques designed to confuse the opponent in combat. The six represent color, voice, taste, smell, touch, and justice. The three represents good, bad, and peace. *Saipai* has a variety of hand, foot, and body techniques that are somewhat unique within *Goju Ryu kata*.

Shisochin means "battle in four directions", and is sometimes called "four fighting monks." It is rumored to have been one *of Chojun Miyagi Sensei's* favorite *kata* in his later years, well suited to his body. This *kata* is unique to *Goju Ryu* and is not used in other *Naha Te* styles.

Sanseiru means "thirty-six hands," based on the formula six times six, and is sometimes called the "dragon kata." It also focuses on fighting in all four directions. The first six in the equation represents eyes, ears, nose, tongue, body, and spirit. The second six represents color, voice, taste, smell, touch, and justice. *Sanseiru* develops low kicks and utilizes many double hand techniques.

Kururunfa means "holding your ground." It is an advanced kata featuring *tai sabaki waza* (moving/shifting techniques) and very quick movement. It contains a wide variety of open-hand techniques, especially hand and hip coordination techniques.

Sanchin means "three battles." It is a moving meditation designed to unify the mind, body, and spirit. Techniques are done in slow motion such that *karateka* can emphasize precise muscle control, breath control, internal power, and body alignment. The movements look simple but are extremely difficult to master.

Chojun Miyagi *Sensei* created *tensho kata*, another moving meditation. *Tensho* means "little heaven" or "heaven's breath." It is a combination of hard dynamic tension with deep breathing and soft flowing hand movements, concentrating strength in the tanden, and is very characteristic of the *Goju Ryu* style.

Suparinpei represents the number 108 (3x36) and has special significance in Buddhism. It is believed that man has 108 evil passions, so in Buddhist temples on December 31, at the stroke of midnight, a bell is rung 108 times to drive away those spirits. The symbolism of 36 is the same as *sanseiru*. *Suparinpei* is *Goju Ryu's* longest *kata*. It utilizes a large number of techniques including breath control and contains the largest number of applications.

Additional Kata:

Some *Goju Ryu* systems add additional *kata* to their curricula. These typically include *taikyoku*, *hookiyu*, *gekiha*, and/or *kakuha*. In our *dojo*, for example, we use the core curriculum above plus *taikyoku* (*jodan*, *chudan*, and *gedan*).

Taikyoku means, "First course." Gichin Funakoshi *Sensei*, the founder of the *Shotokan* karate style, created the original *taikyoku* series. The *Goju Ryu* versions have been modified to reflect elements within our style, such as the *zenkutsu dachi* (front stance) stances. They all follow the basic H pattern and increase slightly in difficulty as more techniques are added.

Hookiyu are universal or unified *kata*, created by Seikichi Toguchi *Sensei*, which introduce the basics of *Goju Ryu* stances and defensive postures. They are sometimes considered a simplified form of *gekisai kata*.

Gekiha translates as "to destroy something large, very hard, or well fortified." Also created by Seikichi Toguchi *Sensei*, *gekiha* expands on the basics introduced in *hookiyu* by adding more complex strikes, counter strikes, body movements, and blocks.

Kakuha represents the three basic traditional schools of karate from the three major port cities in Okinawa—*Goju Ryu, Shorin Ryu,* and *Tomari Te.* It is sometimes translated to represent each school's difference of opinion or separation from each other. It was designed to bring these differences, or representative applications and philosophy, together in one form.

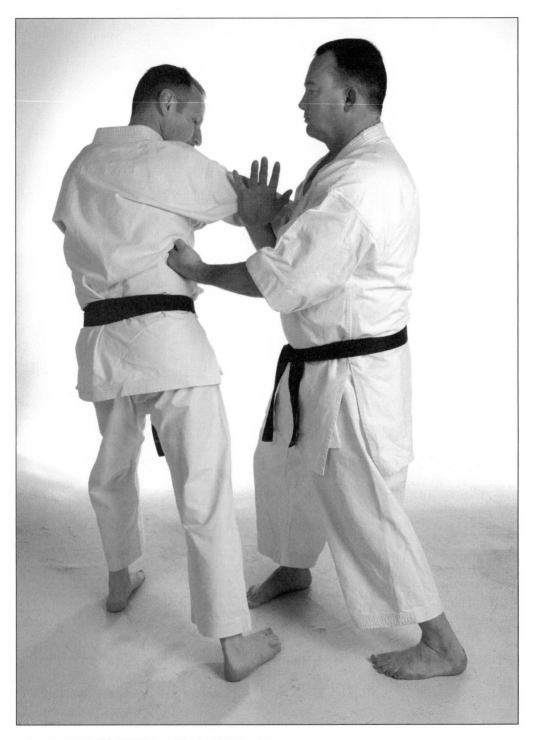

SUPARINPEI ARM LOCK, UPPERCUT. THIS TECHNIQUE IS A SIGNATURE MOVEMENT OF *SUPARINPEI KATA*.

Kata Application Evaluation Checklist

To evaluate a potential kata application, check (✓) the boxes that apply:

Yes	No	Principles	Yes	No	Rules
		1) More than one proper interpretation exists			1) Do not be deceived by the enbusen rule
		2) Every technique should be able to immediately end the fight			2) Advancing techniques imply attack, while retreating techniques imply defense
		3) Strike to disrupt; disrupt to strike			3) There is only one enemy at a time
		4) Nerve strikes are "extra credit"			4) Every movement in kata has martial meaning/significance
		5) Work with the adrenaline rush, not against it			5) A hand returning to chamber usually has something in it
		6) Techniques must work at full speed and power			6) Utilize the shortest distance to your opponent
		7) Application must work on an "unwilling" partner			7) Control an opponent's head and you control the opponent
		8) Understand why it works			8) There is no "block"
		9) Deception is not real			9) Kata demonstrate the proper angles
		10) If you are not there, you cannot get hit			10) Touching your own body in kata indicates touching your opponent
		11) Cross the T to escape			11) Contour the body—strike hard to soft and soft to hard
		12) Stances aren't just for kata			12) There is no pause
		13) Don't forget to breathe	**Yes**	**No**	**Other Considerations**
		14) Use both hands			A) Consistent with style's strategy
		15) A lock or hold is not a primary fighting technique			B) Built on natural physiological reaction

Valid applications should comply with principles, rules, and considerations above. Those that are not applicable should be left blank. If any "no" box is checked your potential application is sub-optimal.

FEEL FREE TO PHOTOCOPY THIS TABLE FOR YOUR OWN USE.

Notes

1. Teruo Chinen *Sensei* the founder of Jundo-Kan International, a karate organization with numerous schools internationally as well as in the United States. Chinen *Sensei* lived three doors away from Chojun Miyagi *Sensei*'s home in Okinawa. He was introduced to the founder of *Goju Ryu* karate (Miyagi) at a very young age and trained under Miyazato *Sensei*, as well as Miyagi *Sensei* himself. This quote is from an interview with Douglas Tran, which took place at the Jundo-Kan International's Spring *Gasshuku* on Sunday, May 31, 1997, in Montclair, New Jersey.

2. From the book *The Heart of Karate-do* by Shigeru Egami, New York, NY: Kodansha International, 1980.

3. Aristotle (384—322 B.C.), Greek philosopher. Aristotle was a major contributor in determining the orientation and content of Western intellectual history. He was the author of a philosophical and scientific system that served as a foundation for scholastic thought until the end of the 17th century.

4. Joe Talbot, Tracy's Karate Studios (St. Louis, MO).

5. Chojun Miyagi (1888—1953), founder of *Goju Ryu* karate. He structured the system of *Naha Te*, which he learned from Kanryo Higashionna *Sensei*, adapted it to the demands of modern society, and made it available to the public as *Goju Ryu*, the first codified form of karate.

6. Ibid.

7. From the article, "The Long and Winding Road," by Paul Okami. *Black Belt Magazine*, January 1983.

8. From the book, *Okinawan Goju Ryu II* by Seikichi Toguchi; Santa Clara, CA: Ohara Publications, 2001.

9. Ibid.

10. Chojun Miyagi (see note 5).

11. Rory A. Miller has been studying martial arts since 1981 and holds *Mokuroku* (teaching certificate) in *Sosuishitsu-Ryu Jujitsu*. He is also trained in fencing and judo. Mr. Miller is a corrections sergeant for a two-thousand bed system. A specialist in defensive tactics and hand-to-hand combat, he is the leader of the Corrections Emergency Response Team.

12. Iain Abernethy has been involved in the martial arts since childhood. He is a senior instructor with the British Karate-Do *Chojinkai* and an instructor with the British Combat Association. Iain regularly writes for the UK's leading martial arts magazines and he is a member of the Combat Hall of Fame. His web site is www.iainabernethy.com.

13. From the article, "Sometimes I play Karatedo like Okinawa Dance Hamachidori: Karatedo and Okinawa Dance is the Same," by Kiyohiko Higa. *Aoi Umi* magazine, February 1978.

14. Marc "Animal" MacYoung teaches experience-based self-defense to police, military, civilians, and martial artists around the world. A former bouncer and street fighter, and all around dangerous guy, his advice is available at www.nononsenseselfdefense.com.

15. Miyamoto Musashi (1584—1645), arguably the greatest swordsman who ever lived. Considered *Kensei*, the sword saint of Japan. Musashi killed more than sixty trained *samurai* warriors in fights or duels during the feudal period where even a minor battle injury could lead to infection and death. Two years before he died, Musashi retired to a life of seclusion in a cave where he codified his winning strategy in the famous *Go Rin No Sho* (*Book of Five Rings*).

16. MacYoung (see note 14).

17. Confucius (551—479 B.C.), Chinese sage. As he traveled widely throughout China, his ideas for social reform made him the idol of the people but made him many powerful enemies as well. His moral teaching stressed the importance of the traditional relations of filial piety and brotherly respect.

18. Miyamoto Musashi (see note 15).

19. From the article, "Strategy vs. Tactics" by Steve Badger, www.playwinningpoker.com.

20. Dwight David Eisenhower (1890—1969), 34th president of the United States. During WWII he successfully commanded the Allied Forces landing in North Africa in 1942 and later in 1944 was the Supreme Commander of Allied troops invading France on D-Day.

21. MacYoung (see note 14).

22. Sigmund Freud (1856—1939), physiologist, medical doctor, psychologist and father of psychoanalysis. Freud is generally considered as one of the most influential and authoritative thinkers of the twentieth century.

23. From the book, *Okinawan Goju Ryu II* (see note 8).

24. Jawaharal Nehru (1889—1964), India's first prime minister. Head of the Indian National Congress (INC), a political party created by Mohandas Gandhi, Nehru led India's fight for independence from Britain. Gandhi chose Nehru to head the transitional government. In the 1947 national election, he was overwhelmingly elected prime minister repeatedly re-elected thereafter until he death on May 27, 1964.

25. Morio Higaonna (1938—), Chief Instructor of the International Okinawan *Goju Ryu* Karate-Do Federation (IOGKF). A direct disciple of Chojun Miyagi *Sensei*, Higaonna is one of *Goju Ryu's* most famous practitioners. He has published numerous books and videos about his art.

26. Sun Tzu (544—496 B.C.), Chinese general who helped the King Ho-Lu capture the city of Ying, bringing about the fall of the Ch'u state in 506 B.C. His collection of essays, *The Art of War*, is one of the best known and most quoted military treatises in the world.

27. From the book, *A Practical Self-Defense Guide for Women* by Paul McCallum; Croaet, VA: Betterway Publications, Inc., 1991.

28. Choki Motobu (1871—1944), one of Okinawa's most feared fighters of that era. Born the third son of a high ranking family at a time when education and privilege were reserved for the first born. Motobu studied karate with several legendary masters including Ankoh Itosu of *Shuri Te* and Kosaku Matsumora of *Tomari Te*.

29. Gichin Funakoshi (1868—1957), founder of *Shotokan* karate. Funakoshi *Sensei* learned both *Shuri Te* and *Naha Te* in Okinawa, combining these styles to form his Shotokan School. He traveled to Japan to demonstrate his art to no lesser dignitaries than the emperor himself, remaining there to teach and promote karate.

30. Nikita Sergeyevich Khrushchev (1894-1971), Soviet Premier. Following the death of Stalin in March 1953, Khrushchev became First Secretary of the All Union Party and, three years later, at the 20th Congress of the Communist Party.

31. Miyamoto Musashi (see note 15).

32. From the book, *Pressure Point Fighting: A Guide to the Secret Heart of Asian Martial Arts* by Rick Clark; North Clarendon, VT: Tuttle Publishing, 2001.

33. From the book, *Secrets of Street Survival—Israeli Style: Staying Alive in a Civilian War Zone* by Eugene Sockut; Boulder, CO: Paladin Enterprises, Inc., 1995.

34. From the book, *Pressure Point Fighting* (see note 32).

35. Marc "Animal" MacYoung (see note 14).

36. Morio Higaonna (see note 25).

37. Miyamoto Musashi (see note 15).

38. Bruce Lee (1940—1973), founder of Jeet Kune Do.

39. Broadside is a collection of pages describing life in Royal Navy in the late eighteenth and early nineteenth century, the time of the Revolutionary and Napoleonic Wars. It is located at www.nelson-snavy.co.uk.

40. Rita Burns, Great Lakes Wushu (Ann Arbor, MI).

41. From the book, *Okinawan Goju Ryu* by Seikichi Toguchi; Burbank, CA: Ohara Publications, 1976.

42. Miyamoto Musashi (see note 15).

43. From the book, *Bunkai Jutsu: The Practical Application of Karate Kata* by Iain Abernethy; Cockermouth, UK: NETH Publishing, 2002.

44. *Pressure Point Fighting* (see note 32).

45. *Okinawan Goju Ryu II* (see note 8).

46. Ibid.

47. Ibid.

48. Ibid.

49. Gichin Funakoshi (see note 29).

50. Victor Smith is a respected teacher of *Isshin Ryu* karate (6th degree black belt) and *tai chi chuan* with over 26 years of training in Japanese, Korean and Chinese martial arts. He is the founder of the martial arts website FunkyDragon.com/bushi and is an associate editor of FightingArts.com.

51. Morio Higaonna (see note 25).

52. Sun Tzu (see note 26).

53. Bunkai Jutsu (see note 43).

54. Ibid.

55. Bertrand Arthur William Russell (1872—1970), British philosopher. He is known for his work in mathematical logic and analytic philosophy.

56. From the book, *Fighter's Fact Book: Over 400 Concepts, Principles, and Drills to Make You a Better Fighter* by Loren Christensen, Wethersfield, CT: Turtle Press, 2000.

57. Christopher Caile is the founder and editor-in-chief of FightingArts.com. He has been a student of the martial arts for over 40 years and holds a 6th degree black belt in *Seido* karate and has experience in judo, aikido, *Diato Ryu*, boxing and several Chinese fighting arts.

58. *Pressure Point Fighting* (see note 32).

59. Miyamoto Musashi (see note 15).

60. *Secrets of Street Survival—Israeli Style* (see note 33).

61. Sir Winston Churchill (1874—1965), British Prime Minister. Churchill became the voice of Britain during WWII, his emotional speeches inspiring his nation to endure hardship and sacrifice necessary to win the war. He also won a Nobel Prize for Literature in 1953 for his six volume history of World War II.

62. Roger Traub, PhD. Professor of Mathematical Neuroscience, Neuroscience Unit, Department of Physiology, University of Birmingham, formerly IBM Research Division, Yorktown Heights, NY.

63. Miyamoto Musashi (see note 15).

64. Gogen Yamaguchi (1909—1989), known as "The Cat" this direct disciple of Chojun Miyagi was the founder of Japanese *Goju-Ryu*—one of Japan's largest and most successful karate organizations.

65. Ben Robinson, master magician. He is considered one of the world's greatest illusionists, and acclaimed consultant in advertising, public relations, and business strategy. An award-winning writer and producer, he gives hundreds of performances a year around the world.

66. *Fighter's Fact Book* (see note 56).

67. Ibid.

68. *Pressure Point Fighting* (see note 43).

69. George Orwell (1903—1950), pen name used by British author and journalist Eric Arthur Blair. Orwell is probably best remembered for two of his novels, *Animal Farm* and *Nineteen Eighty-Four*.

70. Frank Herbert (1920—1986), best selling science fiction writer and author of the *Dune* series. During the WWII he was an accredited photographer with the U.S. Navy. After the war he held a variety of positions including working as a newspaper reporter, oyster-diver, TV cameraman, radio news commentator, jungle survival instructor, and judo instructor.

71. Miyamoto Musashi (see note 15).

72. Admiral Hyman George Rickover (1900—1986), the driving force behind bringing the Navy into the nuclear age with his persistence that the United States build the first atomic-powered submarine, the Nautilus, in 1954.

73. Count Otto von Bismarck (Germany, 1815—1898), Germany's "Iron Chancellor," considered the founder of the German Empire; he is one of the most significant political figures of the 19th century. His primary goal was to unify Germany and once that was achieved he became a master of balancing alliances to keep the European peace, primarily by isolating Napoleon III of France, using him to distract the Austrians in Italy and tempting him with offers of Belgium.

74. Don Sorrel is a teacher of *Isshin Ryu* karate with over 27 years experience in the martial arts. He is the author of the book *Isshin Ryu Karate: The Practical Applications of Seisan Kata*, various articles on applications of *kata*, and frequently gives seminars on the subject of *kata* applications.

75. *Bunkai Jutsu* (see note 43).

76. From the book, *Goju Ryu Karate-Do: Volume 1 Fundamentals for Traditional Practitioners* by Motoo Yamakura, Monroe, MI: G.K.K. Productions, 1989.

77. Napoleon Bonaparte (1769—1821). Born on the island of Corsica, Napoleon rose from obscurity to become Napoleon I, *Empereur des Français* (Emperor of the French) using a combination of military and political ruthlessness.

78. George Foreman (1949—), boxer. Olympic heavyweight boxing champion (1968); world heavyweight boxing champion (1973—1974 and 1994—1995).
79. *Secrets of Street Survival—Israeli Style* (see note 33).
80. Woody Hayes (1913—1987), football coach. As college coach he amassed three national championships and 13 Big Ten titles. He had 241 victories as a college football coach.
81. Dr. W. Edwards Deming (1900—1993). Dr. W. Edwards Deming is known as the father of the Japanese post-war industrial revival and was regarded by many as the leading quality guru in the United States. Trained as a statistician, his expertise was used during World War II to assist the United States in its effort to improve the quality of war materials. At the end of World War II he helped the Japanese become world leaders in producing innovative quality products.
82. Henry Havelock Ellis (1859—1939). Like several members of the Fabian Society, he was a supporter of sexual liberation. His interests in human biology and his own personal experiences led Havelock Ellis to write his six-volume *Studies in the Psychology of Sex*. The books, published between 1897 and 1910 caused tremendous controversy and were banned for several years. Other books written by Havelock Ellis included *The New Spirit* (1890), *Man and Woman* (1894) *Sexual Inversion* (1897) and *The Erotic Rights of Women* (1918). Henry Havelock Ellis died in 1939. His autobiography, *My Life* was published posthumously in 1940.
83. Charles Mingus (1922—1979), musician. An important figure in twentieth century American music, Charles Mingus was a virtuoso bass player, accomplished pianist, bandleader and composer considered easily one of the best jazz bassists of all time.
84. Jim Alan Bouton (1939—), baseball player. Nicknamed "Bulldog," he was a Major League Baseball Pitcher and Author. From 1959 to 1978 he played for the New York Yankees, Seattle Pilots, Houston Astros, Chicago White Sox, and Atlanta Braves.
85. Gilbert K. Chesterton (1874-1936) was a prolific English critic and author. He produced nearly a hundred books, including the classics *Orthodoxy* and *The Man Who Was Thursday*, and biographies of St. Thomas Aquinas and St. Francis of Assisi. He wrote articles for about 125 periodicals, and was also a talented literary critic, mystery writer, economic and political analyst, social commentator, orator, humorist and poet. He was received into the Catholic Church in 1922.
86. Aristotle (see note 3).
87. Iain Abernethy (see note 12).
88. Ibid.

Glossary

Romaji (Romanization) note—We have primarily used the *Hebon-Shiki* (Hepburn) method of translating Japanese writing into the English alphabet and determining how best to spell the words (though accent marks have been excluded), as it is generally considered the most useful insofar as pronunciation is concerned. We have italicized foreign terms such that they can be readily differentiated from their English counterparts (e.g., *dan* meaning black belt rank versus Dan, the male familiar name for Daniel). As the Japanese and Chinese languages do not use capitalization, we have only capitalized those words that would be used as proper nouns in English.

Japanese is a challenging language for many English speakers to pronounce correctly. A few hints—for the most part, short vowels sound just like their English counterparts (e.g., **a** as in f<u>a</u>ther, **e** as in p<u>e</u>n). Long vowels are essentially double-length (e.g., **o** as in <u>oi</u>l, in the word *oyo*). The **u** is nearly silent, except where it is an initial syllable (e.g., *uke*). Vowel combination **e** + **i** sounds like d<u>ay</u> (e.g., *bugeisha*), **a** + **i** sounds like al<u>i</u>ve (e.g., *bunkai*), **o** + **u** sounds like fl<u>oa</u>t (e.g., *tou*), and **a** + **e** sounds like l<u>ie</u> (*kamae*). The consonant **r** is pronounced with the tip of the tongue, midway between **l** and **r** (e.g., *daruma*). Consonant combination **ts** is pronounced like ca<u>ts</u>, almost a **z** (e.g., *tsuki*).

This glossary is split into two sections: a glossary of terms and a glossary of techniques (which are illustrated to facilitate understanding). Although there are a few words here from other languages such as Chinese, Greek, or Latin, the vast majority of words listed in this glossary come from Japanese, hence the header Japanese Terminology.

Glossary of Terms

ashi waza   kicks, leg techniques

atemi waza   pressure point techniques

bo   fighting staff

budo   martial ways (arts); sometimes translated as the "martial way of finding enlightenment, self-realization, and understanding"; evolved from *bugei* at the end of the Japanese feudal era, modern *budo* include such arts as judo, karate, aikido, and kendo

budoka   martial artist, a practitioner of *budo*

bugei   martial arts, specifically classical martial arts as practiced during the time of the *samurai* in feudal Japan

bugeisha   martial artist, a practitioner of *bugei*

bunkai (or *kata bunkai*)   basic or commonly understood applications or fighting techniques found in *kata*

251

bunkai oyo   application of the principles of a *kata*; frequently fighting techniques arranged in a particular flow (logical order) for practice

bushido   "the way of the warrior," the *samurai* philosophy, concepts, and ideals that were generally practiced in feudal Japan. The seven virtues associated with *bushido* include rectitude (right decisions), courage, benevolence, respect, honesty, honor, and loyalty.

Butotu Kai   the institution that groups all martial arts in Japan

Chan Fa   an ancient style of *kung fu*

Ch'Uen Yuan   170 hand and foot positions taught to the monks of *Shaolin* by the monk Bodhidharma

chi   internal energy

chiishi   stone or concrete weight on a stick used for exercise

chudan   chest or middle (for a punch, aim at the solar plexus)

dachi   stance

daito   long sword

dan   black belt rank

daruma   warm-up exercises

Dim Mak   pressure point fighting

dogi (or *gi*)   uniform used for practicing martial arts

dojo   school or training hall; literally a "place to learn the way"; also called *dojang* in Korean or *kwoon* in Chinese

dokko   mastoid process

enbusen   lines of performance in *kata*

fault tolerant   systems that are designed to operate successfully regardless of whether or not an error or defect occurs, as opposed to those that can be broken by a single point of failure or even systems that rarely have problems at all. Like *kata*, they are very robust.

fudoshin   "indomitable spirit" or "warrior heart," a mental edge that makes a personal formidable.

fuku shiki kumite   freestyle sparring with *kata* emphasis

gasshuku   special training; typically extended or intensive coverage of subjects not always covered in general class

gedan   downward (for a punch, aim at the *obi* knot)

gekisai kata   a *Goju Ryu kata* that can be translated as "*attack and smash, destruction*"

gekiha kata   a *Goju Ryu kata* that can be translated as "*to destroy something large, very hard, or well fortified*"

gekon   center of the jaw

geri   kick (or kicking technique)

gi (**or** *dogi*)   uniform used for practicing martial arts

gladius   Latin for short sword, a primarily thrusting weapon used by the ancient Roman foot soldiers

go no sen   to receive an attack then respond

Goju Ryu   an Okinawan form of karate developed by Chojun Miyagi *Sensei*, which focuses ~70 percent on punching, 20 percent on kicking, 5 percent on throwing, and 5 percent on grappling; literally the "hard/gentle way of the infinite fist"

goshin do ippon kumite   self-defense techniques adapted from *kata*

hanshi   model instructor (someone to be modeled after), generally a senior master instructor of 8th degree black belt or higher who has a specialized certification beyond their rank alone

henka waza   commonly translated as variation techniques; applications from a *kata* that vary slightly from the exact way in which they are shown during performance of that *kata*

hichu   larynx

hidari   left

hikite   a push-pull concept that ensures proper body mechanics for maximum quickness and power in any martial technique, literally translates as "pulling hands"

hodoki   unleashing of hands, a trial period for gaining acceptance into a *dojo* in feudal Japan

hojo undo   supplemental training exercises

hookiyu kata   unified *kata*, an elementary *Goju Ryu* form

hosoku joko   supplementary or advanced rules of *kaisai* (method for deciphering *kata*)

hyomengi   apparent movements of fighting techniques

ibuki   breath control; generally hard breathing techniques as typified by *sanchin* or *tensho* *kata*

ippon kiso kumite   prearranged sparring using only the last attack and defense from each *kiso kumite* set followed by freeform attacks

jinchu   intermaxillary suture

jodan   head (for a punch, aim at the chin)

judo   a Japanese martial art developed by Jigoro Kano *Sensei* featuring an emphasis on throwing, grappling, choking, and joint-locking techniques

judoka   judo practitioners (the name of an art form with *ka* on the end refers to its practitioners)

kaisai no genri   method for deciphering *bunkai* (applications) from *kata*; sometimes called the theory of *kaisai kakidameshi*   dueling; ancient custom between *budoka* to test each other's fighting skills in actual combat (similar to that of gunfighters in the old West or *samurai* in feudal Japan)

karate   a (primarily) Japanese or Okinawan martial art which emphasizes weaponless or empty hand striking techniques (e.g., punching/kicking)

karate ni sente nashi   "there is no first strike in karate," a saying made famous by Gichin Funakoshi, the founder of *Shotokan* Karate

karateka   karate practitioners

kata   a pattern of movements containing a series of logical and practical offensive and defensive techniques

keikoku   a warning issued to a tournament competitor for inadvertent rules violations

keppan   blood oath sworn upon entrance to a *dojo* in feudal Japan, a loyalty oath signed and sealed with the applicant's blood

kiai   spirit shout, a loud shout or yell to focus one's energy and off-balance an opponent

ki   spirit and energy

kihon   basic or fundamental techniques such as strikes, blocks, or stances

kihon kata   basic *kata*; in *Goju Ryu* this includes *taikyoku, hookiyu,* and *gekisai.*

kiso kumite   pre-arranged sparring using techniques found in *kata*

kiten point   the physical point from which one originated a *kata* (starting position)

kobudo   a Japanese or Okinawan martial art featuring a variety of weapons forms

koken   wrist

komekami   temple (the body part, not the building)

kumite   sparring

kung fu   (primarily) Chinese martial featuring primarily weaponless or empty hand techniques; literally, "hard work"

kuroi-obi   black belt

koryu kata   old form *kata*; in *Goju Ryu* this includes *saifa, seiyunchin, seisan, saipai, shisochin, sanseiru, kururunfa, suparinpei, and sanchin*

kururunfa   a *Goju Ryu* kata that can be translated as "*holding your ground*"

kyushu   vital areas of the human body; physiologically weak points

kyushu jitsu   vital area techniques

kyoshi   master teaching instructor (teacher of teachers), generally a 6th or 7th degree black belt who has a special certification beyond their rank alone

kyu   colored belt rank (typically white, yellow, green, blue, or brown)

legio   Latin for Roman legions

makiwara   striking post; usually padded with leather, foam, or rope *migi*   right

mikazuki   mandible

miken   *summit of the nose*

mokuso   meditation or empty mind

monjin   person at the gate; someone who had been accepted into the ranks of a *ryu* during feudal Japan

morote   double

mudansha   practitioners within the colored belt or *kyu* ranks (*i kyu* or below); literally "no rank"

muchimi   sticky hands, a method of controlling an opponent through contact and pressure rather than by grabbing him

Naha Te   an Okinawan fighting art influenced by southern style *kung fu*; karate indigenous to the *Naha* region

ne waza   groundwork; ground fighting techniques

nigiri game   gripping jars used for conditioning exercises

nogare   gentle breathing; soft breath control techniques

obi   belt

okuden   hidden teaching; secret techniques of a school or martial style

okuden waza   secret applications intentionally concealed within a *kata*

omote   surface training; the obvious or outer facets of a martial system

oyo   application principles upon which *kata* technique is based

pankration   "all powers fighting" an ancient Greek martial art

pila   Roman javelins (plural); singular is *pilum*

qigong   a Chinese internal art (also known as *chi kung*)

randori   free sparring

renshi   senior expert instructor, generally a 5th or 6th degree black belt who has a specialized certification beyond their rank alone

ryu   system or style of *budo*

sai   a martial arts weapon with a long metal shaft that can be used to stab or strike, and twin forward curving tines in front of the handle that can be used capture an opponent's weapon

saifa kata   a *Goju Ryu kata* that can be translated as "smash and tear"

saipai kata   a *Goju Ryu kata* that can be translated as "*eighteen hands*"

sambo   a Russian military martial art

sanchin kata   a *Goju Ryu kata* that can be translated as "three battles"

sanbon shobu kumite   three point, tournament style fighting *sanseiru*   a *Goju Ryu kata* that can be translated as "*thirty six hands*"

scutum   Latin for shield, specifically those carried by the ancient Roman legionnaires

seidon   circumorbital region

seisan kata   a *Goju Ryu kata* that can be translated as "*thirteen hands*"

seiyunchin   a *Goju Ryu kata* that can be translated as "pull off balance and fight"

sen no sen   intercept an attack once it is underway

sen-sen no sen   pre-emptively cut off an attack before an opponent can translate the mental desire to attack to the physical movement necessary to carry it out

sensei   teacher, literally "one who has come before;" a guide to one's development

shihan   expert instructor, generally a 4th degree black belt or higher who has a specialized certification beyond their rank alone

shikkaku   disqualification issued against a tournament competitor for unsafe behavior or intentional rules violations such hitting with excessive force, making contact with the throat, or attacking the groin, joints or instep.

shime waza   choking techniques

shisochin   a *Goju Ryu kata* that can be translated as "*battle in four directions*"

shodan   first degree black belt; literally "least" or lowest of the *dan* ranks

shomen   front (or place of honor)

Shuri Te   an Okinawan fighting form influenced by the hard techniques of northern *kung fu*

shuyo san gensoko   main or basic rules of *kaisai* (method of deciphering *kata*)

signifer   Latin for standard bearer; officers who carried the legion battle standards in ancient Rome

suparinpei   a *Goju Ryu kata* that can be translated as "*108 hands*"

tachi waza   throwing techniques

tai sabaki waza   movement; shifting, and evasive maneuvers

taikai   public demonstration (e.g., martial arts performance)

Taijiquan   a Chinese martial art also known as *tai chi chuan*

taikyoku kata   a form that can be translated as "*first course*" *kata*

tamashiwara   board breaking

tan   conditioning log

tanden   center of the body, roughly located at a practitioner's *obi* knot (center of *ki* energy) two finger widths below their naval

tatami   practice mat used in traditional grappling arts such as judo

te   hand

te waza   punches, hand techniques

tendo   crown of the head

tento   fontanelle

tensho   a *Goju Ryu kata* that can be translated as *"little heaven"*

Tomari Te   an Okinawan fighting art influenced by both the northern and southern forms of *kung fu*

tori   "attacker" in tandem drills

Tote   "Chinese hand" another name for kung fu as it spread through Okinawa

tsuki   punch; pronounced and sometimes spelled *zuki*

uke   to receive an attack (block); also the term used to describe the "receiver" in tandem drills (i.e., the one being "attacked")

ura waza   inner or subtle way; the essential nuance that makes a martial system or technique work properly

yanjigo   a large diagonal step performed after completing a *kata* to return to the place of origination (*kiten* point) and straighten up the line; literally translated as "45 degrees"

yudansha   practitioners within the black belt or *dan* ranks (*shodan* or higher*)*

yunbi undo   warm-up exercises

zanshin   continuing mind

Glossary of Techniques

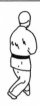 ***bensoku dachi***   cross-foot stance; a transitional stance sometimes performed during a turn

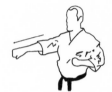 ***choko tsuki***   straight punch

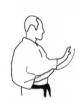 ***chudan hiki uke***   pulling/grasping open-hand chest block

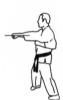 ***chudan tsuki***   chest punch

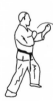 ***chudan uke***   chest block

furi uchi   swing strike

 gedan barai uke   sweeping (open-hand) down block

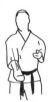 *gedan tsuki*   down punch

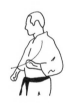 *gedan uke*   down block

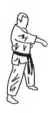 *gyaku tsuki*   reverse punch

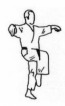 *hakusura dachi*   crane stance

 heiko hiji ate   horizontal elbow strike

 hiji ate   elbow strike

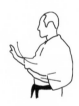 *hiki uke*   open hand chest block

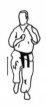 *hiza geri*   knee strike

ippon ken   one-knuckle fist

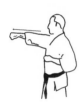

ippon seio nage   one arm shoulder throw

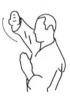

jodan tsuki   head punch

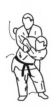

jodan uke   head block

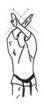

juji uke   cross block

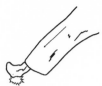

kakato geri   stomping heel kick

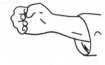

kama-de uchi   bear claw strike

kamae   combative posture—standing in _sanchin dachi_ (hourglass stance), for example, with one hand in chamber (at the side) and one out in front in a chest block

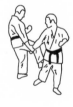

kensetsu geri   joint kick

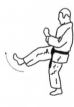

mae geri   front kick

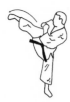

mawashe geri   wheel kick

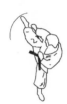

mawashe uke   wheel block

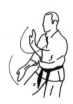

mikazuki geri   hook kick

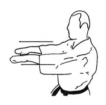

morote kama-de uchi   double bear claw strike

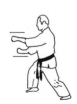

morote seiken tsuki   double punch

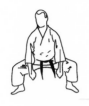 ***naka daka ippon ken***   double downward strike using a one-knuckle fist

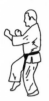 ***neko ashi dachi***   cat stance

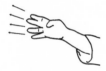 ***nukite***   finger strike

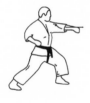 ***oi tsuki***   lunge punch

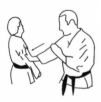 ***osai uke***   press block

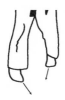

sanchin dachi   hourglass stance

seiken tsuki   fore fist strike; a standard karate punch

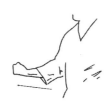

shiko dachi   straddle or *sumo* stance

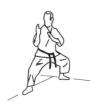

shita tsuki   palm-up center punch (similar to an uppercut but straight in rather than upward angle)

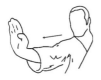

shotei uchi   palm heel strike

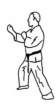

shozenkutsu dachi   half-front stance, a shortened version of *zenkutsu dachi*

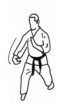

shuto   knife hand strike; also "small" sword

sukui uke   scoop block

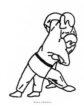

tani otoshi   valley drop throw

tate tsuki   standing fist punch; fist held vertically

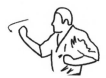 *tetsui uchi*   hammerfist strike

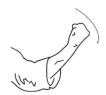 *uchi uke*   inside forearm block

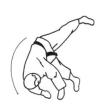 *ukemi waza*   breakfall techniques

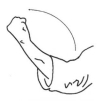 *uraken uchi*   backfist strike

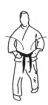 *wa uke*   valley block

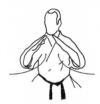

yama uke   mountain block

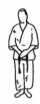

yoi   ready position for beginning a *kata* with hands at waist level, left hand over right, fingers extended together pointing downward, literally translates as *"to prepare"*

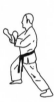

zenkutsu dachi   front forward stance

Bibliography

Books

Abernethy, Iain. *Bunkai Jutsu: The Practical Application of Karate Kata*. Cockermouth, UK: NETH Publishing, 2002.

Abernethy, Iain. *Karate's Grappling Methods: Understanding Kata and Bunkai*. Chichester, UK: Summersdale Publishers, 2001.

Abernethy, Iain. *Throws for Strikers: The Forgotten Throws of Karate, Boxing, and Taekwondo*. Chichester, UK: Summersdale Publishers, 2003.

Ayoob, Massad. *The Truth About Self-Protection*. New York, NY: Bantam Books (Police Bookshelf), 1983.

Burgar, Bill. *Five Years One Kata: Putting Kata Back at the Heart of Karate*. Edinburgh, UK: Martial Arts Publishing Ltd., 2003.

Christensen, Loren. *Fighter's Fact Book: Over 400 Concepts, Principles, and Drills to Make You a Better Fighter*. Wethersfield, CT: Turtle Press, 2000.

Christensen, Loren. *Speed Training: How to Develop Your Maximum Speed for Martial Arts*. Boulder, CO: Paladin Enterprises, Inc., 1996.

Christensen, Loren. *Warriors: On Living With Courage, Discipline and Honor*. Boulder, CO: Paladin Enterprises, Inc., 2004.

Clark, Rick. *Pressure Point Fighting: A Guide to the Secret Heart of Asian Martial Arts*. North Clarendon, VT: Tuttle Publishing, 2001.

Craig, Darrell and Paul Anderson. *Shihan-Te: The Bunkai of Karate Kata*. Boston, MA: YMAA Publication Center, 2002.

DeBecker, Gavin. The *Gift of Fear: Survival Signals That Protect Us From Violence*. New York, NY: Dell Publishing.

Egami, Shigeru. *The Heart of Karate-do*. New York, NY: Kodansha International, 1980.

Funakoshi, Gichin (translated by John Teramoto). *The Twenty Guiding Principles of Karate*. New York, NY: Kodansha International, 2003.

Higaonna, Morio. *Traditional Karatedo—Okinawa Goju Ryu Vol. 1: Fundamental Techniques*. Tokyo, Japan: Minato Research and Publishing Co., Ltd., 1985.

Higaonna, Morio. *Traditional Karatedo—Okinawa Goju Ryu Vol. 2: Performances of Kata*. Tokyo, Japan: Minato Research and Publishing Co., Ltd., 1986.

Higaonna, Morio. *Traditional Karatedo—Okinawa Goju Ryu Vol. 3: Applications of the Kata*. Tokyo, Japan: Minato Research and Publishing Co., Ltd., 1989.

Higaonna, Morio. *Traditional Karatedo—Okinawa Goju Ryu Vol. 4: Applications of the Kata, Part 2*. Tokyo, Japan: Minato Research and Publishing Co., Ltd., 1990.

Kane, Lawrence A. *Martial Arts Instruction: Applying Educational Theory and Communication Techniques in the Dojo*. Boston, MA: YMAA, 2004.

Kaufman, Stephen V. *The Art of War: The Definitive Interpretation of Sun Tzu's Classic Book of Strategy for the Martial Artist*. North Clarendon, VT: Tuttle Publishing, 1996.

Kaufman, Stephen V. *The Martial Artist's Book of Five Rings: The Definitive Interpretation of Miyamoto Mushashi's Classic Book of Strategy*. North Clarendon, VT: Tuttle Publishing, 1994.

Lovret, Fredrick J. *The Way and the Power: Secrets of Japanese Strategy*. Boulder, CO: Paladin Enterprises, Inc., 1987

MacYoung, Marc. *A Professional's Guide to Ending Violence Quickly*. Boulder, CO: Paladin Enterprises, Inc., 1993.

O'Connor, John and Dan Bensky. *Acupuncture: A Comprehensive Text* (Shanghai College of Traditional Medicine, translation). Seattle, WA: Eastland Press, 1981

Rosenbaum, Michael. *Kata and the Transmission of Knowledge: In Traditional Martial Arts*. Boston, MA: YMAA Publication Center, 2004.

Toguchi, Seikichi. *Essence of Karate Textbook No. 1: Okinawa Karate-Do Goju-Ryu Shorei-Kan*, Vancouver, British Columbia, Canada: Shorei-Kan Canada Karate Association, 1993.

Toguchi, Seikichi. *Essence of Karate Textbook No. 2: Okinawa Karate-Do Goju-Ryu Shorei-Kan*, Vancouver, British Columbia, Canada: Shorei-Kan Canada Karate Association, 1993.

Toguchi, Seikichi. *Okinawan Goju Ryu II*. Santa Clara, CA: Ohara Publications, 2001.

Toguchi, Seikichi. *Okinawan Goju Ryu*. Santa Clara, CA: Black Belt Communications, 1979.

Wilder, Kris. *Lessons from the Dojo Floor*. Seattle, WA: Xlibris, 2003.

Wiley, Mark V. *Filipino Martial Culture*. North Clarendon, VT: Tuttle Publishing, 1997.

Wilson, William Scott. *The Lone Samurai: The Life of Miyamoto Musashi*. Tokyo, Japan: Kodansha International, 2004.

Yamakura, Motoo. *Goju-Ryu Karate-Do Volume 1: Fundamentals for Traditional Practitioners*. Monroe, MI: G.K.K. Publications, 1989.

Articles

Abernethy, Iain. Mental Strength. Fightingarts.com

Bishop, Greg. Bruce Lee of NFL Teaches 49ers Martial Arts. *The Seattle Times*, Thursday, September 23, 2004.

Lowry, Dave. The Karate Way: The Earliest Karate Ryu. *Black Belt Magazine*, March, 1998.

Lowry, Dave. The Karate Way: Preparing for Real Violence. *Black Belt Magazine*, February, 2000.

Lowry, Dave. The Karate Way: The Art of Dealing With Doubt. *Black Belt Magazine*, July, 1998.

Lowry, Dave. The Karate Way: The Art of Defending Against Surprise. *Black Belt Magazine*, May, 1998.

Lowry, Dave. The Karate Way: The Art of Overcoming Fear. *Black Belt Magazine*, August, 1998.

Lowry, Dave. The Karate Way: Vital Hip Work of Karate. *Black Belt Magazine*, November, 1997.

Lowry, Dave. The Karate Way: Women are Capable of Kicking Butt in the Real World. *Black Belt Magazine*, March 1999.

Miller, Bruce Everett. Pressure Points 1: Going to the Heart of Pressure Points—What They Really Are. Fightingarts.com

Miller, Bruce Everett. Pressure Points 2: Some Observations on Their Use. Fightingarts.com

Miller, Bruce Everett. Pressure Points 3: Types of Points. Fightingarts.com

Web Sites

Broadside (www.nelsonsnavy.co.uk)

Fighting Arts web site (www.fightingarts.com)

Franco Sanguinetti's web site (www.bushikan.com)

Iain Abernethy's web site (www.iainabernethy.com)

Loren Christensen's web site (www.lwcbooks.com)

Marc "Animal" MacYoung's web site (www.nononsenseselfdefense.com)

The Pacific Martial Arts Federation web site (www.pmakarate.com)

The *Goju Ryu* Karate-do web site (www.gojuryu.net)

The Kenshinkan web site (www.kenshinkan.cl)

Index

Adrenaline, 19, 50, 67, 79-81, 83, 104, 124, 158-160, 184, 234

Aikido, 59, 98, 249, 251

Amygdala, 158-159, 162

archipallium, 80, 164

Atemi Waza (nerve or pressure point attack), 75, 251

Avoidance, 114, 153

Awareness, 90, 98, 149, 151-153, 161-162

Barrier, Language, 10

Bodhidharma, 2-3, 252

Bomb Threats, 151

Boyd's Law (OODA loop), 170, 177

Brain Activity, 145, 160-161

Breathing,
  Breathing, 3, 6, 49, 97-99, 169, 185
  Ibuki (quick energy breath), 99, 105, 253
  Nogare (slow breathing), 99, 105, 255

Bubishi, 8, 172, 239

Budo
  Budo (martial arts), 29-30, 44, 50, 96, 98, 117, 127, 130, 140, 169, 233, 235, 251, 255, 279
  Budoka (martial artists), 20, 29, 32, 114, 117, 133, 190, 233, 251, 254
  Okuden Waza (hidden applications), 15, 29, 68, 88, 96, 101, 103, 105, 181

Bullets, Catching, 145, 164

Bunkai, viv, xxii-xxiv, 2, 14-17, 67-68, 84-88, 109, 134, 181-182, 190, 252
  Bunkai Oyo, 14-15, 17, 84-85, 109, 252
  Henka Waza, 14, 68, 87-88, 103, 181, 234, 253
  Okuden Waza, 15, 29, 68, 88, 96, 101, 103, 105, 181, 232-236, 255

China, 1-3, 5-9, 20, 124, 177, 198, 202, 206, 210, 247
  China, 1-3, 5-9, 20, 124, 177, 198, 202, 206, 210, 247
  Chinese, 2-3, 8, 37, 41, 45, 49, 95,251-252,

Chokes, 16, 18, 58, 60, 63, 94

Criminals, 44, 50, 72, 147, 149, 151, 153, 177
  Amateur, 149, 154
  Drug Addict, 149-150, 177
  Gang Member, 149-150, 177
  Professional, 8, 35, 52, 71, 76, 126, 147-149, 161, 269, 277, 279

Psychopath, 149-150, 177
  Sex Predator, 149, 150, 177
  Terrorist, 147, 151

Decision Stick, 43-44, 64, 170

Dojo, 57, 97, 99, 117, 146, 157, 186-187, 190-191, 231, 252

Drills, 14, 72, 84, 119, 152, 167, 188, 190, 249, 257, 269
  4 to1 vs. 2 to 1 vs. 1 to 1 Tandem Drill, 84, 121
  Bomb Threat/Suspicious Package Drill, 150-152
  Flow Drill, 14
  Invading Personal Space, 46
  Line Sparring Drills, 190
  Roman Shield Drill (aggressive blocking), 126-128
  Tandem Sparring Drills, 84
  Tap Drill, 72-73
  Up Against the Wall Drill, 167

Enbusen (lines of performance), 110-112, 130, 236

Escalation, 90-91, 105, 154, 165

Fight, 13-15, 17-20, 40-43, 49, 54, 60, 64, 67-70, 103, 105, 121-123, 128, 134, 139-140, 145-148, 178, 233-238

Fighting Environment, 157

Goju Ryu, xxiii, 4, 7-9, 45-47, 50-57, 59-64, 189, 239,

Higashionna, Kanryo, 4-7, 9, 15, 210, 247

Imbalance, 45-51, 56, 60, 64, 102, 169, 182
  Happo No Kuzushi (8 directions of imbalance), 47
  Imbalance, 45-51, 56, 60, 64, 102, 169, 182

Indomitable Spirit, 116, 252

Inner Circle, 21, 29, 233

Japan, 1, 4-5, 8, 21, 57, 113, 124, 177, 247-249, 251-255, 269-270
  Japan, 1, 4-5, 8, 21, 57, 113, 124, 177, 247-249, 251-255, 269-270
  Japanese, 4, 14-15, 251

Judo, 9, 18, 23, 26, 40, 58-59, 62, 64, 102, 114, 116, 247, 249, 251, 253, 256, 277

Kaisai, Theory of, 109, 139, 253

Karate, history of, xiii, xiv, 9-11, 21, 233

Karateka (karate practitioner), 7, 21, 40, 112, 130, 138, 242, 254

Kata,
  Core *Kata*, 35, 60, 64, 241
  Gekiha, 242, 252
  Gekisai, 51, 53, 84-85, 111, 118, 181, 226-229, 241-242, 252, 254
  Hookiyu, 23-24, 45, 53, 242, 253-254
  Kakuha, 242-243
  Koryu, 124, 254
  Kururunfa, 107, 212, 214-217, 241-242, 254
  Saifa, 15, 22-23, 46, 65, 85, 124-125, 130-132, 137-138, 194-197, 241, 254-255
  Saipai, 23, 134-136, 206-209, 241, 254-255
  Sanchin, 6, 8, 13, 21, 47-48, 51, 99, 169, 185-186, 241-242, 253-255, 262, 265
  Sanseiru, 23, 218-221, 241-242, 254, 256
  Seisan, 120-121, 132, 202-205, 241, 249, 254, 256
  Seiyunchin, 87-89, 112, 119, 133, 198-201, 241, 254, 256
  Shisochin, 23, 143, 210-213, 241, 254, 256
  Suparinpei, 55, 222-225, 241-242, 244, 254, 256
  Taikyoku, 242, 254, 256
  Tensho, 7-8, 99, 241-242, 253, 257
Kendo, 9, 98, 251, 279
Kensetsu Waza, 101
Kihon, 13, 24, 53, 86, 118, 182, 187, 254
Kobudo, 7-8, 45, 98, 254, 277
Kumite (sparring), 16-18, 68, 81, 98, 110, 113, 117, 163, 187-188, 252-255
  Kiso Kumite (prearranged sparring), 16-18, 110, 253-254
  Kumite (sparring), 16-18, 68, 81, 98, 110, 113, 117, 163, 187-188, 252-255
  Randori (freestyle sparring), 18-19, 188, 190, 255
  Sanbon Shobu Kumite (three point tournament style), 17-18, 255
Kung Fu, 2-4, 28, 56, 95, 252, 254-257, 280
Kyushu, 7, 61-62, 171-172, 178, 254
  Vital Area Chart, 173
  Vital Area Descriptions, 172
Magellan, 41-42, 58
Meiji Restoration, 5, 124
Miyagi, Chojun, 2-3, 7-9, 12, 20-22, 40, 45, 64, 109, 169, 226, 241-242, 247-249, 253
Mushin (no mind), 92

Okinawa, 1, 3-10, 13, 15, 20, 29, 60, 113, 124, 177, 226, 232-233, 241, 243, 247-248, 257, 269-270, 278-279
  Okinawa, 1, 3-10, 13, 15, 20, 29, 60, 113, 124, 177, 226, 232-233, 241, 243, 247-248, 257, 269-270, 278-279
  Okinawan, 3, 5, 15, 21, 49, 90, 92, 109, 247-248, 253-257, 270
Omote, 86, 104, 233, 235, 255
Phalanx, 168
Physiological Damage, 46, 50-51, 55-56, 60, 62, 64, 70, 79, 104, 146, 157, 164, 171, 182, 234
Principles,
  Principle 1, 182
  Principle 2, 116, 119, 182
  Principle 3, 51, 101-102, 124, 183
  Principle 4, 63
  Principle 5, 124, 184
  Principle 6, 183
  Principle 7, 183
  Principle 8, 183, 189
  Principle 9, 70
  Principle 10, 113, 116, 128, 182
  Principle 12, 185
  Principle 13, 6, 185
  Principle 14, 118, 183
Roman, 35-36, 126-128, 253-256
Rules,
  Advanced Rules, 110, 139, 236, 253
  Basic Rules, 109-110, 139, 236, 256
  Rule 1, 130, 182
  Rule 2, 110, 112
  Rule 3, 186
  Rule 4, 101, 185
  Rule 5, 100, 184
  Rule 6, 123, 129, 182
  Rule 7, 184
  Rule 8, 58, 69, 112-113, 119, 123, 182
  Rule 9, 182
  Rule 10, 88, 141
  Rule 11, 61, 185
  Rule 12, 55, 184
Self-Defense, xxvii, 16, 19, 97, 102, 154, 178, 238
Stances, 16, 36, 41, 45-47, 52, 68, 73, 88, 95-97, 104-105, 116, 122, 185, 189, 235, 241-242

Bensoku Dachi, 133, 258
Hakusura Dachi, 137
Neko Ashi Dachi, 45, 47, 49, 118, 165, 226, 228
Sanchin Dachi, 13, 47-48, 51, 185-186, 262, 265
Shiko Dachi (*sumo* stance), 47-49, 53, 97, 112, 122, 241, 265
Zenkutsu Dachi (front stance), 47-48, 51, 53, 96, 101, 130, 135, 168, 242, 266
Stealing Time, 145, 166
Strategy, xxv, 35-43, 45-61
Tactics, 37-40, 60
Tae Kwon Do, 55, 134, 137, 277
Tai Chi, 37, 95, 98, 248, 256, 279-280
The Tell, 91-92, 128
Throws, 24, 26, 60, 62-64, 84, 102, 114,
Timing, Awareness of, 151-152
Uke, xxi, xxiii, 58, 72, 113, 121, 126, 167, 190
Ura Waza, xxi, 86-87, 104, 232-235
Violence, Types of, 147-148
    Criminal, 102, 147-150, 157-158, 177
    Frenzy, 147-148, 177
    Tantrum, 147-148, 177
Zanshin (continuing mind), 145, 161-162, 257

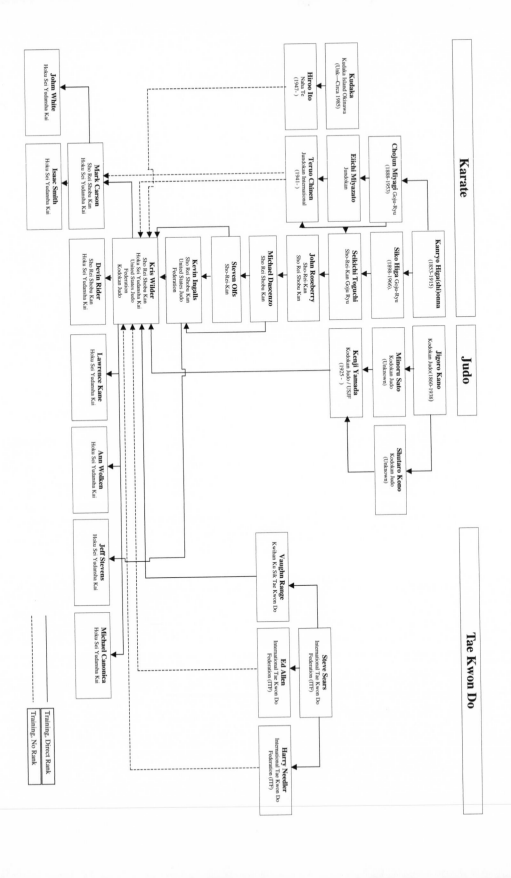

Karate

Judo

Tae Kwon Do

Kudaka
Kudaka Island Okinawa
(Unk.—Circa 1985)

Hiroo Ito
Naha Te
(1947–)

John White
Hoku Sei Yudansha Kai

Chojun Miyagi Goju-Ryu
(1888–1953)

Eiichi Miyazato
Jundokan

Teruo Chinen
Jundokan International
(1941–)

Isaac Smith
Hoku Sei Yudansha Kai

Mark Carson
Sho Rei Shobu Kan
Hoku Sei Yudansha Kai

Kamryo Higa(shi)onna
(1853–1915)

Siko Higa Goju-Ryu
(1898–1966)

Seikichi Toguchi
Sho-Rei-Kan Goju Ryu

John Roseberry
Sho-Rei-Kan
Sho Rei Shobu Kan

Michael Dascenzo
Sho-Rei-Kam
Sho Rei Shobu Kan

Steven Olfs
Sho-Rei-Kan

Kevin Ingalls
Sho Rei Shobu Kan
United States Judo
Federation

Kris Wilder
Sho Rei Shobu Kan
Hoku Sei Yudansha Kai
United States Judo
Federation
Kodokan Judo

Devin Rider
Sho Rei Shobu Kan
Hoku Sei Yudansha Kai

Jigoro Kano
Kodokan Judo (1860–1938)

Minoru Sato
Kodokan Judo
(Unknown)

Kenji Yamada
Kodokan Judo / USJF
(1925–)

Shutaro Kono
Kodokan Judo
(Unknown)

Lawrence Kane
Hoku Sei Yudansha Kai

Ann Wolken
Hoku Sei Yudansha Kai

Jeff Stevens
Hoku Sei Yudansha Kai

Vaughn Range
Kwihan Ku Sik Tae Kwon Do

Steve Sears
International Tae Kwon Do
Federation (ITF)

Ed Allen
International Tae Kwon Do
Federation (ITF)

Harry Needler
International Tae Kwon Do
Federation (ITF)

Michael Canonica
Hoku Sei Yudansha Kai

Training, Direct Rank
Training, No Rank

About the Authors

Lawrence Kane

Lawrence Kane is the author of *Martial Arts Instruction: Applying Educational Theory and Communication Techniques in the Dojo* (YMAA 2004). Over the last 30 or so years, he has participated in a broad range of martial arts, from traditional Asian sports such as judo, arnis, kobudo, and karate to recreating medieval European combat with real armor and rattan (wood) weapons. He has taught medieval weapons forms since 1994 and *Goju Ryu* karate since 2002. He has also completed seminars in modern gun safety, marksmanship, handgun retention and knife combat techniques, and he has participated in slow-fire pistol and pin shooting competitions.

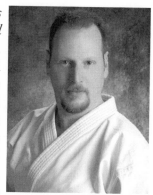

Since 1985 Lawrence has supervised employees who provide security and oversee fan safety during college and professional football games at a Pac-10 stadium. This job has given him a unique opportunity to appreciate violence in a myriad of forms. Along with his crew, he has witnessed, interceded in, and stopped or prevented literally hundreds of fights, experiencing all manner of aggressive behaviors as well as the escalation process that invariably precedes them. He has also worked closely with the campus police and state patrol officers who are assigned to the stadium and has had ample opportunities to examine their crowd control tactics and procedures.

Lawrence lives in Seattle, Washington with his wife Julie and his son Joey. He can be contacted via e-mail at lakane@ix.netcom.com.

Kris Wilder

Kris Wilder is the author of *Lessons from the Dojo Floor* (Xlibris 2003). He started practicing the martial arts at the age of fifteen. Over the years, he has earned black belt rankings in three styles, *Goju-Ryu* karate (4th *dan*), tae kwon do (2nd *dan*), and judo (1st *dan*), in which he has competed in senior national and international tournaments.

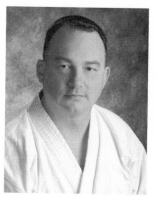

He has had the opportunity to train under skilled instructors, including Olympic athletes, state champions, national champions, and gifted martial artists who take their lineage directly from the founders of their systems.

Kris has trained across the United States and Okinawa. He is a founding member of the *Hokusei Yudanshakai*.

Kris lives in Seattle, Washington. He can be contacted via e-mail at kwilder@quidnunc.net or through the West Seattle Karate Academy web site at www.westseattlekarate.com.

BOOKS FROM YMAA

6 HEALING MOVEMENTS	B050/906
101 REFLECTIONS ON TAI CHI CHUAN	B041/868
108 INSIGHTS INTO TAI CHI CHUAN—A STRING OF PEARLS	B031/582
ANCIENT CHINESE WEAPONS	B004R/671
ANALYSIS OF SHAOLIN CHIN NA 2ND ED.	B009R/0002
ARTHRITIS RELIEF—CHINESE QIGONG FOR HEALING & PREVENTION 3RD ED.	B015R/0339
BACK PAIN RELIEF—CHINESE QIGONG FOR HEALING & PREVENTION 2ND ED	B030R/0258
BAGUAZHANG	B020/300
CARDIO KICKBOXING ELITE	B043/922
CHIN NA IN GROUND FIGHTING	B064/663
CHINESE FAST WRESTLING—THE ART OF SAN SHOU KUAI JIAO	B028/493
CHINESE FITNESS—A MIND / BODY APPROACH	B029/37X
CHINESE TUI NA MASSAGE	B057/043
COMPLETE CARDIOKICKBOXING	B038/809
COMPREHENSIVE APPLICATIONS OF SHAOLIN CHIN NA	B021/36X
DR. WU'S HEAD MASSAGE—ANTI-AGING AND HOLISTIC HEALING THERAPY	B075/0576
EIGHT SIMPLE QIGONG EXERCISES FOR HEALTH, 2ND ED.	B010R/523
ESSENCE OF SHAOLIN WHITE CRANE	B025/353
ESSENCE OF TAIJI QIGONG, 2ND ED.	B014R/639
EXPLORING TAI CHI	B065/424
FIGHTING ARTS	B062/213
HOW TO DEFEND YOURSELF, 2ND ED.	B017R/345
INSIDE TAI CHI	B056/108
KATA AND THE TRANSMISSION OF KNOWLEDGE	B071/0266
LIUHEBAFA FIVE CHARACTER SECRETS	B067/728
MARTIAL ARTS ATHLETE	B033/655
MARTIAL ARTS INSTRUCTION	B072/024X
MARTIAL WAY AND ITS VIRTUES	B066/698
MIND/BODY FITNESS	B042/876
MUGAI RYU	B061/183
NATURAL HEALING WITH QIGONG - THERAPEUTIC QIGONG	B070/0010
NORTHERN SHAOLIN SWORD, 2ND ED.	B006R/85X
OKINAWA'S COMPLETE KARATE SYSTEM—ISSHIN RYU	B044/914
OPENINGS	B026/450
POWER BODY	B037/760
PRINCIPLES OF TRADITIONAL CHINESE MEDICINE	B053/99X
PROFESSIONAL BUDO	B023/319
QIGONG FOR HEALTH & MARTIAL ARTS 2ND ED.	B005R/574
QIGONG FOR LIVING	B058/116
QIGONG FOR TREATING COMMON AILMENTS	B040/701
QIGONG MASSAGE—FUNDAMENTAL TECHNIQUES FOR HEALTH AND RELAXATION	B016R/0487
QIGONG MEDITATION - EMBRYONIC BREATHING	B068/736
QIGONG, THE SECRET OF YOUTH	B012R/841
ROOT OF CHINESE QIGONG, 2ND ED.	B011R/507
SHIHAN TE—THE BUNKAI OF KATA	B055/884
TAEKWONDO—ANCIENT WISDOM FOR THE MODERN WARRIOR	B049/930
TAEKWONDO—SPIRIT AND PRACTICE	B059/221
TAO OF BIOENERGETICS	B018/289
TAI CHI BOOK	B032/647
TAI CHI CHUAN	B019R/337
TAI CHI CHUAN MARTIAL APPLICATIONS, 2ND ED.	B008R/442
TAI CHI CONNECTIONS	B073/0320
TAI CHI SECRETS OF THE ANCIENT MASTERS	B035/71X
TAI CHI SECRETS OF THE WU & LI STYLES	B051/981
TAI CHI SECRETS OF THE WU STYLE	B054/175
TAI CHI SECRETS OF THE YANG STYLE	B052/094
TAI CHI THEORY & MARTIAL POWER, 2ND ED.	B007R/434
TAI CHI WALKING	B060/23X
TAIJI CHIN NA	B022/378
TAIJI SWORD, CLASSICAL YANG STYLE	B036/744
TAIJIQUAN, CLASSICAL YANG STYLE	B034/68X
TAIJIQUAN THEORY OF DR. YANG, JWING-MING	B063/432
TRADITIONAL CHINESE HEALTH SECRETS	B046/892
THE WAY OF KATA—A COMPREHENSIVE GUIDE FOR DECIPHERING MARTIAL APLICATIONS	B074/0584
THE WAY OF KENDO AND KENJITSU	B069/0029
WILD GOOSE QIGONG	B039/787
WISDOM'S WAY	B027/361
WOMAN'S QIGONG GUIDE	B045/833
XINGYIQUAN, 2ND ED.	B013R/416

VIDEOS FROM YMAA

ADVANCED PRACTICAL CHIN NA - 1	T059/0061
ADVANCED PRACTICAL CHIN NA - 2	T060/007X
ANALYSIS OF SHAOLIN CHIN NA	T004/531
ARTHRITIS RELIEF—CHINESE QIGONG FOR HEALING & PREVENTION	T007/558
BACK PAIN RELIEF—CHINESE QIGONG FOR HEALING & PREVENTION	T028/566

more products available from...
YMAA Publication Center, Inc. 楊氏東方文化出版中心
4354 Washington Street Roslindale, MA 02131
1-800-669-8892 • ymaa@aol.com • www.ymaa.com

VIDEOS FROM YMAA (CONTINUED)

CHINESE QIGONG MASSAGE—SELF	T008/327
CHINESE QIGONG MASSAGE—PARTNER	T009/335
COMREHENSIVE APPLICATIONS OF SHAOLIN CHIN NA 1	T012/386
COMREHENSIVE APPLICATIONS OF SHAOLIN CHIN NA 2	T013/394
DEFEND YOURSELF 1—UNARMED	T010/343
DEFEND YOURSELF 2—KNIFE	T011/351
EMEI BAGUAZHANG 1	T017/280
EMEI BAGUAZHANG 2	T018/299
EMEI BAGUAZHANG 3	T019/302
EIGHT SIMPLE QIGONG EXERCISES FOR HEALTH 2ND ED.	T005/54X
ESSENCE OF TAIJI QIGONG	T006/238
MUGAI RYU	T050/467
NORTHERN SHAOLIN SWORD—SAN CAI JIAN & ITS APPLICATIONS	T035/051
NORTHERN SHAOLIN SWORD—KUN WU JIAN & ITS APPLICATIONS	T036/06X
NORTHERN SHAOLIN SWORD—QI MEN JIAN & ITS APPLICATIONS	T037/078
QIGONG: 15 MINUTES TO HEALTH	T042/140
SCIENTIFIC FOUNDATION OF CHINESE QIGONG—LECTURE	T029/590
SHAOLIN KUNG FU BASIC TRAINING - 1	T057/0045
SHAOLIN KUNG FU BASIC TRAINING - 2	T058/0053
SHAOLIN LONG FIST KUNG FU—TWELVE TAN TUI	T043/159
SHAOLIN LONG FIST KUNG FU—LIEN BU CHUAN	T002/19X
SHAOLIN LONG FIST KUNG FU—GUNG LI CHUAN	T003/203
SHAOLIN LONG FIST KUNG FU—YI LU MEI FU * ER LU MAI FU	T014/256
SHAOLIN LONG FIST KUNG FU—SHI ZI TANG	T015/264
SHAOLIN LONG FIST KUNG FU—XIAO HU YAN	T025/604
SHAOLIN WHITE CRANE GONG FU— BASIC TRAINING 1	T046/440
SHAOLIN WHITE CRANE GONG FU— BASIC TRAINING 2	T049/459
SHAOLIN WHITE CRANE GONG FU— BASIC TRAINING 3	T074/0185
SIMPLIFIED TAI CHI CHUAN—24 & 48	T021/329
SUN STYLE TAIJIQUAN	T022/469
TAI CHI CHUAN & APPLICATIONS—24 & 48	T024/485
TAI CHI FIGHTING SET	T078/0363
TAIJI BALL QIGONG - 1	T054/475
TAIJI BALL QIGONG - 2	T057/483
TAIJI BALL QIGONG - 3	T062/0096
TAIJI BALL QIGONG - 4	T063/010X
TAIJI CHIN NA	T016/408
TAIJI CHIN NA IN DEPTH - 1	T070/0282
TAIJI CHIN NA IN DEPTH - 2	T071/0290
TAIJI CHIN NA IN DEPTH - 3	T072/0304
TAIJI CHIN NA IN DEPTH - 4	T073/0312
TAIJI PUSHING HANDS - 1	T055/505
TAIJI PUSHING HANDS - 2	T058/513
TAIJI PUSHING HANDS - 3	T064/0134
TAIJI PUSHING HANDS - 4	T065/0142
TAIJI SABER	T053/491
TAIJI & SHAOLIN STAFF - FUNDAMENTAL TRAINING - 1	T061/0088
TAIJI & SHAOLIN STAFF - FUNDAMENTAL TRAINING - 2	T076/0347
TAIJI SWORD, CLASSICAL YANG STYLE	T031/817
TAIJI WRESTLING - 1	T079/0371
TAIJI WRESTLING - 2	T080/038X
TAIJI YIN & YANG SYMBOL STICKING HANDS–YANG TAIJI TRAINING	T056/580
TAIJI YIN & YANG SYMBOL STICKING HANDS–YIN TAIJI TRAINING	T067/0177
TAIJIQUAN, CLASSICAL YANG STYLE	T030/752
WHITE CRANE HARD QIGONG	T026/612
WHITE CRANE SOFT QIGONG	T027/620
WILD GOOSE QIGONG	T032/949
WU STYLE TAIJIQUAN	T023/477
XINGYIQUAN—12 ANIMAL FORM	T020/310
YANG STYLE TAI CHI CHUAN AND ITS APPLICATIONS	T001/181

DVDS FROM YMAA

ANALYSIS OF SHAOLIN CHIN NA	D0231
CHIN NA IN DEPTH COURSES 1 - 4	D602
CHIN NA IN DEPTH COURSES 5 - 8	D610
CHIN NA IN DEPTH COURSES 9 - 12	D629
EIGHT SIMPLE QIGONG EXERCISES FOR HEALTH	D0037
ESSENCE OF TAIJI QIGONG	D0275
QIGONG MASSAGE	D0592
SHAOLIN KUNG FU FUNDAMENTAL TRAINING - 1&2	D0436
SHAOLIN LONG FIST KUNG FU - BASIC SEQUENCES	D661
SHAOLIN WHITE CRANE GONG FU BASIC TRAINING 1 & 2	D599
SUNRISE TAI CHI	D0274
TAIJIQUAN CLASSICAL YANG STYLE	D645
TAIJI PUSHING HANDS	D0495
TAIJI SWORD, CLASSICAL YANG STYLE	D0452
WHITE CRANE HARD & SOFT QIGONG	D637

more products available from...
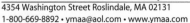
YMAA Publication Center, Inc. 楊氏東方文化出版中心
4354 Washington Street Roslindale, MA 02131
1-800-669-8892 • ymaa@aol.com • www.ymaa.com